W0106262

*Presented
with the compliments
of
Weddel
Pharmaceuticals
Ltd*

Thromboembolism
Aetiology, Advances in
Prevention and Management

Thromboembolism
Aetiology, Advances in Prevention and Management

Edited by A. N. Nicolaides

MTP

Medical and Technical Publishing Co. Ltd.

Published by

MTP
MEDICAL AND TECHNICAL
PUBLISHING CO LTD
PO Box 55, St Leonard's House,
St Leonardgate,
Lancaster, Lancs

Copyright 1975 A. N. Nicolaides
Softcover reprint of the hardcover 1st edition 1975

*No part of this book may be reproduced
in any form without permission from the publisher
except for the quotation of brief passages
for the purposes of review*

ISBN-13: 978-94-011-6146-6   e-ISBN-13: 978-94-011-6144-2
DOI: 10.1007/978-94-011-6144-2

First Published 1975

Blackburn Lancs., **BB2 1AB**

Contents

List of Contributors

Norma Alkjaersig, Ph.D.,
Research Associate Professor of Medicine,
Department of Internal Medicine,
Washington University School of Medicine,
St Louis, Missouri, U.S.A.

John Bonnar, M.D., F.R.C.O.G.,
Clinical Reader, Nuffield Department of Obstetrics and Gynaecology,
University of Oxford,
The John Radcliffe Hospital, Oxford.

Jay W. Constantine, Ph.D.,
Assistant Director, Department of Pharmacology,
Pfizer Medical Research Laboratories,
Groton, Connecticut, U.S.A.

Lennart Diener, M.D.,
Assistant Professor, Department of Radiology,
Stureby Sjukhus, Enskede, Stockholm, Sweden.

John A. Dormandy, F.R.C.S.,
Consultant Surgeon, St. James' and St. George's Hospitals,
London.

Pierre A. Dupont, F.R.C.S.,
Lecturer in Surgery, Surgical Unit,
St. Mary's Hospital Medical School, London W.2.

W. Robert Felix, Jr., M.D.,
Department of Surgery,
The Medical College of Pennsylvania and Veterans Administration Hospital,
Philadelphia, Pennsylvania, U.S.A.

Anthony P. Fletcher, M.D., M.R.C.P.,
Associate Professor of Medicine,
Washington University School of Medicine,
St Louis, Missouri, U.S.A

A. S. Gallus, B.S., F.R.C.P.(C), F.R.A.C.P.,
Assistant Professor, Department of Pathology,
Faculty of Medicine, McMaster University,
Department of Hematology, St Joseph's Hospital,
Hamilton, Ontario, Canada.

Robert J. Gibson, M.S.,
Consultant, Franklin Institute Research Laboratories,
Philadelphia, Pennsylvania, U.S.A.

Ian Gordon-Smith,
Senior Registrar, Surgical Unit,
St. Mary's Hospital Medical School, London W.2.

Gerald N. Grumet, M.D.,
Associate Professor Department of Medicine,
Northwestern University Medical School.
Associate Chief of Hematology Service,
Veterans Administration Research Hospital,
Chicago, Illinois, U.S.A.

Jack Hirsh, M.D., F.R.A.C.P., F.R.C.P.(C),
Professor, Department of Pathology and Medicine,
McMaster University Medical Centre,
Hamilton, Ontario, Canada.

Johannes Ipsen, M.D.,
Department of Community Medicine,
University of Pennsylvania School of Medicine,
Philadelphia, Pennsylvania, U.S.A.
(Presently at Institute for Social Medicine, Arhus University, Denmark).

Doreen Irving, B.Sc., D.I.C.,
Lecturer in Medical Statistics,
London School of Hygeine and Tropical Medicine and St. Mary's Hospital,
Medical School, London.

Jeffrey R. Justin,
Department of Surgical Research, The Medical College of Pennsylvania,
Philadelphia, Pennsylvania, U.S.A.

Hau C. Kwaan, M.D., F.R.C.P. (Edin), F.A.C.P.,
Professor of Medicine, Hematology Section,
Veterans Administration Research Hospital,
Chicago, Illinois, U.S.A.

John D. Lewis, M.B., F.R.C.S.,
Consultant Vascular Surgeon,
Northwick Park Hospital and Clinical Research Centre,
Harrow, Middlesex.

Raymond Mark, M.D.,
Department of Pathology, The Medical College of Pennsylvania,
Philadelphia, Pennsylvania, U.S.A.

Judith Mausner, M.D.,
Department of Community and Preventive Medicine,
The Medical College of Pennsylvania, U.S.A.

Jeanette Meadway, M.B., M.R.C.P.,
Registrar, Department of Cardiology,
St. Mary's Hospital Medical School, London W.2.

A. N. Nicolaides, M.B., F.R.C.S., F.R.C.S.E.,
Lecturer in Surgery, Surgical Unit,
St. Mary's Hospital Medical School, London W.2.

J. D. O'Connell, M.B., B.Ch., B.A.O.,
Consultant Radiologist, St. Finbar's Hospital,
Cork, Eire.

Janet A. Parker, M.D.,
Department of Nuclear Medicine, The Medical College of Pennsylvania,
Philadelphia, Pennsylvania, U.S.A.

George L. Popky, M.D.,
Department of Radiology, The Medical Centre of Pennsylvania,
Philadelphia, Pennsylvania, U.S.A.

Irene M. Purcell, M.A.,
Research Assistant, Pfizer Medical Research Laboratories,
Groton, Connecticut, U.S.A.

J. G. Sharnoff, M.D.,
Associate Professor of Clinical Pathology,
New York Medical College, Valhalla, New York,
Pathologist, Department of Pathology,
The Mount Vernon Hospital, New York, U.S.A.

Bernard Sigel, M.D.,
Professor of Surgery, Department of Surgery, The Medical College of
*   Pennsylvania,*
Philadelphia, Pennsylvania, U.S.A.

John A. Sirs, B.Sc., Ph.D.,
Reader, Head of Biophysics Department,
St. Mary's Hospital Medical School, London W.2.

Gwendolyn J. Stewart, Ph.D.,
Associate Research Professor of Medicine,
Temple University Hospital, Health Sciences Centre,
Philadelphia, Pennsylvania, 19140, U.S.A.

George C. Sutton, M.D., M.R.C.P.,
Senior Lecturer in Cardiology, Cardiothoracic Institute,
London S.W.3; Consultant Cardiologist, Hillingdon Hospital, Uxbridge,
*   Middlesex.*

Stanford Wessler, M.D.,
Professor of Medicine,
New York University School of Medicine,
New York, New York 10016, U.S.A.

Jimmie Williams,
Department of Surgical Research,
The Medical College of Pennsylvania,
Philadelphia, Pennsylvania, U.S.A.

Foreword

When Mr. Nicolaides told me he was editing a book on Thromboembolism I was constrained to say "not another" for there have been a number of recent contributions to this field. Yet venous thromboembolism is a major accompaniment of nearly all forms of medical and surgical illness. All clinicians should know about it; all should be able to integrate their knowledge into clinical management. The problems remain of what to know and where to find it, particularly in a field which draws increasingly on other areas for its fundamentals and which is also changing fast. This volume is a brave endeavour to provide a view over the whole subject. It could not possibly succeed absolutely and both editor and contributors undoubtedly realise this. Nevertheless they have put at our disposal knowledge of a wider kind than that available before and thus made it possible for the relatively inexpert such as myself to perceive how complex are the disturbances we produce by surgery or are produced by illness and where we can hope for advances in understanding and therapy in the future. A text of this kind hardly needs a foreword—it is of self evident value, although I expect the pace set by its writers and others in the field will, with the additional stimulus provided by this synthesis of ideas that has been achieved, soon require another volume. In the meantime it is a timely venture.

H. A. F. Dudley

Preface

The problem of thromboembolism occurs in all branches of Medicine and Surgery. During the last five years many advances have been made particularly in the field of prevention. The contributors of this book report a series of research observations which they believe will lead to a better understanding of the cause and better practice of prevention and management of thromboembolism.

In a volume such as this it is not possible to cover all topics that merit inclusion. The emphasis has been on subjects where advance is rapid, on new concepts and on results which point the direction which research should follow.

The book is aimed both at research workers and clinicians who are anxious to incorporate the conclusions of recent work into their practice. The aim is to bridge the gap between established textbooks and original Papers and to provide an assessment on depth of certain aspects of the subject.

I am very grateful to the authors for their contributions and the care they have taken with their manuscripts; Professor H. A. F. Dudley for his guidance in editing the book; Mr. C. Russell for his advice on chapters written by colleagues from St Mary's Hospital; Mrs Rosemary Bowers for her editorial assistance; finally the editorial staff of Medical and Technical Publishing Company, Particularly Mr. P. M. Lister and Mr. D. G. Bloomer for their understanding and help in overcoming the problems of preparing this book.

Andrew N. Nicolaides

1

The problem of deep venous thrombosis and pulmonary embolism

P. A. Dupont

INTRODUCTION

Although thromboembolism was first described by Rudolph Virchow in 1846 (Virchow, 1846), it was not until 1894 that the first case of postoperative deep venous thrombosis was noted (Strauch, 1894). Since then the diagnosis of venous thrombosis has been made with increasing frequency. It is now recognised as one of the major hazards of medical and surgical patients, predisposing to the often unrecognised complication of pulmonary embolism which is also increasing. Pulmonary embolism may produce sudden death, hypotension with progressive deterioration ending in death or may give rise to pulmonary hypertension which may eventually result in heart failure. Occasionally there may be complete resolution with no resultant symptoms or signs. Locally the thrombotic process may resolve completely, may fail to recanalise, or, should recanalisation occur, may produce extensive valve damage. Both of the latter conditions may lead to chronic venous insufficiency.

Although it is impossible to state categorically the incidence of deep venous thrombosis and pulmonary embolism, there is evidence that despite the greater awareness and more frequent diagnosis, there is a definite increase in the incidence of both of these closely related conditions (Registrar General's Statistical Reviews of England and Wales, 1941-1971). This increase has become more evident since the late 1940s and early 1950s and it is probably the result of the introduction of safer methods of anaesthesia, antibiotics and blood transfusion which led to the undertaking of complex operations especially on older patients. With the introduction of intensive care, more patients survive serious trauma to succumb eventually to pulmonary embolism. An interesting example in terms of absolute increase in frequency is shown in an early retrospective report (Morrell *et al.*, 1963) of the incidence of pulmonary embolism at postmortem in a hospital group, in which over 90 per cent of the hospital deaths came to necropsy. This study revealed a progressive increase from 33 recorded cases of embolism in 1952 to 154 in 1961. The annual deaths from embolism increased from 18 to 72 in the same period.

INCIDENCE OF DEEP VENOUS THROMBOSIS
The clinical diagnosis of deep venous thrombosis may be obvious in extreme cases but in the majority of patients it is inaccurate (Haeger, 1969; Kakkar, 1971; Nicolaides *et al.*, 1971; Nicolaides, 1972). By using venography as a routine diagnostic test, it has become apparent that one-third of the patients with symptoms and signs suggestive of thrombosis have normal deep veins (Kakkar, 1971); when the clinical signs are confined below the knee, half of the patients have normal veins (Nicolaides *et al.*, 1971). When the diagnosis of deep venous thrombosis was made by scanning the patient's legs with the ^{125}I-fibrinogen test, one-half of the patients with thrombosis had no symptoms or signs (Kakkar, 1971).

The overall incidence of deep venous thrombosis based on postmortem studies in unspecified groups of medical and surgical patients has been estimated to be between 34 and 60 per cent respectively (Hunter *et al.*, 1945; McLachlin and Paterson, 1951; Gibbs, 1957); for elderly patients and in the presence of trauma, figures of 80 to 86 per cent have been quoted (Sevitt and Gallagher, 1959; 1961). Probably the most accurate figures available are those from studies with the ^{125}I-fibrinogen test in postoperative patients. The incidence of thrombosis detected by this test varied from 15 per cent in patients having gynaecological operations, (Bonnar *et al.*, 1972) to 75 per cent in patients with pertrochanteric fractures (Field *et al.*, 1972). In general surgical patients the incidence varied from 24 per cent (Nicolaides *et al.*, 1972) to 35 per cent (Flanc *et al.*, 1968).

INCIDENCE OF PULMONARY EMBOLISM
The Registrar General's figures for deaths from pulmonary embolism are probably gross underestimates. Figures for 'pulmonary embolism and infarction' are classified under category 450 of the International Classification of diseases (I.C.D), but a large number of deaths from pulmonary emboli are also classified under 'other venous emboli and thromboses'

2

(I.C.D. 453) (Hume *et al.*, 1970) indicating a source of inexactitude. The Registrar General's figures (see Table 1.1) for England and Wales are 687 deaths for I.C.D. category 450 and 3028 for I.C.D. 453 making a total of 5715 or if converted for the total population, 117 deaths per million. Using data made available during a sample analysis of multiple causes of death mentioned in death certificates in 1966, it has been calculated (Hume *et al.*, 1970) that instead of a total of 4700 deaths (I.C.D. 450 plus 452) the probable true estimate was in the region of 21 000 deaths. Therefore the low figure of 4700 in 1966 and similary 5715 in 1971 may be due to inaccuracies in diagnosis, partly because postmortem examination is limited to deceased inpatients which leads to inaccuracies in the filling in of death certificates.

Table 1.1. Yearly deaths from pulmonary embolism and death rates per million population—derived from Registrar General's Stastistical Reviews of England and Wales, Part I, Table 7 (Eighth revision of I.C.D.)

Year	Pulmonary embolus and infarction I.C.D. 450	Other venous emboli and thromboses I.C.D. 453	Total	Death rate per million population		
				I.C.D. 450	I.C.D. 453	Total
1961	1645	*	*	36	*	*
1962	1711	*	*	37	*	*
1963	1906	*	*	41	*	*
1964	1976	*	*	42	*	*
1965	2006	*	*	42	*	*
1966	2195	*	*	46	*	*
1967	2408	2558	4966	50	53	103
1968	2410	2783	5193	50	57	107
1969	2447	3057	5504	50	63	113
1970	2659	3287	5946	54	67	121
1971	2687	3028	5715	55	62	117

*Prior to 1967 I.C.D. categories 450 and 453 were grouped together.

VENOUS THROMBOEMBOLISM AND OESTROGEN COMPOUNDS

In 1961 a young girl receiving an oestrogen–progesterone compound for endometriosis developed pulmonary embolism (Jordan, 1961). Subsequently a number of case reports appeared linking oral contraceptives, especially preparations high in oestrogen content, with thromboembolic disease in young women (Vessey and Doll, 1969). Furthermore men receiving oestrogen compounds for the treatment of prostatic cancer showed an increased incidence of thromboembolic disease (Veterans Administration Cooperative Urological Research Group, 1967). In young women un-

3

dergoing surgery, preoperative oral contraception increased the risk of postoperative deep venous thrombosis or pulmonary embolism by 3.5–6 times (Vessey *et al.*, 1970; Greene and Sartwell, 1972). In a prospective study of 885 women aged 20-44 years the estimate of the relative risk for thromboembolism in those using oral contraceptives as compared to non-users was 11 (Report from the Boston Collaborative Drug Surveillance Program, 1973).

A survey of 25 086 pregnant women (Aaro *et al.*, 1966) at the Mayo Clinic revealed an incidence of deep venous thrombosis of 0.36 per 100 in the antepartum period and 1.5 per 1000 in the first 4 weeks after delivery. That the increased incidence in the postpartum period was due to the suppression of lactation by oestrogens was suggested by Daniels *et al.*, (1967) and confirmed by Jeffcoate who also showed that the incidence of thromboembolism was three times greater in mothers who did not breast feed (Jeffcoate et al., 1968).

RECURRENCE OF VENOUS THROMBOEMBOLIC DISEASE

The risk of recurrence of venous thrombosis is at its highest immediately after discharge from hospital if anticoagulant therapy were discontinued (Coon and Willis, 1973). The risk gradually decreases to reach a plateau after three years. Therefore, it is suggested that anticoagulant therapy should be maintained for a prolonged period, ideally for three years. Practically and economically this is difficult, and a minimum of four months has been suggested with extension of this period when a history of previous deep venous thrombosis or pulmonary embolism exists (Coon and Willis, 1973).

Six years after the completion of a study of venous thromboembolism in young women on the Pill (Vessey and Doll, 1969) the majority of the group and controls were investigated (Badaracco and Vessey, 1974) with regard to recurrence. A significant smaller number of the former contraceptive users had developed a recurrence in comparison with the control group. This suggests that the risk is diminished after discontinuing oral contraceptives.

THE POSTTHROMBOTIC SYNDROME

The majority of thrombi start in the calf (Chapters 10, 11, 14). Seventy-eight per cent of these either remain localised to the calf or lyse spontaneously, but the remaining 22 per cent extend into the popliteal and more proximal veins (Kakkar *et al.*, 1969). Some of the latter produce the typical phlegmasia alba dolens, phlegmasia caerulea dolens or venous gangrene if there is arterial insufficiency. Unless there is rapid resolution of the thrombus, the process of organisation and recanalisation will result in venous insufficiency because of the destruction of valves (Kakkar *et al.*, 1969; Field *et al.*, 1972). Failure of recanalisation, particularly in the proximal veins in the presence of valvular damage, is often responsible for the most severe venous hypertension. This venous hypertension leads to valvular incompetence of the perforating veins, which results in capillary stasis, tissue necrosis and ulceration of the skin especially if trauma, superficial thrombophlebitis or cellulitis are also present (Hobbs, 1973). Estimated figures for the resultant postthrombotic syndrome in England and Wales suggest an incidence of 5 per 1000 persons most of whom are middle-aged or elderly people (Boyd *et al.*, 1952). A study of the postthrombotic syndrome in Sweden (Gjores, 1956) suggested an incidence which ranged from 1.87 to 3.13 per cent in different districts. This was based on a questionnaire sent to 15 000 people with a subsequent examination of 1453 of these, all over the age of eighteen. The breakdown of events immediately preceding the development of thrombosis was: 41 per cent obstetric, 21 per cent postoperative, 18 per cent unknown, 13 per cent following medical illness and 6 per cent after injury.

The management of patients with the postthrombotic syndrome is a major problem. So far, surgery has been disappointing although since the introduction of the crossed bypass using the contralateral saphenous vein (Palma and Esperon, 1960) enthusiasts have reported that a large proportion of the transplanted veins have remained patent with relief of lower limb swelling (Harris, 1965; Izquierdo, 1965; Dale, 1966; 1969; Husni, 1971). At the moment the only effective treatment appears to be the elimination of perforating veins by injection compression therapy or operation, and by elastic bandages and stockings which alleviate the venous hypertension in the superficial veins (Hobbs, 1971).

RECENT ADVANCES AND THE FUTURE
Research workers realise that if the mortality due to pulmonary embolism and the morbidity due to the postthrombotic syndrome are to be significantly reduced several requirements have to be fulfilled. The incidence should be reduced by preventive measures (Chapters 14–16); the diagnosis should be made early and accurately (Chapters 17, 19, 21); treatment should provide rapid resolution of the thrombus with preservation of valvular function (Chapters 18–21). A better understanding of the aetiology (Chapters 2–9) and pathogenesis of deep venous thrombosis (Chapters 10, 11 and 14) and the ability to select the patients at risk (Chapters 12 and 13) will assist in fulfilling these requirements.

Thromboembolism

References

Aaro, L. A., Johnson, M. R. and Ivergens, J. L. (1966). Acute deep vein thrombosis associated with pregnancy, *Obstet, Gynecol.*, **28,** 553.

Badaracco, M. A. and Vessey M. P. (1974). Recurrence of venous thromboembolic disease and use of oral contraceptives. *Brit. Med. J.*, **1,** 215.

Bonnar, J. and Walsh, J. (1972). Prevention of thrombosis after pelvic surgery by Dextian 70. *Lancet,* i, 614.

Boston Collaborative Drug Surveillance Program. (1973). Oral contraceptives, venous thromboembolic disease, surgically confirmed gall bladder disease and breast tumours. *Lancet,* i, 1399.

Boyd, A. M., Jepson, R. P., Ratcliffe, A. H. and Rose, S. S. (1952). Logical management of chronic ulcers of the leg. *Angiology,* **3,** 207

Coon, W. W. and Willis, P. W. (1973). Recurrence of venous thromboembolism. *Surgery,* **73,** 823

Dale, W. A. (1966). Chronic iliofemoral venous occlusion including seven cases of crossover vein grafting. *Surgery,* **59,** 117

Dale, W. A. and Harris, J. (1969). Crossover vein grafts for il ac and femoral venous occlusion. *J. Cardiovasc. Surg.*, **10,** 458

Daniels, D: G., Campbell, H. and Turnbull, A. C. (1967). Puerperal thromboembolism and suppression of lactation, *Lancet,* ii, 287

Field, E. S., Nicolaides, A. N., Kakkar, V. V. and Crellin, R. Q. (1972). Deep vein thrombosis in patients with fractures of the femoral neck. *Brit. J. Surg.*, **59,** 377

Field E. S., Flanc, C. Kakkar, V. and Clarke, M. (1968). The detection of venous thrombosis of the legs using   I-labelled Fibrinogen. *Brit. J. Surg.*, **55,** 742

Gibbs, N. M. (1967). Venous thrombosis of the lower limbs with particular references to bed rest. *Brit. J. Surg.*, **45,** 209

Gjores, J. E. (1956). Value of anticoagulant therapy in the prevention of the post-thrombotic syndrome (Transl.). *Sven. Lak. Tidan.*, **53,** 3006

Greene, G. R. and Sartwell, P. E. (1972). Oral contraceptive use in patients with thromboembolism following surgery, trauma, or infection, *Amer. J. Pub. Health.*, **62,** 680

Haeger, K. (1969). Problems of acute deep venous thrombosis 1. The interpretation of signs and symptoms. *Angiology,* **20,** 219

Harris, J. (1965). Cross leg venous graft for the relief of unilateral lower limb venous obstruction. *Surg. Gynaecol. Obstet.*, **120,** 1232

Hobbs, J. T. (1971). *Proceedings of Stoke Mandeville Symposium, pp 29* and *84*

Hobbs, J. T. (1971). The problem of the post-thrombotic syndrome, *Postgrad Med. J.,* **49,** (Suppl. & 48).

Hume, M., Sevitt, S. and Thomas, D. P. (1970). *Venous Thrombosis and Pulmonary Embolism,* (Oxford University Press)

Hunter, W. C., Krygrer, J. J., Kennedy, J. C. and Sneedon, V. D. (1945). Etiology and prevention of thrombosis of the deep leg veins *Surg,* **17,** 178

Husni, E. A. (1971). Venous reconstruction in post-phlebitic disease. *Circulation,* **43,** (Suppl. 1), 147

Izquierdo, G. F. (1965). Homologous vein transplants surgical treatment of the post-phlebitic sequelae. *J. Cardiovasc. Surg.*, **6,** 188

Jeffcoate, T. N. A., Miller, J. and Roos, R. F. (1967). Puerperal thromboembolism in relation to the inhibition of lactation by oestrogen therapy. *Brit. Med., J.*, **4,** 19

6

Thromboembolism

Jordan, W. M. (1961). Pulmonary embolism. *Lancet,* **ii,** 1146

Kakkar V. V., Howe, C. T., Flanc, C. and Clarke, M.B. (1969). Natural history of postoperative deep vein thrombosis. *Lacnet,* **ii,** 230

Kakkar, V. V., (1971). Medical treatment of deep vein thrombosis. *Brit. J. Hosp. Med.,* **6,** 741

McLachlin, J. and Paterson, J. C. (1951) Some basic observations on venous thrombosis and pulmonary embolism. *Surg. Gynaecol. Obstet.,* **93,** 1

Morrell, M. L., Trulove, S. C. and Barr. A. (1963). Pulmonary embolism. *Brit. Med. J.,* **2.** 530

Nicolaides, A. N. (1972). The prevention of postoperative deep venous thrombosis, Jacksonian Prize Essay

Nicolaides, A. N., Kakkar. V. V., Field, E. S. and Renney, J. T. G. (1971). The origin of deep vein thrombosis: a venographic study, *Brit. J. Radiol.,* **44,** 635

Palma, E. C. and Esperon, R. (1960). Vein transplants and grafts in the surgical treatment of the post-phlebitic syndrome. *J. Cardrorasc. Surg.* **1,** 94

Registrar General's staistical reviews of England and Wales. (1941—1971) (Her Majesty's Stationery Office)

Seritt, S. and Gallagher, N. G. (1959). Prevention of venous thrombosis and pulmonary embolism in injured patients. *Lancet, i,* 981

Seritt, S. and Gallagher, N. G. (1961). Venous thrombosis and pulmonary embolism: A clinicapathological study in injured and burned patients. *Brit. J. Surg.,* **48,** 475

Strauch, M. von. (1894). Ueber Venenthrombose dur unteren Extremitaten nach Koliotomien bei Bechenhochlagerung und Athernarkose. *Gynak.,***18,** 304

Vessey, M. P. and Doll, R. (1969). Investigation of relation between use of oral contraceptives and thromboembolic disease. A further report. *Brit. Med. J.,* **2,** 651

Vessey, M. P. Doll, R. and Fairbairn, A. S. (1970). Postoperative thromboembilism and the use of oral contraceptives. *Brit. Med. J.,* **3,** 123

Veterans Administration Cooperative Urological Research Group (1967). Treatment and survival of patients with cancer of the prostate. *Surg. Gynaecol. Obstet.,* **124,** 1011

Virchow, R. (1846). Die Verstopfung der Lungenarterie und ihre Folgen. *Beitr. Exp. Path. Physiol.,* **2,** 1

2

Factors in the initiation of deep venous thrombosis

Stanford Wessler

INTRODUCTION

Deep venous thrombosis of the lower extremities is a common, age-related condition manifest by focal intravascular coagulation in which the mechanism is obscure, the clinical recognition elusive, the recurrence rate high and mortality unpredictable yet infrequent relative to the high prevalenee of the lesion.

Since the time of Virchow (1856) it has been widely assumed that hypercoagulability, vessel wall injury and retarded blood flow are causally related singly or together to the initiation of thrombosis anywhere in the circulation. In this chapter a thesis will be developed that in venous thrombosis, in contradistinction to the arterial lesion, increased coagulability of the blood is the prime initiating factor in thrombogenesis and that the role of the vascular intima and of stasis are important but secondary factors.

HYPERCOAGULABILITY

Clotting factors

The identification of each new clotting factor has raised the possibility that abnormalities in that factor might be found among patients with thromboembolism. Data have yet to be presented, however, demonstrating a causal relationship between intravascular coagulation and an alteration, either quantitative or qualitative, in any of the 13 clotting factors recognised internationally as specific coagulation activities. This observation is valid not only for intact zymogens but also for derivative portions of these

Supported in part by the National Heart and Lung Institute through a Specialised Centre of Research (SCOR) in Thrombosis (HL 14147), by a National Heart and Lung Institute Grant (5 RO1 HL 11470): and bv a Grant-in-Aid from the American Heart Association.

molecules as measured by a variety of sophisticated physicochemical techniques.

Some of the clotting factors essential for the formation of fibrin become activated during the coagulation of mammalian blood *in vitro*. Two of these zymogens, activated Factor X (Xa or autoprothrombin-C) and thrombin, are absent from serum, while others, such as Factors XII and XI, persist in serum in their activated form. Fibrinogen is the natural substrate for thrombin and their reaction product, fibrin, is a potent antithrombin. At least 85 per cent of the thrombin formed during blood coagulation is immediately adsorbed by fibrin, whereas the remaining thrombin is more slowly neutralised by a substance in blood known as antithrombin III. This plasma activity, moreover, can also neutralise a large quantity of preformed thrombin in a slow progressive manner in the absence of fibrin. Activated Factor X (the enzyme responsible for the converersion of prothrombin to thrombin) does not clot fibrinogen, has not shown to be adsorbed by fibrin and does not lose its activity in the presence of thrombin. Therefore, the rapid disappearance of activated Factor X within minutes after plasma clots, may be attributed to the presence in blood of a naturally occurring blood clotting antagonist. The disappearance of actived Factor X upon its addition to bovine serum was initially reported by Seegers and Marciniak (1962). In pursuing this subject it was decided to examine the role of the Factor X molecule first identified as an activity missing from the blood of certain patients with haemorrhagic states (Telfer *et al.*, 1956; Hougie *et al.*, 1957). In the past 15 years, it has become increasingly clear that the activation of Factor X represents a focal point in both the intrinsic and extrinsic clotting pathways, being located at the beginning of the final pathway to thrombin formation and hence to both platelet aggregation and fibrin deposition. Activated Factor X is an essential component of prothrombin activator and is also formed by the direct action of Russell's viper venom and of trypsin on precursor Factor X. It has been demonstrated that whereas non-activated Factor X is inert *in vivo,* activated Factor X is thrombogenic and more potently so than purified thrombin itself (Wessler and Yin, 1968; Yin and Wessler, 1968).

Plasma inhibitors

Although plasma inhibitors of *in vitro* blood coagulation had been recognised at the beginning of the century (Morawitz, 1905), few investigators have attempted to include any inhibitory factors in the overall formulation of blood clotting reactions (Grannis and Kazal, 1966). Recent studies have, in fact, centered largely on the forward reaction.

Two of the most useful formulations, often referred to as the Waterfall (Davie and Ratnoff, 1964) or the 'cascade' (Macfarlane, 1964) schemes, did not make any specific provision for the role of the naturally occurring inhibitors of blood coagulation. Subsequently, proposals have been made to modify these schemes so as to include a postulated inhibitor that might influence prothrombin activation by prothrombin activator (Hemker *et al.,* 1965; Hemker *et al.,* 1967; Hemker and Hemker, 1968; Hemker *et al., 1968).*

For many years antithrombin III (progressive antithrombin) has been considered by numerous investigators to be the principal circulating inhibitor to thrombin. However, Seegers reported that a fraction of antithrombin III from bovine plasma was capable of neutralising autoprothrombin-C (activated Factor X) and postulated that the capacity of this fraction to neutralise both activated Factor X and thrombin belonged to a single proteinase inhibitor termed antithrombin III. (Seegers and Marciniak, 1962).

It had been suggested that antithrombin III is identical with heparin cofactor (antithrombin II), a plasma protein that, in conjunction with heparin, exerts an instant antithrombin effect. A number of other investigators, however, have claimed a lack of identity for these two activities.

It has also been observed that antithrombin III levels vary considerably with age and that there are differences between health and disease (Von Kaulla, 1967; Abildgaard, 1968). Congenital deficiencies in antithrombin III have been reported and members of these families have been found to be thrombophilic (Ekberg, 1965). Finally, antithrombin III levels have been reported to be reduced in women on oral contraceptive agents (Von Kaulla and Peterson *et al.,* 1970; Von Kaulla, 1970).

From a chance clinical observation we were able to demonstrate in man and then *in vitro* that heparin, in trace amounts, markedly potentiates the rate of activated Factor X neutralisation by its natural inhibitor (Yin and Wessler, 1970). This inhibitor, an α_2 globulin with a small molecular weight, was partially purified and entirely separated from all other known coagulation activities (Yin *et al.,* 1971b). It was established at an early stage that heparin was reacting with the inhibitor rather than with another plasma component to cause the rapid inhibition of activated Factor X (Yin and Wessler, 1970). Furthermore, while heparin alone cannot inhibit activated Factor X, this drug, *in vitro,* markedly potentiates the activity of the zymogen's inhibitor (Yin *et al.,* 1971b; 1971c).

These findings strongly suggested that the primary role of heparin in

11

retarding intravascular coagulation was the potentiation of the neutral-isation of Factor X by its inhibitor. This plasma globulin also inhibits thrombin but is without effect on precursor X. The inhibitor is on a weight basis 30 times more active against activated Factor X than against thrombin.

Since 1 μg of inhibitor can neutralise 32 units of activated Factor X, it can indirectly prevent the potential generation of 1600 NIH units of thrombin. Thus to neutralise this amount of thrombin itself would require 1330 μg of inhibitor, more than a 1300-fold increase in the quantity of inhibitor protein (Yin et al., 1971b). Seegers, had, in fact, found that to inactivate 222 units of previously formed thrombin in 60 min, 500 μg of antithrombin III were required (Seegers, 1968).

Subsequently, we demonstrated that the biological activities variously termed activated Factor X inhibitor, antithrombin III and heparin cofactor all belong to a single plasma proteinase with broad specificity (Yin et al., 1971c). Some of these findings have been confirmed by other groups (Biggs et al., 1970; Marciniac and Tsujamura 1972).

The coagulation system and lipid
One of the key functions of phospholipid in blood coagulation is its role in accelerating the conversion of prothrombin to thrombin by activated Factor X in the presence of Factor V and calcium ions. In animal and in vitro experiments we have observed evidence that the thrombogenicity of activated Factor X infused into rabbits is enhanced several fold when either crude or purified phospholipid is added to activated Factor X infusates. Thus, the duration of the thrombogenic stimulus induced by infusions of activated Factor X alone is prolonged from ten seconds to four minutes when appropriate lipid is added to the infusate (Barton et al., 1970).

The brief duration of the thrombotic state induced by infusions of activated Factor X is caused by the rapid inactivation of the enzyme by its plasma inhibitor. When, however, activated Factor X forms a complex with phospholipid, the neutralisation of the zymogen by its inhibitor is retarded, thus facilitating the rapid formation of the prothrombin activator complex.

These data suggest that under pathological conditions the presence of an excess of phospholipid or related compounds in conjunction with retarded blood flow will favour the accumulation of any Factor X that becomes activated. This result leads, in turn, to the formation of the potent prothrombin activator that, via thrombin, causes both platelet aggregation and fibrin deposition. Heparin can overcome this lipid inhibition of activated Factor X neutralisation by its inhibitor. However, the amount of heparin required to accelerate this neutralisation in the presence of phospholipid is greater than when lipid is omitted from the reaction mixture (Yin *et al.*, 1973a).

The coagulation system and platelet aggregation

Aggregation of platelets *in vitro* can be induced by at least three important physiological agents: adenosine diphosphate (Gardner *et al.*, 1961; Kazer-Glanzman and Luscher, 1962), thrombin (Fonio, 1940), and activated Factor X (Jevons and Barton, 1971). Adenosine diphosphate is released from platelets by the action of thrombin (Haslam, 1969). Thrombin, however, is evolved from prothrombin as a result of its proteolytic cleavage of activated Factor X.

It has been shown that when 0.05 units of activated Factor X were added to a freshly washed standard platelet suspension, aggregation invariably resulted. If 30 μg of inhibitor were added to an identical suspension, platelet aggregation was totally abolished. This did not occur when only 3 μg of the inhibitor were introduced into the same test system. Platelet aggregation induced by 0.05 units of activated Factor X was, however, completely prevented when 3 μg of plasma inhibitor, mixed with 0.05 units of heparin, were added to the reaction mixture. This amount of heparin alone failed to inhibit platelet aggregation induced by 0.05 units of activated Factor X. Furthermore, for the inhibitor alone to be effective in preventing platelet aggregation, it must react with activated Factor X more rapidly than do platelets (Yin *et al.*, 1973b).

The key step in the *in vitro* aggregation of washed platelets by activated Factor X is, of course, the formation of minute amounts of thrombin, insufficient to clot a standard fibrinogen fraction in several hours. Similarly, for the efficient conversion of prothrombin to thrombin, Factor V, calcium ions and phospholipid must also be present. The platelet membrane thus can substitute for phospholipid as an effective surface upon which both of these reactions can occur. Barton and Hanahan (1967) have demonstrated the binding of Factor II to phospholipid *in vitro*. It is possible that Factors II and V adsorb more effectively to a platelet membrane that is altered of traumatised to provide a more active surface than exists in the normal intact platelet population. This membrane alteration presumably can be achieved by ageing or physical injury. Such an hypothesis for the availability of platelet factor 3 has in fact. been suggested (Surgenor and Wallach, 1961; Marcus and Zucker, 1965).

These comments invite the further speculation that intact circulating platelets may normally lack coagulation proteins such as Factor II attached to their surfaces, but, under pathologic condition *in vivo* or, when removed from the circulation, they may undergo biochemical or physical changes that provide ideal surfaces for binding some of the clotting proteins. If this thesis should prove to be valid, then the data indicating that the surface membranes of isolated washed platelets contain clotting factors, such as Factor II, may reflect a pathological rather than a physiological phenomenon.

A new concept of hypercoagulability

Women on the Pill have a slight, but significantly increased incidence of thromboembolic episodes as compared with their matched controls (Royal College of General Practitioners, 1967; Inman and Vessey, 1968; Vessey and Doll, 1969; Sortwell et al., 1969). Fagerhol and his associates who detected, immunologically, low levels of antithrombin III in women on the Pill stated that patients with a 50 per cent reduction in antithrombin III were thrombophilic—a claim based on their experience with two thrombophilic families who exhibited an hereditary 50 per cent decrease in antithrombin III (Fagerhol et al., 1970).

In collaboration with Dr David Rothman we measured the inhibitor levels of an unselected group of 450 premenopausal women who were on oral contraceptive agents from six weeks to eight years. Twenty-six per cent had levels ranging from 76 to 100 per cent; 39 per cent had levels from 51 to 75 per cent; 30 per cent had levels from 26 to 50 per cent and 5 per cent, or 20 women, had inhibitor levels between 12 and 25 per cent of normal. None of these 20 subjects had oedema or other signs or symptoms of venous thromboembolism. Six, who had leg pains, were examined and three of these six had venograms all of which were normal.

We would interpret these fiindings differently than might Fagerhol and suggest that these women with very low inhibitor levels are not thrombotic, but have a lowered defense mechanism against proteolytic reactions capable of activating coagulation zymogens so that a smaller quantity of clot initiator is effective than would be the case in normal individuals. In short, unless such a minimal inciter of coagulation enters the blood stream these women will not develop thrombosis.

These studies of the possible relation of the inhibitor and the Pill suggested to us the first operational definition of hypercoagulability since this concept was initially described in 1676 by an English physician (Wiseman, 1676). *Hypercoagulability may be represented as an altered state of circulating blood that requires a smaller quantity of a clot initiating substance to induce intravascular coagulation than is required to produce comparable thrombosis in a normal subject.* One of the attractive features of this definition is that it is susceptible to experimental verification.

Accordingly, we initiated a collaborative study, presently ongoing with

Mr V. V. Kakkar and his surgical team at Kings College Hospital Medical School in London, England. The preliminary data, obtained without concomitant inhibitor levels, have been encouraging. The London team did the ^{125}I-fibrinogen test on eight young women on the Pill subjected to emergency surgery, and on 12 matched control women not on the Pill but exposed to the same operative intervention. Positive post-operative venous limb scans were noted in three of the eight women on the Pill, but in none of the 12 controls. On the basis of these preliminary suggestive findings, it can be proposed that some women on the Pill can be considered hypercoagulable but not thrombotic, and that under the stimulus of surgery their hypercoagulability facilitates the development of deep venous thrombosis that did not occur in their matched controls. The thromboembolic risk of surgery for women on the Pill has been noted by others (Vessey *et al.*,1970; Greene and Sortwell, 1972).

Endotoxin—an inducer of thrombosis
One of the critical unanswered questions concerning the mechanism of intravascular coagulation is the nature of the biological substance that can activate a clotting protein—a proteolytic step necessary to initiate thrombosis. It has been demonstrated in many laboratories over a long span of years that the infusion into animals of one or more activated clotting zymogens will induce intravascular coagulation regardless of whether the infused material is in a crude (Hayem, 1923; Feissly, 1935; Warner *et al.*, 1939; Wessler, 1955; Penick *et al.*, 1958; Henderson and Rapaport 1962) or in a highly purified form (Wessler and Yin, 1968; Yin and Wessler, (1968).

Thrombosis may also be induced experimentally by substances that are not themselves activated clotting proteins including tissue thromboplastin (Penick *et al.*, 1958) trypsin (Taylor *et al.*, 1954; Wessler *et al.*, 1961), fatty acids (Connor *et al.*, 1963; Henderson and Rapaport, 1962; Thomas *et al.*,1963), ellagic acid (Botti and Ratnoff, 1963) and endotoxin (Thomas and Wessler, 1964; Makay *et al.*, 1968).

Endotoxin is suitable for study as a thrombogenic trigger because Gram-negative infections are common in Western Society, because endotoxin produces thrombosis in both animals (Thomas and Wessler, 1964; Corrigan *et al.*, 1967) and in man (Abilgaard *et al.*, 1967; McGehee *et al.*, 1967), and because bacterial endotoxins may enter the systemic circulation during shock (Ravin and Fine, 1962). In experimental animals activation of the blood coagulation mechanism is initiated by endotoxins released from bacteria (Thomas and Wessler, 1964; Corrigan *et al.*, 1967), and in areas of retarded blood flow endotoxin may produce stasis thrombi immediately following a single injection of endotoxin (Thomas and Wessler, 1964).

It has not been clear, however, at precisely what site in the recipient animal's coagulation mechanism endotoxins act, although many possible loci have been suggested (Shimamoto *et al.*, 1958; Des Prez *et al.*, 1961; Spink and Vick, 1961; Born and Cross, 1964; McKay *et al.*, 1968; Alexander *et al.*, 1969).

VESSEL WALL INJURY

The formed elements of the blood

Acceptance of the causative role of vessel injury in deep venous thrombosis has been supported historically by experimental observations, particularly in the microcirculation, ever since Bizzozero (1882) demonstrated that injury to a vein wall resulted in the adherence of platelets to the endothelium of the injured area and that aggregation occurred at the injured site. Since these early investigations of thrombosis and haemostasis in living animals, the platelet has continued to be regarded as having a dominant role in this complex biological reaction to various types of injury (Chapters 7 and 8). However, apart from preliminary vasomotor changes, the first tissue response in acute inflammation, produced by noxious agents, is the sticking of leukocytes to endothelium (Cohnheim, 1889; Cappell, 1958; Payling-Wright, 1958; Florey, 1962) and in these descriptions platelet sticking is not mentioned. This variation in response may be accounted for by a difference in the intensity of injury (Silver and Stehbens, 1965; Stehbens, 1965), yet the discrepancy in the literature indicates the extent of our ignorance of the essential difference in the role of platelets, leukocytes and erythrocytes in vessel injury.

The detailed behaviour of platelets in the microcirculation, other than the observation of aggregation in advanced thrombosis, has to a large extent been overlooked until recent times. Extensive observations in non-inflamed ear chambers have demonstrated that platelets rarely adhere to the vessel wall and, contrary to popular belief, the presence of a platelet in the plasma zone is not necessarily an indication that it is about to stick to the endothelium. When platelets adhere, they do so at very localised points of attachment and are easily washed away. Other platelets may adhere to those already fixed to the vessel wall though they do not adhere to one another in the cirulation or in stagnant vessels. Platelets do not stick to circulating erythrocytes, but it is not unusual for one or two platelets to adhere to a leukocyte which is rolling along the vessel wall. However not all leukocyte sticking is associated with this phenomenon (Silver and

16

Stehbens, 1965; Stehbens, 1966; 1969).

In the microcirculation, after mild trauma, an accentuation of the tendency of platelets to adhere to leukocytes results in the gradual build-up of platelet-leukocyte thrombi which shed embolic fragments. This process may be quite localised and even confined to a single vessel with minimal trauma. Considering the innumerable small vessel injuries that must occur in man constantly, it seems reasonable to believe that such leukocyte-platelet aggregation must be reversible.

The experimental introduction of substances to increase platelet aggregation is accompanied to a varying degree by accentuation of this platelet-leukocyte response, although in some instances massive red cell aggregation also occurs (Stehbens, 1966; Stehbens and Biscoe, 1967). In the latter circumstance, large red cell masses of sludged blood have been seen impeding or completely obstructing blood flow (Knisely, 1965). By definition, such red cell aggregates must be considered a type of thrombus.

Platelet ultrastructure
Examination of the ultrastructure of early platelet aggregation has shown that platelets initially do not exhibit deformity in shape and that the areas of contact between the platelets are limited (Stehbens, 1966; Stehbens and Biscoe, 1967). With subsequent changes the adjoining platelets gradually become applied to one another with consequent alteration in shape, but dendritic forms, degranulation and rearrangement of granulomere location are not observed in these early stages. In the aggregation of platelets and the formation of a tightly packed mass, it is now known that fusion of the platelets does not occur. With electron microscopy it is seen that platelets ultimately form a tightly packed mosaic and it has been suggested that the close approximation of platelets to one another may be related to the known property of platelets to spread on a 'foreign' surface—in this instance an altered platelet surface.

Stehbens has concluded from a study of early *in vivo* changes that pseudopod formation and dendritic forms can be artifacts induced by the separation and handling of the platelets prior to fixation for electron microscopy (Stehbens and Biscoe, 1967). Therefore, if platelets have already undergone considerable morphologic change, as evidenced by many published electron micrographs of 'normal' platelets separated prior to fixation, they may have also undergone considerable biochemical change initiated by the alteration in the environment. These findings, in fact, raise a serious question as to how relevant *in vitro* data on platelets are to the observed *in vivo* phenomena.

In regard to the artifacts in studies of platelets *in vitro*, examination of the endothelium *en face* has illustrated how readily the endothelium is damaged in the handling of vessels. It had been claimed that stigmata along the silver-stained endothelial cell borders were platelet thrombi (Samuels and Webster, 1952); electron microscopy, however, has failed to substantiate this interpretation (Majno and Palade; 1961), and similar staining reactions can be induced *in vitro* in the absence of blood (Stehbens, 1965). Platelets adhere to severely damaged endothelium at the edges of areas of desquamation and where the endothelium is denuded, but not to normal endothelium (Stehbens, 1965). Others have found thrombi adherent to amorphous remnants of endothelium or to the basement membrane (Poole *et al.*, 1963).

Vascular response to injury

On the basis of his own investigation and his survey of the literature, Spaet has concluded that thrombosis is primarily a vascular lesion in which the blood haemostatic components are responding normally (Spaet and Erickson, 1966). This thesis maintains that different pathologic processes converge to give an initial 'final common pathway' resulting in' the appearance at the endothelial surface of denuded collagen to which platelets adhere. Although the entire chemical mechanism underlying platelet thrombus formation is not fully understood, it is presently believed that following the adhesion of platelets to collagen fibres, there is a release of ADP with reversible platelet aggregation. Subsequently, irreversible platelet aggregation is mediated by local thrombin formation. It has been clearly shown that fibrin deposition follows the formation of platelet thrombi which can occur even in incoagulable afibrinogenaemic or heparinised blood.

Whereas intimal damage may underlie the initiation of most thrombi, investigators have repeatedly experienced difficulty in producing routinely grossly visible thrombi by means of severe local trauma (Jacques, 1951). Moreover, when experimental thrombi do form, they tend to remain limited to the area of local injury, even though the endothelial damage is greater than that frequently found clinically. These observations suggest that thrombosis induced by purely local vascular injury can be readily contained by normal compensatory mechanisms; only when these mechanisms are overwhelmed or destroyed by some more generalised reaction can thrombosis proceed.

Role of platelet in venous thrombosis

Venous thrombi often begin at valve cusps and the venous plexi in the soleus and gastrocnemious muscles (Chapters 10 & 11). Such sites reflect anatomical factors and the flow condition of a slowed venous stream including the production of local eddy currents The absence of a recognisable intimal lesion with venous thrombi is in striking contrast to the overt endothelial lesion usually associated with arterial thrombi.

The presence of platelets in a valve cusp may be primarily a rheological phenomenon. Silting of platelets into valve pockets probably results directly from local turbulence and eddies promoted by venous stasis (Cotton and Clark, 1965). There is no direct morphological evidence in man that the initial thrombus in a valve cusp, or elsewhere, is a purely platelet nidus. Platelets and fibrin are intermixed in thrombi examined early and it may be impossible to determine which came first. (Paterson and McLachlin, 1954; Hume *et al.,* 1970).

Platelets, as has been already mentioned, do not adhere to normal endothelium: it is only when the endothelium is removed, exposing the subendothelium that a definite platelet thrombus develops (French *et al.,* 1974). The extent of injury required to produce a platelet thrombus appears to be fairly substantial. Thus, Ashford and Freiman (1967) found that platelets accumulated over an altered endothelial surface only when the endothelial barrier was interrupted and the underlying connective tissue exposed. Even injury sufficient to produce extreme vacuolisation of the endothelial cell failed to produce platelet aggregation if the plasma membrane remained intact (Ashford and Freiman, 1967; Johnson, 1971; Baumgartner and Handenschild, 1972). It must be appreciated that whereas platelet aggregation usually precedes fibrin deposition as the first anatomical evidence of thrombus formation, the visualised platelet aggregate results from trace amounts of thrombin that cannot be recognised by morphological techniques. Baumgartner and Haudenschild (1972) have shown, moreover, that platelets are less likely to adhere to a damaged vessel wall under conditions of low blood flow than under conditions of high flow, reinforcing the view that platelet aggregation in veins where there is no obvious intimal damage is not necessarily the result of endothelial injury.

It is from these lines of evidence and from what has been stated above in the section under hypercoagulability that leads us to suspect that in venous thrombosis, irreversible platelet aggregation is a phenomenon that follows activation of clotting zymogens. Important as platelet aggregation is for the eventual evolution of the venous thrombus, the data are consistent with the view that it is a secondary rather than an initiating factor in the formation of deep venous thrombosis. (Chapter 7).

RETARDED BLOOD FLOW

Stasis can be demonstrated to occur under physiological conditions in normal man during varying degrees of immobilisation or during pregnancy, and in diverse pathological states such as polycythaemia vera, the dysproteinaemias, shock and congestive heart failure, some of which are associated with increased viscosity (Wells and Merrill, 1962; Faney et al., 1965; Putnam et al., 1965). In many of these clinical situations a greater than normal incidence of thrombosis has been recorded.

Numerous reports have implicated stasis in the precipitation of clinical phlebitis following prolonged sitting in air-raid shelters, automobiles, airplanes and during television programmes (Simpson, 1940; Homans, 1954; Naide, 1957). These are, of course, uncontrolled observations and do not reflect any greater immobilisation in patients developing phlebitis than occurs in other individuals who do not demonstrate intravascular coagulation clinically.

Although this cumulative association of stasis and thrombosis appears valid, data both in animals and man suggest that retarded blood flow alone does not initiate thrombosis. It is an old observation that blood trapped between two ligatures in the canine jugular vein remains fluid for more than three hours (Hewson, 1771; Glenard, 1875; Baumgarten, 1877; Lister, 1893; Wessler, 1952).

Roentgenographic studies in man have shown that profound retardation of blood flow can occur in the deep veins of the leg unassociated with thrombosis. If radio-opaque fluid is introduced into the dorsal foot vein of elderly supine subjects, it is retained in venous valve pockets, on occasion, for as long as 60 min and immediately leaves the veins when the subject's legs are elevated slightly from the horizontal plane (Stanton et al., 1949; McLachlin et al., 1960).

Taken together, these observations on the remarkable intravascular resistance to coagulation of a static column of blood suggest that retarded blood flow alone cannot initiate thrombosis. Therefore, in the presence of a normal intima, some alteration in the circulating constituents of the blood must be present to trigger intravascular coagulation.

Rheology and thrombosis

In relating rheology to thrombosis certain terms used in fluid dynamics require definition. These terms are frequently expressed through the analogy of the movement of playing cards, one across the other, in a clean pack on a table. Shear stress refers to the horizontal pushing force against the playing card divided by the area of the card. Shear rate, on the other hand refers to the horizontal distance of displacement per second of a given card beyond its immediate neighbour, divided by its thickness. The term viscosity, expressing the friction between playing cards, is then defined as the ratio of shear stress to shear rate. When the viscosity of a fluid remains the same at all shear rates, it is known as a Newtonian fluid. When viscosity is not constant, but changes in relation to shear stress or shear rate, flow is termed non-Newtonian. At low flow rates, such as occur in veins, human blood behaves like a non-Newtonian fluid, whereas at the high flow rates found in arteries, its fluid characteristics are Newtonian. In order to slip one card over another the horizontal thrust required to start the slip process is defined as the yield stress (Merrill, 1969). Yield stress thus refers to a shearing force below which no flow occurs.

The most significant non-Newtonian characteristics of blood are produced by the interaction of red reclls and fibrinogen. Fibrinogen is essential in producing the red cell structures which are responsible for the special rheological properties of blood in areas of retarded flow. Except for the effect of β-lipoprotein (and for macroglobulins and cryoglobulins which produce bizarre rheological effects), the ordinary globulins have little if any influence on rheological properties (Merill *et al.*, 1965).

The experimental data on the non-Newtonian viscosity of blood clearly suggest that native fibrinogen is absorbed onto the red cell membrane and acts as a reversible adhesive agent for red cells. Thus, the non-Newtonian viscosity of blood near or at zero shear rate would appear to have relevance to irregular, slow, or stalled circulation anywhere in the vasculature, but especially in the veins. If a platelet or other thrombus is effective in halting the flow of blood, or nearly halting it, the stalled or slowly flowing blood will facilitate the thrombotic process by mechanically protecting it from being 'washed out' by fluid blood.

In areas of retarded flow there is adhesion of adjacent red cells to create a three-dimensional random structure, the evolution of contiguous, adherent rouleaux from the original structure, and densification of the red cell structure with syneresis of plasma (Merrill, 1965). These events are all manifestations of the 'bridging' of red cell surfaces by non-activated fibrinogen (Merrill, 1965). From these data it may be proposed that in areas of retarded blood flow, thrombus evolution would be favoured in the plasma phase within the static red cell network, because thrombin is protected against dilution to subcritical concentration and nascent fibrin is protected against premature dispersion.

A more intriguing, though more speculative, consequence of the rheology of stalled blood is in the area of the chemical kinetics of thrombosis. The red cell 'structure', of which yield stress is direct evidence, will retard dilution of the activated clotting factors by fresh plasma. It will also favour increases in the concentration of each of the clotting factors to the critical level for activation of the next in the series of clotting reactions. In respect to the red cell thrombus, it is possible that fibrinogen adsorbed onto the red cell surfaces has the additional function of facilitating the incorporation of red cells as 'quanta' in the red thrombus. On this account, the mechanical strength of the thrombus should increase at a greater rate than if the red cells were absent.

It is even conceivable that the activated clotting factors might adsorb preferentially onto the red cell membrane adjacent to fibrinogen molecules and that the activation of fibrinogen as adsorbed on a red cell membrane may be kinetically far more rapid than fibrinogen in plasma solution (Merrill, 1965).

All these observations and speculations lead to the conclusion that whereas stasis is an important factor in thrombogenesis, it is a facilitating rather than an initiating factor in deep venous thrombosis.

SUMMARY

Our understanding of the mechanism of thrombus formation in veins has been significantly changed in recent years. On the basis of presently available evidence it appears likely that hypercoagulability of the blood is the key initiating factor in this pathological process. Platelets play an important early role in thrombogenesis by providing a surface upon which the coagulation reactions can proceed with increased efficiency. In addition, when trace amounts of thrombin are formed, platelets undergo irreversible aggregation contributing to the original substance of the thrombus. When more thrombin is evolved, fibrin is formed which, together with entrapped erythrocytes, causes both enlargement and stability of the original platelet mass. Throughout, retarded blood flow serves, by a variety of mechanisms, only as a facilitator of thrombus formation.

The pivotal role of activated Factor X in the generation of thrombin has now been well-defined and the inhibition of this reaction by a normal plasma globulin has been clarified. The interplay of activated Factor X, its plasma inhibitor, phospholipid and heparin has provided an increased understanding of the significance of several reactions that determine whether or not irreversible platelet aggregation and fibrin deposition will occur. These data have had a gratifiyingly rapid spin-off for clinical medicine.

Thromboembolism

They have, for example, contributed to a biochemical rationale for the action of heparin, to a possible use of this drug in preventing postoperative deep venous thrombosis without risk of haemorrhage and to an understanding of the failures as well as the successes of heparin as an anticoagulant (Wessler and Yin, 1973). These findings have also led to the development of an improved assay for plasma heparin with its attendant clinical implications (Yin et al., 1973c).

Finally, studies of the activated Factor X inhibitor have stimulated advances in our appreciation of one mechanism whereby endotoxin can induce the essential proteolytic event required to initiate prothrombin activation: this work has also led to a new definition of hypercoagulability that has among its attributes a ready susceptibility to experimental verification in animals and in man.

References

Abilgaard, C. F., Corrigan, J. J., Jr, Seder, R. A., Simone, J. V. and Schulman, I. (1967). Meningococcemia associated with intravascular coagulation. *Pediatrics,* **40,** 78

Abildgaard, U. (1968). Highly purified antithrombin 3 with heparin cofactor activity prepared by disc electrophoresis. *Scan. J. Clin. Invest.,* **21,** 89

Alexander, B. Kliman, A., Colman, R., Scholtz E. and Francesco, A. (1969) *New 'Hemophilid' defects: some clinico-laboratory and experimental abnormalities in thromboplastin generation. Hemophilia and other Hemorrhagic States,* 137 (Chapel Hill, Univ.: North Carolina Press)

Ashford, T. P. and Freiman, D. G. (1967). The role of the endothelium in the initial phases of thrombosis. *Ame. J. Pathol.,* **50,** 257

Barton, P. G. and Hanahan, D. J. (1967). The preparation and properties or a stable Factor V from bovine plasma. *Biophys.* **Biochem.** *Acta, 133,* 506

Barton, P. G., Yin, E. T. and Wessler, S. (1970). Reactions of activated Factor X: Phosphatide mixtures *in vitro* and *in vivo. J. Lipid Res.,* **11,** 87

Baumgarten, P. (1877). *Die Sogennaute Organization Des Thrombus. (Leipzig: Otto Wigand)*

Baumgartner H. R. and Haudeschild, C. (1972). Adhesion of platelets to subendothelium. **In** *Platelets and their role in hemostasis,* **201,** 22, *(Ann. N. Y. Acad. Sci)*

Biggs, R., Denson, K. W. E., Akman, N., Borrett, R. and Hadden, M. (1970). Antithrombin III, antifactor Xa and heparin. *Brit. J. Haemat.* **19,** 283

Bizzozero, J. (1882). Wever einen neuen formbestandtheil des blutes and dessen rolle bei der thrombose und der blutgerinnung. *Arch. Path. Anat.,* **90,** 261

Born, G. V. R. and Cross, M. J. (1964). Effects of inorganic ions and of plasma proteins on the aggregation of blood platelets by adenosine diphosphate. *J. Physiol.,* **170,** 397

Botti, R. E. and Ratnoff, O. D. (1963). The clot-promoting effect of soaps of long-chain saturated fatty acids. *J. Clin. Invest.,* **42,** 1569

Cappell, D. F. (1958). In: *Muir's Textbook of Pathology,* (London: Edward Renold Ltd)

Thromboembolism

Cohnheim, J, (1889). In: *Lectures on General Pathology*. Vol. I, 249 A. B. McKee, editor (London New Sydenham Society)

Connor W. E., Hoak J. C. and Warner, E. D. (1963). Massive thrombosis produced by fatty acid infusion. *J. Clin. Invest.,* **42,** 860

Corrigan, J. J., Jr. Abilgaard, C. F., Vander Weiden, J. F. and Schulman, I. (1967). Quantitative aspects of blood coagulation in the generalized Shwartzman reaction. *Ped. Res.,* **1,** 39

Cotton, L. T. and Clark, C. (1965). Anatomical localization of venous thrombosis. *Ann. Royal Coll. Surg.,* **36,** 214

Davie, E. W. and Ratnoff, O. D. (1964). Waterfall sequence for intrinsic blood clotting. *Science,* **145,** 1310

Des Prez, R. M., Horowitz, H. I. and Hook, E. W. (1961). Effects of bacterial endotoxin on rabbit platelets. O. Platelet aggregation and release of platelet factors in vitro. *J. Exp. Bio.,* **114,** 857

Ekberg, O. (1965). Inherited antithrombin deficiency causing thrombophilia. *Thromb. Diath. Haemorrh.,* **13,** 576

Fagerhol, M. K. Abilgaard, U., Bergshe, P. and Jacobsen, J. H. (1970). Oral contraceptives and low antithrombin-III concentration. *Lancet,* **i,** 1175

Fahey, J. L., Barth, W. F. and Solomon, A. (1965). Serum hyperviscosity syndrome. *J. Amer. Med. Ass.,* **192,** 464

Feissly, R. (1925). La Stabilite du fibrinogine in vivo. Compt. Rend. Soc. Biol., **92,** 319

Florey, H. W. (1962). *General Pathology,* (London: Floyd-Luke)

Fonio, A. (1940). Beobachtungen uber den Gerrinungs und den Thrombo-sevorgang in Dunhelfeldnativpraparat. *Schweiz. Med. Wschr.* **70,** 510

French, J. E., Macfarlane, R. G. and Sanders, A. G. (1964). The structure of haemostatic plugs and experimental thrombi in small arteries. *Brit. J. Exp. Pathol.,* **45,** 467

Gaardner, A., Jansen, J., Laland, S., *et al.,* (1961) Adenosine diphosphate in red cells as a factor in the adhesiveness of human blood platelets. *Nature* London, **192,** 531

Glenard, F. (1875). Contribution a l'etude des causes de la coagulation spontanee du sang a son issue de l'organisme, application a la transfusion. *Paris Thesis—46*

Grannis, G. F. and Kazal, L. A. (1966). Prothrombin and antithrombin: their opposing functions in blood coagulation. *Thromb. Diath. Haemorrh.,* **16,** 497

Greene, G. R. and Sortwell, P. E. (1972). Oral contraceptive use in patients with thromboembolism following surgery, trauma or infection. *Amer. J. Public Health,* **62,** 680

Haslam, R. J. (1969). Mechanisms of blood platelet aggregation. In: *The Physiology of Haemostasis and Thrombosis* 88—172. S. A Johnson and W. H. Seegers, Editors, Springfield, Illinois: Charles C. Thomas

Hayem, G. (1923). *Hamatoblaste,* 120 (Paris: Les Presses Universitaries de France).

Hemker, H. c., Esnouf, M. P., Hemker, P. W., Smart, A C. and Macfarlane, R. G. (1967). Formation of prothrombin converting activity. *Mature,* **215,** 248

Hemker, H. C. Hemker P. W. and Loeliger, E. A. (1965). Kinetic aspects of the interaction of blood clotting enzymes. I. Derivation of basic formulas *Thromb, Diath. Haemorrh.,* **13,** 155

Hemker, H. C., Veltkramp, J. J. and Loeliger, E. A. (1968). Kinetic aspects of the interaction of blood clotting enzymes. 3. Demonstration of an inhibitor of prothrombin conversion in vitamin K deficiency. *Thromb. Diath. Haemorrh.,* **91,** 346

Thromboembolism

Hemker, H. C. and Hemker, P. W. (1968). Kinetic aspects of the interaction of blood clotting enzymes. IV. Kinetics of competitive inhibition in clotting tests. *Thromb. Diath. Haemorrh.*, **19**, 364

Henderson, E. S. and Rapaport, S. I. (1962). The thrombotic activity of activation product. *J. Clin. Invest.*, **41**, 235

Hewson, W. (1771). *Experimental inquiries*. 1. An inquiry into the properties of the blood, with some remarks on some of its morbid appearances, and an appendix relating to the discovery of the lymphatic system in birds, fish and the animals called amphibians (London: T. Cadell)

Homans, J. (1954). Thrombosis of deep leg veins due to prolonged sitting. *New Eng. J. Med.*, **250**, 148

Hougie, C., Barrow, E. M. and Graham, J. B. (1957). Stuart clotting defect. 1 Segregation of an hereditory hemorrhagic state from the heterogeneous group heretofore called stable factor (SPCA proconvertin, Factor VII) deficiency. *J. Clin. Invest.*, **36**, 485

Hume, M., Sevitt, S. and Thomas, D. P. (1970). Venous thrombosis and pulmonary embolism (Cambridge, Mass.: Harvard Univ. Press)

Inman, W. H. W. and Vessey, M. P. (1968). Investigation of deaths from pulmonary, coronory, and cerebral thrombosis and embolism in women of child-bearing age. *Brit Med. J.*, **2**, 193

Jacques, L. B. (1951). In: *Blood clotting and allied problems*, 42 Trans. Fourth Conf. (J. E. Flynn, editor) (New York: Josiah Macy, Jr Foundation)

Jevons, S. and Barton, P. G. (1971). Biochemistry of blood platelets. I. Interaction of activated Factor X with platelets. Biochem., **10**, 428

Johnson, S. A. (1971). Platelets in hemostasis and thrombosis In: *The Circulating Platelet*, 356. (S. A. Johnson, editor) New York: Academic Press

Kazer-Glanzman, R. and Luscher, E. F. (1962). The mechanism of platelet aggregation in relation to hemostasis. *Thromb. Diath. Haemorrh.*, **7**, 480

Knislely, M. H. (1956). In: Handbook of Physiology, Section 2, Circulation 3 Lister, J. (1893). The Croonian Lecture on the coagulation of the blood. *Lancet*, **ii**, 149

Macfarlane, R. G. (1964). An enzyme cascade in the blood clotting mechanism and its function as a biochemical amplifier. *Nature (London)*, **202**, 498

Majno, G. and Palade, G. E (1961). Studies on inflammation. 1 The effect of histamine and seotonin on vascular permeability: an electron microscopic study. *J. Biophys. Biochem. Cytol.*, **11**, 571

Marciniak, E. and Tsukamura, S. (1972). Two progressive inhibitors of Factor Xa in human blood. *Brit. J. Haematol.*, **22**, 341

Marcus, A. J. and Zucker, M. B. (1965). In: The Physiology of Blood Platelets, 21 (New York: Grune and Stratton)

McGehee W. G., Rapaport, S. I and Hjort, P. F. (1967). Intravascular coagulation in fulminant meningococcemia. *Ann. Int. Ked*, **67**, 250

McKay, D. G., Shapiro, S. and S. and Shanberge, J. N. (1968) Alterations in the blood coagulation system induced by bacterial endotoxin. *J. Exp. Med.*, **107**, 369

McLachlin, A. D., McLachlin, J. A., Jory, T. A. and Rawling, E. G. (1960). Venous stasis in the lower extremities. *Ann. Surg.*, **152**, 678

Merrill, E. W., Morgetts, W. G., Cokelet, G. R., Britten, A., Salzman, E. W., Pennell, R. G. and Melin, M. (1965). Influence of plasma proteins on the rheology of human blood. In: *Proc. Fourth Int. Cong. Rheology*, 601(Wiley)

Thromboembolism

Merrill, E. W. (1969). Rheology of human blood: *in vitro* observations and theoretical considerations. *In Thrombosis*, 477 (S. Sherry, K. M. Brinkhouse, E. Genton and J. Stengle, editors) (Washington D. C.: Nat. Acad. Sci.)

Morawitz, P. (1905). Die chemie der blutgerinnung. *Erghen. Physiol.* **4,** 307

Naide, M. (1957). Prolonged television viewing as cause of venous and arterial thrombosis in legs. *J. Amer. Med. Ass.,* **165,** 681

Paterson, J. C. and McLachlin, J. A. (1954). Precipitating factors in venous thrombosis. *Surg. Gynalcol. Obstet.,* **98,** 96

Payling-Wright, G. (1958). *An Introduction to Pathology.* (London: Longmans Green and Co.)

Penick, G. D., Roberts, H. P., Webster, W. P. and Brinkhous, K. M. (1958). Hemorrhagic states secondary to intravascular clotting: an experimental study of their evolution and prevention. *Arch. Pathol.,* **66,** 708

Peterson, R., Krull, P. E., Finley, O. and Ettinger, M. G. (1970). Changes in antithrombin III and plasminogen induced by oral contraceptives. *Amer. J. Clin. Pathol.,* **53,** 468

Poole, J. C. F., French, J. E. and Cliff, W. J. (1963). The early stages of thrombosis. *J. Clin. Pathol.,* **16,** 523

Putnam, T. C., Kevy, S. V. and Replogle, R. L. (1965). Factor affecting the viscosity of blood *Surg. Forum,* **16,** 126

Ravin, H. A. and Fine, J. (1962). Biological implications of intestinal endotoxins. *Fed. Proc.,* **21,** 65

Royal College of General Practitioners. (1967). Oral contraception and thromboembolic disease. *J. Coll. Gen Practit.,* **136,** 267

Samuels, P. B. and Webster, D. R. (1952). The role of venous endothelium in the inception of thrombosis. *Ann. Surg.,* **136,** 422

Seeger, W. H. and Marciniak, E. (1962). Inhibition of autoprothrombin C activity with plasma. *Nature (London),* **193,** 1188

Seegers, W. H. (1968). Antithrombin a proteinase inhibitor. *Ann. N. T. Acad. Sci.,* **146,** 593

Schimamoto, T., Yamazaki, H., Sagawa, N., Iwakara, S., Koniski, T. and Mawzawa, H. (1958). Effect of bacterial endotoxins on platelets and release of serotonin (5-hydroxytryptamine). II. Appearance of platelet-agglutinating substance and serotonin (5-hydroxytryptamine) in the plasma of rabbits by administration of bacterial endotoxin. *Proc. Japan Acad.,* **34,** 450

Silver, M. D. and Stehbens, W. E. (1965). The behavior of platelets *in vivo. Quart, J. Expt. Phsiol.,* **50,** 241

Simpaon, K. (1940). Sheter deaths from pulmonary embolism. *Lancet,* **ii,** 744

Sortwell, P. E., Masi, A. J., Arthes, F. G., Greene, G. R. and Smith, H. D. (1969). Thromboembolism and oral contraceptives: an epidemiologic case-control study. *Amer. J. Epid.,* **905,** 365

Spaet, T. H. and Erickson, R. B. (1966). The vascular wall in the pathogenesis of thrombosis. *Thromb. Diath. Hawmorrh.,* **Suppl. 21,** 67

Spink, W. W. and Vick, J. (1961). A labile serum factor in experimental endotoxin shock: cross-transfusion studies in dogs. *J. Exp. Med.,* **114,** 501

Thromboembolism

Stanton, J. R., Freis, E. D. and Wilkins, R. W. (1949). The acceleration of linear flow in the deep veins of the lower extemity of man by local compression *J. Clin. Invest.*, **28,** 553

Stehbens, W. E. (1965). Reaction of venous endothelium to injury. Lab. Invest., **14,** 449

Stehbens, W. E. (1966) *Proc. Fourth Eur. Conf. Microcirculation,* (Basel: S. Karger).

Stehbens, W. E. (1967). Observations on the microcirculation in the rabbit ear chamber. *Quart. J. Exp., Phsiol.,* **52,** 150

Stehbens, W. E. and Biscoe, T. J. (1967). The ultrastructure of early platelet aggregation *in vivo. Amer. J. Pathol.,* **50,** 219

Surgenor, D. M. and Wallach, D. F. H. (1961). In: *Blood Platelets: 289, S. A. Hohnson, Rebuck Monto, R. W. and J. W., (editors) (Boston Little, Brown)*

Taylor, A., Overman, R. S. and Wright, I. S. (1954). Studies with crystalline trypsin. Results and hazards of intravenous administration and its postulated role in blood coagulation. *J. Amer. Med. Ass.,* **155,** 347

Telfer, T. P., Denson, K. W. and Wright, D. R. (1956). A 'new' coagulation defect. *Brit. J. Haematol,* **2,** 308

Thomas, D. P., Wessler, S. and Reimer, S. M. (1963). The relation of Factors XII, XI, and IX to hypercoagulable states. *Thromb. diath, Haemorrh.,* **9,** 90

Thomas, D. P. and Wessler, S. (1964). Stasis thrombi induced by bacterial endotoxin. *Circ. Res.,* **14,** 486

Vessey, M. P. and Doll, R. (1969). Investigation of relation between use of oral contraceptives and thromboembolic disease. A further report. *Brit. Med. J.,* **2,** 651

Vessy, M. P., Doll, Fairbairn, A. S. and Glaber, G. (1970). Postoperative thrombembolism and the use of oral contraceptives. *Brit. Med. J.,* **3,** 123

Virchow, R. (1856). *Gaesmmelte Abhandhingen zur Wissen-Schaftlichen Medicine,* 219 (Frankfurt: Meidinger Sohn)

VonKaulla, E. and VonKaulla K. N. (1967). Antithrombin III and diseases. *Amer. J. Clin. Pathol.,* **48,** 69

VonKaulla, E. and VonKaulla, K. M. (1970). Oral contraceptives and low antithrombin-3 activity. *Lancet,* **I,** 36

Warner, F. D., Brinkhous, K. M., Seegers, W. H. and Smith, H. P. (1939). Further experience with the use of thrombin as a hemostatic. *Proc. Soc. Exp. Biol. Med.,* **41,** 655

Wells, R. E., Jr. and Merill, E. W. (1962). Influence of flow properties of blood on viscosity-hematocrit relationships. *J. Clin. Invest.,* **41,** 1591

Wessler, S. (1952). Studies in intravascular coagulation. I. Coagulation changes in isolated venous segments. *J. Clin. Invest.,* **31,** 1011

Wessler, S. (1955). Studies in intravascular coagulation. III. The pathogenesis of serum-induced venous thrombosis. *J. Clin. Invest.,* **34,** 647

Wessler, S., Reimer, S. M., Freiman, D. G. and Thomas, D. P. (1961). Factors involved in the imitiation of thrombosis. In: *Anticoagulants and Fibrinolysis,* 108, (Toronto)

Wessler, S. and Yin, S. M. (1968). The experimental hypercoagulable state induced by Factor X: a comparison of the non-activated and activated forms. J. Lab. Clin. Med., **72,** 256

Wessler, S. and Yin, E. T. (1973). The theory and practice of mini-dose heparin: a status report. *Circulation,* **47,** 671

Thromboembolism

Wiseman, R. (1676). *Several Chirurgical Treatises*, Ed. 2, 64 (London: Norton and Macock)

Yin, E. T. and Wessler, S. (1968). Investigation of the apparent thrombogenicity of thrombin. *Thromb. Diath. Haemorrh.* **20,** 465

Yin, E. T. and Wessler, S. (1970). Heparin-accelerated inhibition of activated Factor X by its natural inhibitor. *Biochem. Biophys. Acta.,* **201,** 387

Yin, E. T., Wessler, S. and Stoll, P. (1971). Rabbit plasma inhibitor of the activated species of blood coagulation Factor X: purification and some properties. *J. Biol. Chem.,* **246,** 3694

Yin, E. T., Wessler, W. and Stoll, P. (1971a). Biological properties of the naturally occurring plasma inhibitor to activated Factor X *J. Biol. Chem.,* **246,** 3703

Yin, E. T., Wessler, S. and Stoll P. J. (1971b). Identity of plasma-activated Factor X inhibitor with antithrombin III and heparin cofactor. *J. Biol. Chem.,* **246,** 3712

Yin, E. T., Chen, J. S. and Wessler, J. V. (1973a). Effect of lipid on neutralization of activated Factor X by its plasma inhibitor. (Abst.) *Amer. Soc. Hematol.,* Dec

Yin, E. T., Giudice, L. C. and Wessler, S. (1973b). Inhibition of activated Factor X induced platelet aggregation: The role of heparin and the plasma inhibitor to activated Factor X. *J. Lab. Clin, Med.,* **82,** 390

Yin, E. T., Wessler, S. and Butler, J. V. (1973c). Plasma heparin: a unique, practical submicrogram-sensitive assay. *J. Lab. Clin. Med.,* **81,** 298

3

The nature of fibrinogen and fibrinogen-fibrin degradation products

H. C. Kwaan

INTRODUCTION

Among the plasma proteins, fibrinogen is perhaps unique in its properties, its distribution within the body, and its metabolism. The protein is present in both the intravascular and extravascular compartments and in many conditions can be broken down without the need to be first converted to fibrin (Hammond and Verle, 1959; Fletcher et al., 1962; Takeda, 1966). The primary physiological function of fibrinogen is the provision of a fibrin network in haemostasis. In addition, it forms a fibrin barrier in inflammatory tissues for the localisation of infections, foreign bodies or possibly even tumour cells (O'Meara, 1958; Kwaan, 1964). The conversion of fibrinogen to fibrin is achieved in the body by the action of thrombin formed as a result of a series of enzymatic reactions involving the blood coagulation factors (McFarlane, 1964). Under certain unusual pathological circumstances such conversion may also take place in the body through the action of other proteolytic enzymes such as trypsin (Pechet and Alexander, 1962). After completion of its function, the fibrin barrier is removed mainly by the process of fibrinolysis in which fragments of different weights and different sizes of the fibrin molecule are formed. They are known as fibrin degradation products (FDP) and may be found in the blood, urine and other body fluids (Kowalski, 1968). When there is excessive fibrinolysis, fibrinogen can also be broken down into fibrinogen degradation products. These are similar in properties to the degradation products derived from fibrin. The products from both sources are referred to in this article interchangeably as FDPs unless specifically stated

29

otherwise. The amounts of FDPs present in various sites reflects the pathophysiological processes which lead to excessive fibrin formation and fibrin breakdown. Thus, the identification and quantification of the FDPs serves as a useful diagnostic aid. In this chapter the clinical significance of fibrinogen and its degradation products will be discussed.

THE STRUCTURE OF FIBRINOGEN
Considerations of the structure of fibrinogen are necessary for the proper understanding of the nature of FDP. Mammalian fibrinogen consists of a molecule having a molecular weight of 340 000 made up of three peptide chains, a (A), β (B) and γ (Blomback, 1967; Blomback *et el.*, 1968). It has a dimeric structure and thus can be represented by the formula $(a(A)\ \beta(B)\gamma)^2$ (Figure 3.1). Two symmetrical monomers of 170 000 unit weight are joined by disulphide bonds located between respective a (A) and γ chains.

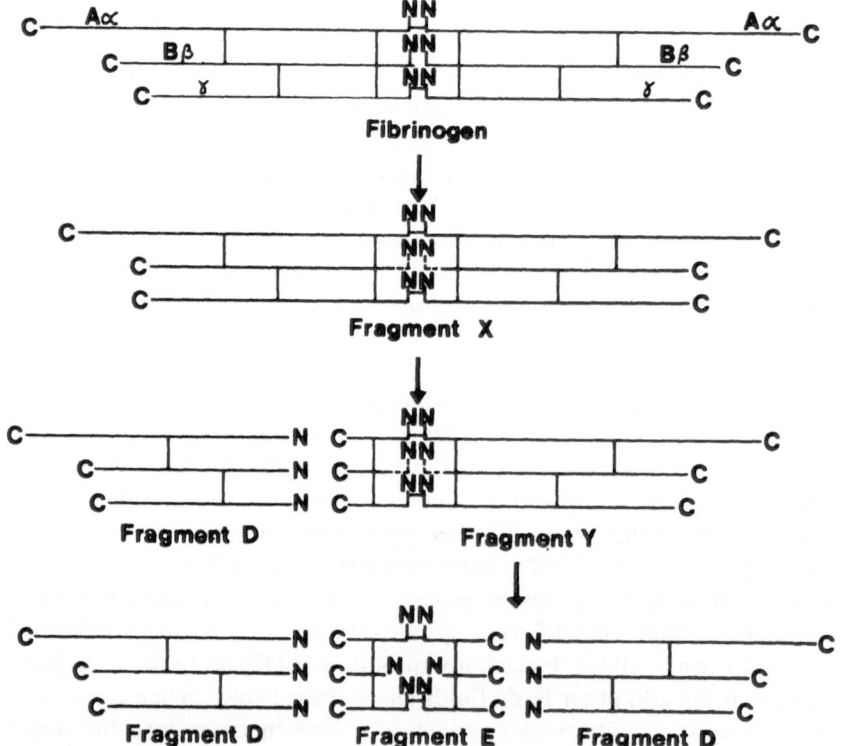

Figure 3.1 Marder's scheme of sequential plasmin degradation of fibrinogen (reproduced by courtesy of *J. Biol. Chem.* Marder *et al.*, 1972). N and C denotes the NH_2 and COOH ends of the polypeptide chains

During the conversion of fibrinogen to fibrin by thrombin, a part of the α B chain at the N-Terminal end, known as fibrinopeptide A is split off along with another part of the N-Terminal portion of the β (B) chain known as fibrinopeptide B. The cleavage of these two fibrinopeptides occurs at the arginyl-glycyl bonds linking the fibrinopeptides to their respective chains on the fibrinogen molecule. As a result, the release of negative charges induces a conformational change in the molecule leading to polymerisation of the molecule into fibrin. In addition to thrombin, fibrinogen may be converted to fibrin by trypsin, papain, ficin and various snake venoms (Blomback, 1958; Blomback, 1967). Two of the latter have been refined; they are Ancrod (also known as Arvin and Venacil) from the venom of *Agkistrodon rhodostoma,* and Reptilase (also known as Defibrase) from that of *Bothrops atrox.* They differ from thrombin in that they remove only fibrinopeptide A from fibrinogen. The fibrin polymer formed by these two snake venom preparations is structurally different from that formed by thrombin (Laurent and Blomback, 1958; Kwaan and Barlow, 1971). As a result, the Ancrod and the Reptilase-induced fibrin is more susceptible to plasmin proteolysis than the thrombin-induced fibrin. An interesting enzyme has been isolated from the venom of another viper, *Agkistrodon contortrix* (Herzig *et al.,* 1970), which hydrolyses fibrinopeptide B faster than the fibrinopeptide A. In this case, no clotting occurs until sufficient fibrinopeptide A is removed, showing the necessity for cleavage of peptide A in fibrinogen-fibrin conversion.

FORMATION OF FDP
Either fibrinogen or fibrin may be broken down by the proteolytic action of many proteases. However, the biological significance is confined to the peptide fragments derived from proteolysis by plasmin. Several stages of fragmentation of fibrinogen have been identified. Although the detailed sequences are still being worked out, the process may be depicted diagrammatically (Marder *et al.,* 1972) in Figure 3.1. The earliest fragment derived from a parent molecule is termed fragment X with a molecular weight of 240 000. This particular FDP is also known as the first intermediate product and the first fibrin derivative. Fragment X derived from fibrinogen retains the fibrinopeptides A and B. Thus, when fragment X is acted upon by thrombin, it is still clottable, though at a much slower rate than that of the clotting of fibrinogen.

The next states of digestion is characterised by the formation of fragment Y, also known as the second intermediate product, having a molecular weight of 155 000. At the same time, a smaller fragment termed fragment D with a molecular weight of 83 000 is formed. The final stage is indicated by a further breakdown of fragment Y into a second fragment D and a fragment E with a molecular weight of 50 000. The digestion process is associated with loss of about 20 per cent of the peptides because of the formation of minor fragments A, B and C.

Recent studies indicate that fragment E is located at the N-Terminal of the molecule and contains the fibrinopeptide A (Latallo *et al.*, 1970). Thus, the fragment E derived from fibrinogen would be different from that derived from fibrin. Fragment D is located at the COOH-Terminal and therefore has the same structure whether it is derived from fibrin or fibrinogen. Fragment D also contains the site for fibrin cross-linking (Gaffney, 1973).

Various FDPs may form soluble complexes with one another, the parent fibrinogen molecule or the fibrin monomer either individually or in groups (Kowalski, 1968; Fletcher *et al.*, 1970). These complexes are described in Chapter 4.

IMMUNOLOGICAL CONSIDERATIONS

Since the identification of FDPs is performed frequently by immunological methods, a clear understanding of the antigenic determinants on each of the FDP fragments is essential. One common antigenetic determinant is present in fibrinogen, fibrin and fragments X, Y, D and E (Nussenzweig and Seligman, 1960; Fisher *et al.*, 1967) thus these components react and form precipitating anti-antibody complexes with anti-fibrinogen serum. When fragments D and E are formed during proteolysis of fibrinogen, one antigenic determinant from the parent molecule stays on each of these fragments. An additional antigenic site is present in fragment D and is immunologically distinct from that of fragment E. Thus, while fragments D and E would both react with antifribrinogen (or antifragment X or antifragment Y) serum, there is no cross reaction between fragments D or E and their antiserum. It also follows that if one uses antifibrinogen serum, one would get a stronger reaction with fibrinogen fragments X and Y than with fragments D and E. Conversely, certain commercially available test systems, such as the Wellcotest (prepared by the Burroughs Wellcome Company) which utilises a mixture of anti-D and anti-E sera, would be more sensitive to fragments D and E.

BIOLOGICAL PROPERTIES

The most pronounced biological effect of FDP of clinical significance is a marked anticoagulant activity. This activity is responsible for much of the defective haemostatic function in patients with disseminated intravascular coagulation. Fibrin formation is inhibited by FDP in several ways, including a competitive inhibition of the action of thrombin. This property of FDP is also identified as antithrombin 6 effect, and is more pronounced with fragment Y than with fragment X, but weak with fragments D and E (Marder and Shulman, 1969). The polymerisation of the fibrin monomer is also inhibited by FDP (Bang *et al.*, 1962). As a result, the monomer may either form soluble complexes with FDP or weakly polymerised fibrin with faulty structure.

The haemostatic function may also be interferred with by an inhibitory effect on platelet function (Niewiarowski *et al.*, 1970). Platelet adhesiveness, aggregation and release reactions are impaired by the action of FDPs of small molecular sizes, while the larger FDP and the FDP-fibrinogen-fibrin complexes have the opposite effect. In the presence of a mixture of FDP of varying sizes, the net effect on platelet function would very much depend on the composition of the FDP. Thus, in disseminated intravascular coagulation, increased platelet aggregation may be encountered; whereas, during therapeutic defibrination with Ancrod therapy, when only the smaller FDP fragments are present, a distinct impairment of platelet function can be demonstrated (Prentice *et al.*, 1969).

Other less clearly defined biological effects of FDP include action such as induction of smooth muscle contraction, enhancement of the contractive action of bradykinin, increase in capillary permeability and chemotaxis of granulocytes (Buluk *et al.*, 1966; Maliofiejew and Buluk, 1968).

METHODS OF DETECTION
Collection of samples: When dealing with the assay of FDP, one should always be reminded that proteolytic activity including that of plasmin is frequently present in test samples such as blood, urine and other body fluids. It follows that artifactual production of FDP may occur *in vitro* unless a protease inhibitor is added to the collection tubes. It is common practice to use soybean trypsin inhibitor, aprotinin or epsilon aminocaproic acid for this purpose.

When dealing with blood samples, either serum or plasma is obtained for the assay. Plasma, containing fibrinogen as well as the FDPs, is not suitable for immunological methods, because the fibrinogen will mask the immunoreactivity of the FDPs. On the other hand, because the larger peptides such as fragment X and the larger complexes are thrombin-clottable, and are thus removed from the plasma during clotting, serum does not contain the whole spectrum of FDPs. Serum is used when assaying only for fragments Y, D, and E and the smaller peptides.

Immunological methods: Fibrinogen, or its major degradation products, carries with it the antigenic component that will react with antifibrinogen

33

serum. The smaller particles, D and E, have additional antigenic sites so that antifragment D and the antifragment E will not cross react with each other and both are partially cross reacting with antifibrinogen serum. Specific anti-D and E sera are thus preferably used for the detection of these two respective fragments. A number of immunological methods are available but the most sensitive is the tanned red cell haemagglutination inhibition immunoassay (TRCHII) (Merskey *et al.*, 1969). It can detect as little as $0.6\,\mu$g per ml of fragment X or Y or $1.2\,\mu$g per ml of fragment D. This method is relatively insensitive in detecting fragment E. A modification using latex particles instead of tanned red cells is also available commercially. One such preparation (Hoq and Cash, 1973), the Thrombo-Wellcotest, utilises a mixture of anti-D and E and is thus suitable for detection of fragments D and E as well as the larger fragments and complexes. Precipitating reactions also occur, and the immuno-diffusion method is also frequently used. The latter suffers from the drawback of being a lengthly procedure in contrast to the quicker methods mentioned above which are more suitable for emergency clinical situations. For the identification of individual fragments, immuno-electrophoresis is necessary. A less sensitive but rapid method is the direct observation of flocculation on adding the test sample to antifibrinogen serum.

Anticoagulation methods: As indicated above, the FDPs have an antithrombin action and interfere with the polymerisation of fibrin monomers. This inhibition of fibrinogen-fibrin conversion can be detected by the thrombin time assay which has long been used as an indicator of FDP activity. Its usefulness, however, is limited because of the relative insensitivity of the test particularly for the detection of fragment E. The antipolymerisation action is directed against the fibrin monomers formed not only by the action of thrombin but also by that of Ancrod or Reptilase. Thus, in addition to thrombin time, the Ancrod time or the Reptilase time are also prolonged in the presence of FDP and may be used as diagnostic methods (Funk *et al.*, 1971). Because heparin interferes with the action of thrombin, the thrombin time cannot be used for the detection of FDPs in clinical situations when the patient is heparinised e.g. during treatment for disseminated intravascular coagulation. Ancrod and Reptilase, on the other hand, are not affected by heparin and should be used instead.

Staphylococcal clumping method: Fibrin and its derivatives produce clumping of a suspension of staphylococci *(Staphylococcus aureus* of the Newman D_2 C strain) and because of the simplicity of the test, it is commonly used in the detection of FDP (Hawiger *et al.*, 1970). However, this test is sensitive only to the larger fragments and does not react with fragments D and E. One has to remember the difference in the sensitivity of this test when compared with that of the immunological techniques especially in those clinical situations when only the small fragments are predominant in the blood. Examples of this can be seen during therapeutic defibrination with Ancrod or Reptilase.

Paracoagulation methods: When fibrin monomers or fragment X dissociate from FDP complexes, gel or fibrin-strand formation occurs spontaneously or on the addition of ethanol or protamine sulphate (Niewiarowski and Gurewich, 1971). This phenomenon is called paracoagulation and is the basis of the ethanol gelation test (Breen and Jullis, 1968) and the protamine sulphate test (Niewiarowski and Gurewich 1971). These tests are frequently positive in plasma obtained from patients with acute disseminated intravascular coagulation. They are, however, negative in pathological fibrinolytic disorders. Their use in the differential diagnosis of these conditions will be discussed later.

The relative merits and sensitivity of the different methods have been investigated in recent comparative studies (Marder *et al.,* 1971). For acute clinical situations, the thrombin time, the direct flocculation test and the 'Thrombo-Wellcotest' can provide a quick and roughly quantitative answer. These tests are simple to set up and easy to perform. They are recommended for use in smaller community hospitals with limited laboratory facilities. A comparison of different methods is seen in Table 3.1.

Table 3.1 Comparative sensitivity of fibrinogen and the various FDPs to the commonly used methods of detection.*

	fibrino-gen	X	Y	D	E
Anticoagulation assay	−	+++	+++	++	+
Thrombin clottability	+++	+++	+	−	−
Staphycococcal clumping	+++	++	++	−	−
Immunodiffusion	++	++	++	++	++
Flocculation	++	++	++	++	++
TRCHII	+++	+++	++	+	+
Latex agglutination 'Thrombo-Wellcotest'	+++	+++	++	+	+

*Levels of sensitivity are indicated by +++ for most sensitive; +, least sensitive and −, insensitive.

CLINICAL CONSIDERATIONS

Because FDP can be derived from the breakdown of fibrinogen or fibrin, either intravascularly or 'extravascularly', the finding of excessive FDP in blood can occur in a wide variety of pathological conditions. During the course of catabolism of fibrinogen, a small amount of FDP is present in the blood even under physiological conditions. Observations by various investigators indicated that FDP values up to 8 μg per ml are not abnormal in blood under basal conditions (Das *et al.*, 1967). Exercise can significantly increase the serum FDP levels as much as four-fold, probably due to a concurrent physiological increase of fibrinolytic activity. Normal urine does not contain sufficient FDP to give a positive test; however, when it is concentrated at least fifty times, a trace quantity can be detected, (Rayner *et al.*, 1969).

Abnormally high levels of FDP in blood may be found in a wide variety of disorders in which fibrin or fibrinogen is broken down at a rate in excess of the capacity for their removal by the reticulo-endothelial system. Intravascular breakdown of fibrin or fibrinogen is not usually localised to one particular part of the body. Extravascular fibrin breakdown can also result in the production of high levels of intravascular FDP even though the source of such fibrin is limited to one part of the body. A list of the clinical conditions in which FDP levels in blood are significantly elevated can be seen in Table 3.2.

PATHOLOGICAL FIBRINOLYSIS (Primary Fibrinolysis)

Primary fibrinolytic disorder is seen when there is an increase in the release of plasminogen activator, a decrease in the normal clearing mechanism for plasminogen activator, or a decrease in the inhibitors of fibrinolysis. This has been observed in patients with liver disease, during a variety of surgical operations and in certain cases of leukaemia (Kwaan, 1972).The excessive activity of plasminogen activator in blood will lead to the following chain reaction: the plasminogen in the plasma will be activated, resulting in increased plasmin activity that will overcome the circulating antiplasmin; a direct proteolytic action on plasma fibrinogen will follow leading to the production of large amounts of FDP. Because intense plasmin activity is present in such situations, an active progression of the digestion process of the FDP would be taking place, so that there is a fairly rapid breakdown of the larger fragments. The amount of detectable FDP in blood will be proportional to the excessive plasmin activity. Smaller fragments will also be excreted in the urine.

Table 3.2 Clinical disorders in which FDPs may be present in abnormally high quantities in the blood

THOSE OF intravascular origin:
    Derived from Fibrinogen
        Pathologic fibrinolysis
        Thrombolytic therapy
    Derived from Fibrin
        Disseminated intravascular coagulation
        Pulmonary embolism
        Extensive deep vein thrombosis
        Therapeutic defibrination with Ancrod or Reptilase

THOSE OF extravascular origin:
        Large haematoma
        Tumour
        Sepsis
        After extensive surgery
        Pregnancy
            Normal labour
            Abruptio placentae
            Toxaemia of pregnancy
    Renal Diseases
        Acute glomerulonephritis
        Proliferative glomerulonephritis
        Renal homograft rejection
        Nephrotic syndrome
        Lupus nephritis
        Schonlein–Henoch nephritis

THROMBOLYTIC THERAPY

During the course of treatment with urokinase or streptokinase, sufficient plasmin may be generated to cause proteolysis of fibrinogen. This would result in the production of FDP as in the case of primary fibrinolysis. A greater activation of circulating plasminogen is seen with streptokinase therapy than with urokinase therapy. In the latter case, unless prolonged intravenous infusion is given, plasminogen activation is limited locally to the thrombus. Apparently, the thrombus has an affinity for urokinase and until the infused urokinase has thoroughly 'saturated' all the intravascular thrombi, there will be no free urokinase available to'activate the circulating plasminogen. However, this is not so with streptokinase infusion in which an early fall in the circulating plasminogen level is consistently seen. Frequently, the circulating plasminogen may be completely depleted rendering streptokinase inactive as a fibrinolytic agent. Furthermore, any plasmin already formed that may be available for fibrinogenolysis may be taken up by the streptokinase to form a streptokinase-plasmin complex. The complex is inactive as a proteolytic agent for fibrinogen, though it is a potent activator of plasminogen. Because of these difficulties, fibrinolytic assay methods are unsuitable for the clinical control of treatment with streptokinase; the thrombin time is used instead because it measures the amount of FDP released from fibrinogenolysis. A thrombin time twice that of the control value is considered an indication of satisfactory treatment.

DISSEMINATED INTRAVASCULAR COAGULATION (Secondary Fibrinolysis)

In this syndrome, the primary event is intravascular fibrin formation which is often accompanied by varying degrees of secondary increase in plasma fibrinolytic activity. The breakdown of such fibrin leads to FDP production (Kwaan, 1972). The amount of FDP generated is thus determined by the intensity of the intravascular coagulation and, to a much lesser extent, by the degree of plasma fibrinolytic activity. Because the therapeutic approaches to primary fibrinolytic disorders and to disseminated intravascular coagulation are very different, attempts have been made to distinguish the two syndromes by means of identification of the plasma FDP. In primary fibrinolysis, the FDP is derived from the plasmin digestion of fibrinogen; and as mentioned earlier, the amount of FDP formed is proportional to the increase in fibrinolytic activity. In disseminated intravascular coagulation, the FDP generated is in excess of the level of plasma fibrinolytic activity, because the latter is a secondary phenomenon. The paracoagulation methods, such as the protamine sulphate or the ethanol gelation tests have also been used to distinguish between the FDPs which occur in the two syndromes. The degradation products derived from fibrinogen breakdown (in the case of primary fibrinolytic disorders) still carry with them the fibrinopeptides (e.g. fragment X^{fp}): these fragments do not paracoagulate. By contrast, in disseninated intravascular coagulation the FDPs are formed from the breakdown of fibrin and are devoid of the fibrinopeptides (e. g. fragment X^{o}) and produce positive paracoagulation results. In addition, when intravascular coagulation occurs, fibrin monomers are produced by the action of thrombin. They, too, paracoagulate. The ethanol gelation test is relatively insensitive and frequently gives negative results in desseminated intravascular coagulation, while the protamine sulphate test is reported to be quite reliable.

PULMONARY EMBOLISM AND DEEP VENOUS THROMBOSIS

The need for improved diagnostic methods for these conditions led to a number of studies of FDP in the blood of these patients. Though increases in the blood FDP levels were reported in many patients with deep venous thrombosis, particularly during the immediate postoperative period, the degree of increase was variable and commonly insufficient to give this test a diagnostic value. This finding is not unexpected as the FDPs are derived from the fibrinolysis of the thrombus, and would thus vary with the extent and stage of its resolution. Of interest are the observations that the peak FDP values were always seen one or more days before the appearance of clinical features of deep venous thrombosis, but that in acute pulmonary embolism, a consistently raised FDP level in blood was observed in all the reported series (Ruckley et al., 1970). A good correlation between positive pulmonary angiographic findings and elevated FDP levels was seen (Wilson et al., 1971: Rickman et al., 1973) and the FDP values were increased in proportion to the degree of pulmonary resistance (Rickman et al., 1973). Again, the FDP concentration is highest early in the disease, with values at their maximal levels within one day of the onset of the symptoms. The difference in the results in these two conditions may be explained by a greater fibrinolysis of pulmonary emboli than of venous thrombi. This concept is supported by the observation of an increase in the local activity of plasminogen activator in pulmonary arteries where emboli were lodged (Kwaan et al., 1973). By contrast, where the venous intima is injured in the formation of a thrombus, the local intima plasminogen activator activity may be absent (Kwaan and Astrup, 1965).

THERAPEUTIC DEFIBRINATION WITH ANCROD OR REPTILASE

The use of these two defibrinating agents in thromboembolic disorders has led to the study of their effect on FDP levels. After the intravenous injection of Ancrod or of Reptilase, almost all of the circulating fibrinogen in blood is converted to fibrin. The latter is rapidly removed before extensive microthrombosis takes place because of an increased susceptibility of Ancrod and Reptilase-induced fibrin to proteolysis, with rapid breakdown of fibrin particles to small FDP fragments (Kwaan and Barlow, 1970; Kwaan et al., 1973). An early rise of FDP levels is seen after an intravenous injection of Ancrod; the result is a profound anticoagulant effect as reflected in a prolonged thrombin time. However, the effect does not persist if defibrination is continued with repeated doses of Ancrod because of a rapid degradation of the FDP to smaller fragments which are not as sensitive to the anticoagulant methods of assay. Fragments D and E were reported to be increased in plasma during prolonged Ancrod therapy (Barlow *et al.*, 1973).

Another pharmacological effect of the smaller FDP fragments is the inhibition of platelet aggregation. This impaired platelet function has been observed during Ancrod therapy and contributes to the antithrombotic efficacy of this form of therapy.

EXTRAVASCULAR PRODUCTION OF FDP

Frequently the presence of fibrin locally in a haematoma or a pathological lesion can result in the production of sufficient amounts of FDP to cause an increased amount in the blood levels. This source of FDP accounts for the increased blood levels in postoperative patients, and those with large haematomas. Increased FDP levels found in small numbers of patients with ovarian tumours are believed to be partly explainable on the basis of extravascular breakdown of fibrin by tumour cells (Astedt *et al.*, 1971).

PREGNANCY

FDP levels slightly in excess of normal have veen reported in normal pregnancy, particularly in the second and third trimesters culminating in a sharp increase at the onset of labour. The large amounts of fibrin formed in the placenta during labour and the high uterine fibrinolytic activity is believed to be the reason for a substantial local production of FDP. This state of affairs continues after delivery for the first week of puerperium. Higher blood FDP levels may be seen if labour is complicated by post partum haemorrhage, eclampsia, abruptio placentae or intrauterine foetal death (Bonnar *et al.*, 1969). The higher FDP levels in these complications reflect the greater degree of fibrin deposition and lysis beyond the confines of the uterus. In the more severe instances, they represent examples of disseminated intravascular coagulation.

RENAL DISEASES

FDP may be derived from two sources, the breakdown of intraglomerular fibrin deposits or the lysis of fibrinogen lost in the urine. Examples of the first instance may be seen in various forms of glomerulonephritis (Clarkson *et al.*, 1971), particularly in the proliferative form (Stiehm and Trygstadt, 1969), in experimentally-induced renal disease (Humair *et al*, 1969), in renal homograft rejection (Braun and Merrill, 1968; Clarkson *et al.*, 1970), lupus nephritis and Schonlein-Henoch nephritis (Ramner *et al.*, 1969). An increased fibrinolytic activity in the glomeruli is believed to be responsible for lysis of the intraglomerular fibrin deposits. However, the degree of such lysis is unpredictable in that no correlation could be found between the presence of immunofluorescent identifiable fibrin in the glomerular lesions and the appearance of urinary FDP (Cortes *et al.*, 1973). Because considerable quantities of FDPs are excreted in the urine, repeated assay of urinary FDP concentration may be of value is assessing the severity and progress of the renal lesions, especially in proliferative glomerulonephritis.

In nephrotic syndrome, most of the fibrinogen lost in the urine is broken down by the urinary plasmin activity derived from urokinase (Cortes *et al.*, 1973). It is uncommon to find thrombin-clottable fibrinogen in the urine in these cases. The presence of urinary FDP without a concurrent increase of serum FDP is characteristic of nephrotic syndrome with heavy proteinuria of low selectivity. A disappearance of urinary FDP in these patients may signal an increased selectivity of the proteinuria and clinical improvement seen with steroid therapy.

CONCLUSION

As metabolites of fibrinogen and fibrin, FDPs are recognised to be of use in the clinical diagnosis of a wide variety of disorders associated with abnormal fibrin deposition and increased fibrinolysis. An understanding of the clinical significance of a finding of abnormal FDP level requires knowledge not only of the metabolism of fibrinogen, but also of the degree of involvement of fibrin in the particular pathological lesion concerned. When properly evaluated, the results of FDP assay can be of great assistance to the clinician in both the initial diagnosis and the subsequent follow-up of many pathological processes in addition to thromboembolism.

References

Astedt, B. Svanberg, L. and Nisson, J. M. (1971). Fibrin Degredation Products and Ovarian Tumors. *Brit. Med. J.*, **4**, 458

Bang, N. U., Fletcher, A. P., Alkjaersig N. and Sherry, S. (1962). Pathogensesis of the coagulation defect developing during pathological plasma proteolytic (fibrinolytic) states. III. Demonstration of abnormal clot structres by electron microscopy. *J. Clin. Invest.*, **41**, 935

Barlow, G. H., Lazer, S. L., Finley, R., Kwaan, H. C. and Donahoe, J. F. (1973). Some studies on proteins in the defibrinated state during Ancrod (A-38414). Studies in normal humans. *Thromb. Res.*, **2**, 115

Blomback, B. (1958). Studies on the action of thrombic enzymes on bovine fibrinogen as measured by N-Terminal analysis. *Arkiv Kemi,*12, 321

Blomback, B. (1967). Fibrinogen to fibrin transformation. In: *Blood Clotting Enzymology*, −143-215. (*W. H. Seegers, editor* New York, Academic Press)

Blomback, M. Blomback, B., Hessel, B., Iwanaga, S. and Woods, K. R. (1968). N-Terminal disulphide knot of human fibrinogen. *Nature (London)*, **218**, 130

Braun, W. E. and Merrill, J. P. (1968). Urine Fibrinogen Fragments in Human Renal Allografts. A Possible Mechanism of Renal Injury. *New. Eng. J. Med.,***278**, 1355

Thromboembolism

Breen, F. A., Jr and Tullis, J. L. (1968). Ethanol gelation. A rapid screening test for intravascular coagulation. *Ann. Int. Med.,* **69,** 7

Bonnar, J., Davidson, J. F., Pidgeon, C. F., McNicol, G. P. and Douglas, A. S. (1969) Fibrin Degradation Products in Normal and Abnormal Pregnancy and Parturition. *Brit. Med. J.,* **5,** 137

Buluk, K., Malofiejew, M. and Czokalo, M. (1966). Unkown prperties of the products of plasmin degradation of fibrinogen and fibrin. *Bull. Acad. Pol. Sci.,* **14,** 193

Clarkson, A. R., Morton, J. B. and Cash, J. D. (1970). Urinary Fibrin Fibrinogen Degradation Products after Renal Homotransplantation. *Lancet,* **2,** 1220

Clarkson, A. R., MacDonald, M. K., Petrie, J. J. B., Cash, J. D. and Robson, J. S. (1971). Serum and Urinary Fibrin/Fibrinogen Degradation Products in Glomerulonephritis. *Brit. Med. J.,* **21,** 447

Cortes, P., Potter, E. V., and Kwaan, H. C. (1973). Characterization and significance of urinary fibrin degradation products, *J. Lab. Clin. Med.,* **82,** 277

Das, P. C., Allen, A. G. E., Woodfield, D. G., *et al.* (1976). Fibrin degredation products in sera of normal subjects. *Brit. Med. J.,* **4,** 718

Fisher, S., Fletcher, A. P., Alkjaersig, N. and Sherry, S. (1967). Immunoelectrophoretic characterization of plasma fibrinogen derivatives in patients with pathological plasma proteolysis. *J. Lab. Clin. Med.,* **70,** 903

Fletcher, A. P., Alkjaersig, N. and Sherry, S. (1962). Pathogenesis of the coagulation defect developing during pathological plasma proteolytic (fibrinolytic) states. The significance of fibrinogen proteolysis and correlating fibrinogen breakdown products. *J. Clin. Invest.,* **41,** 869

Fletcher, A. P. Alkjaersig, N. O'Brien, J. R. and Tulevski, V. G. (1970). Blood hyper-coagulativity and thrombosis. *Trans. Ass. Amer. Phys.,* **3,** 159

Fund, C., Gnur, J., Herold, R., and Straub, P. W. (1971). Reptilase. A new reagent in blood coagulation. *Brit. J. Haematol.* **21,** 41

Gaffney, P. H. (1973). Subunit relationships between fibrinogen and fibrin degradation products. *Thromb. Res.,* **2,**201

Hammond, J. D. S. and Verle, D. (1959). Observations on the distribution and biological half-life of human fibrinogen. *Brit. J. Haematol,* **5,** 431

Hawiger, J., Niewiarowski, S., Gurewich, V., and Thomas, D. P. (1970). Measurement of fibrinogen and fibrin degradation products in serum by staphylococcal clumping test. *J. Lab. Clin. Med.,* **75,** 93

Herzig, R. N., Ratnoff, O. B., and Shinoff. J. R. (1970). Studies on the procoagulant factor of southern copperhead snake venom: The preferential release of fibrinipeptide *Brit. J. Lab. J. Lab. Clin. Med.,* **76,** 451

Hog, M. S. and Cash, J. D. (1973). Studies on a direct latex agglutination technique for the semiquantitation fibrin/fibrinogen degradation products. *Thromb. Res.,* **2,** 21

Humair, L., Potter, E. V. and Kwaan, H. C. (1969). The role of fibrinogen in renal disease I. Production of experimental lesions in mice. *J. Lab. Clin. Med.,* **74,** 60

Kowalski, E. (1968). Fibrinogen derivatives and their biological activities. *Seminars in Hematol.* **5,** 45

Kwaan, H. C. (1964). Fibrinolytic activity of reparative connective tissue. *J. Pathol. Bacteriol.,* **87,** 409

Kwaan, H. C., and Astrup, T. (1965). Fibrinolytic activity in thrombosed veins. *Circulation Res.,* **17,** 477

Kwaan, H. C. and Barlow, G. H. (1971). The mechanism of action of Arvin and Reptilase. *Tromb. Diath. Haemorrh.,* **Suppl. 47,** 361

Thromboembolism

Kwaan, H. C. (1972). Disorders of fibrinolysis. *Med. Clen. N. Amer.* **56**, 163

Kwaan, H. C. (1972). Disseminated intravascular coagulation. *Med. Clin. N. Amer.,* **56,** 177

Kwaan, H. C., Barlow, G. H. and Suwanwela, N. (1973). Fibrinogen and its derivatives in relationship to Ancrod and Reptilase. *Thromb. Res.,* **2,** 123

Latallo, Z. S., Teisseyre, E., Wegrzynowicz, Z. and Kipec, M. (1970). Degradation of fibrinogen by protceolytic enzymes. *Scand. J. Haematol.* **Suppl.** **13,** 15–19

Macfarlane, R. G. (1946). An enzyme cascade in the blood clotting mechanism, and its function as a biochemical amplifier. *Nature (London),* **202,** 498

Maliofiejew, M. and Buluk, K. (1968). Effect of products plasmin degradation of fibrinogen on the permeability of capillaries. *Pol. Tyg. Lek.,* **17,** 619

Marder, V. J. and Shulman, N. R. (1969). High molecular weight derivatives of human fiibrinogen produced by plasmin. II. Mechanism of their anticoagulant activity. *J. Biol. Chem.,* **244,** 2120

Marder, V. J., Matchett, M. O. and Sherry, S. (1971). Detection of serum fibrinogen and fibrin degradation products. Comparison of six techniques using purified products and application in clinical studies. *Amer. J. Med.,* **51,** 71

Marder, V. J., Budzynski, A. Z. and James, H. L. (1972). High Molecular Weight Derivatives of Human Fibrinogen Produced by Plasmin., III. Their NH –Terminal Amino Acids and Comparison with the NH_2–Terminal Di–sulfide Knot. *J. Biol. Chem,* **24,** 4775

Merskey, C., Lalezare, P. and Johnson, A. J. (1960). A rapid, simple sensitive method for measuring fibrinolytic split products in human serum. *Proc. Soc. Exp. Biol. Med.,* **131,** 871

Niewiarowski, S., Rean, V. J. and Thomas, D. P. (1970). Effect of fibrinogen derivatives on platelet aggregation. *Thromb. Diath. Haemorrh.* **Suppl. 42,** 49

Niewiarowski, S. and Gurewich, V. (1971). Laboratory identification intravascular coagulation. The serial dilution protamine sulfate test for the detection fo fibrin monomer and degradation products. *J. Lab. Clin. Med.,* **77,** 665

Nussenzweig, V. and Seligman, M. (1960). Analyse par des methodes immunochimiques de la degradation par la plasmine du fibrinogene hamain et de la fibrine a differents stades. *Rev. Haematol.,* **15,** 451

O'Meara, R. A. Q. (1958). Coagulation properties of cancer. *Irish J. Med. Sci.,* **394,** 474

Pechet, L. and Alexander, B. (1962). The effect of certain proteolytic enzymes on the thrombin-fibrinogen interaction. *Biochemistry,* **1,** 875

Prentice, C. R. N., Hassanein, A. A., Turpie, A. G. G. and Douglas, A. S. (1969). Changes in platelet behaviour during Arvin Therapy. *Lancet,* **i,** 644

Rayner, H., Parasheras. F., Isaels, L. G. and Israels, E. D. (1969). Fibrinogen breakdown products identification and assay in serum and urine. *J. Lab. Clin. Med.,* **74,** 586

Rickman, F. D., Handin, R., Howe, J. P. Alpert, J. S., Dexter, L. and Dalen, J. E. (1973). Fibrin Split Products in Acute Pulmonary Embolism., *Ann. Int. Med.,* **74,** 664

Ruckley, C. V., Das, P. C. Leitch, A. G., *et al.,* (1970). Serum fibrin/fibrinogen degradation products associated with postoperative pulmonary embolus and venous thrombosis. *Brit. Med. J.,* **4,** 395

Stiehm, C. R. and Trygstadt, C. W. (1969). Split products of fibrin in human renal diseases. *Amer. J. Med.,* **46,** 774

43

Thromboembolism

Takeda, Y. (1966). Studies of the metabolism and distribution of fibrinogen in healthy men with autologus 125 I-labelled fibrinogen. *J. Clin. Invest.*, **45**, 103

Wilson, J. E. III. Frenkel, E. P., Pierce A. K., *et al.*, (1971). Spontaneous fibrinolysis in pulmonary embolism. *J. Clin. Invest.*, **50**, 484

4

Plasma fibrinogen chromatography, blood viscosity and venous thrombosis

A. P. Fletcher and Norma Alkjaersig

INTRODUCTION

There has long been a need for the development of blood assay methods capable of detecting the presence of an *in vivo* thrombus. Plasma fibrinogen chromatography* fulfils this by quantification of specific fibrinogen-fibrin derivatives which occur in plasma secondary to the presence of a thrombus or intravascular fibrinous deposit. As will be described later in this chapter, these new methods are sensitive to the presence of very small thrombi and thus equal or better the use of the ^{125}I-fibrinogen test in the diagnosis of venous thrombosis in the lower limb. While specific for the pathological event, a thrombus or intravascular fibrinous deposit, the method is not specific for the detection of deep venous thrombosis, because it does not provide information on the location or size of the thrombus. Nevertheless, even at its present stage of development, this technique provides, in defined clinical circumstances, data not obtainable by any other means.

Most blood coagulation tests used in the clinical laboratory are for assay of blood coagulation factors and tests of overall coagulation function; that is, these assays are designed for the detection and quantification of blood coagulation system *reactants*. Development of assays for *specific reaction end-products* has been technically difficult and indeed, until recently, despite improvement and newer methods not feasible. Since

*It should be emphasised that plasma fibrinogen chromatography is wholly dissimilar in principle from serum FDP methods in use by routine clinical laboratories. Plasma fibrinogen chromatography quantifies thrombin clottable protein in plasma, whereas only non-clottable moieties are assayed in the serum FDP.

Supported by HL 03745, NS 06833 and NICHHD—71-2302

growth of the concept in this field has been of recent origin, and has largely been spurred by clinical study and observation, a summary of the initial clinical studies is provided below before consideration of the equally necessary, but generally more abstruse, biochemical background.

Some years ago, we demonstrated (Fisher *et al.*, 1967) that plasma assay for a specific thrombin clottable fibrinogen derivative (fibrinogen first derivative (Fletcher *et al.*, 1966); molecular weight 267 000 directly formed from uncomplexed fibrinogen of 330 000 MW by plasmin action) was a more sensitive method than any other for the diagnosis of incipient pathological plasma proteolysis. In the development of the reaction end-product approach, a method was devised, based on the work of Allison and Humphrey (1960), which quantified the molecular weight of the predominant fibrinogen-fibrin derivative present in plasma (determined as protein diffusion constant or $D_{20.w}$). Thus, it could be ascertained whether plasma thrombin clottable protein 'fibrinogen' was uncomplexed, 'fibrinogen' with a larger $D_{20.w}$ value (2.5 for fibrinogen first derivative), or whether 'fibrinogen' was present in a large molecular weight complexed form with a smaller $D_{20.w}$ value (usually of approximately 1.5).

In the summer of 1967, 200 patients, the majority middle-aged or older, were admitted to St. Louis City Hospital with heatstroke (Alkjaersig, 1967; Bachmann, 1969). Fifty-five patients died acutely from heat stroke, but a further 25 died unexpectedly 10-18 days after admission, during a phase of apparent clinical recovery, from pulmonary embolism or acute myocardinal infarction. Data were available on 4 patients dying wholly un-expectedly from catastrophic pulmonary embolism and in two additional patients developing non-fatal pulmonary embolism. In each instance, sub-stantial concentration of high molecular weight fibrinogen complexes, $D_{20.w}$ 1.5, were detected in their plasma for several days before death. While other patients, who recovered without incident, also showed the sporadic presence of fibrinogen complexes with a $D_{20.w}$ of 1.5 the evidence suggested that the detection of high molecular weight fibrinogen complexes in plasma was consequent upon the presence of clinically-silent thrombosis.

Unfortunately, the relatively simple methods used during this study were not readily applicable to the clinical problem, because: (a) they required 3-7 days for their performance and (b) were essentially qualitative methods, inadequate to provide other than rough quantification of the various 'fibrinogen' components in plasma. Consequently, important technical changes in method were needed. However, the principles which emerged were (a) the use of plasma rather than serum, (b) the identification and quantification of fibrinogen-fibrin products in plasma by the use of monospecific fibrinogen-fibrin antisera and (c) the classification by molecular weight, (specifically in the later studies by protein Stokes radius determinations).

PATHOPHYSIOLOGY OF INTRAVASCULAR COAGULATION AND THROMBOSIS

Figure 4.1 displays a schema of the pathophysiological reactions of the blood coagulation and plasma fibrinolytic enzyme system. Triggering the blood coagulation cascade system initiates a series of reactions which, depending on the intensity and nature of the initiating stimulus and the effect of plasma inhibitors, chiefly antithrombin III, etc, results in thrombin formation. Thrombin cleaves peptides A and B from fibrinogen, forming fibrin monomer and also activates plasma factor XIII (fibrinogen stabilising factor or FSF).

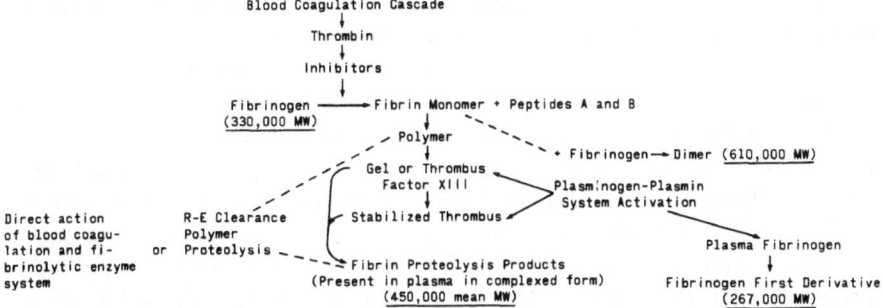

Figure 4.1 Pathophysiology of intravascular coagulation. Those components, whose molecular weight is given and underlined can be quantified by plasma fibrinogen chromatography. The reaction end-products of main importance are fibrin proteolysis products, present in complex form in plasma with· a mean molecular weight of 450 000, fibrinogen first derivative 267 000 MW and fibrinogen dimer 610 000 MW. Fibrinogen derivatives of lower molecular weight may also be quantified.

Quantification of these reaction end-products permits diagnosis of thrombotic. blood hypercoagulable and fibrinolytic states occuring *in vivo*.

Normally, fibrin monomer in plasma spontaneously polymerises and may later gel to form a thrombus or intravascular deposit which, *in vivo,* is then cross-linked by the actions of plasma coagulation Factor XIII (FSF). When the concentration of fibrin monomer is low it combines with fibrinogen to form dimer (610 000 MW). Where either thrombosis or intravascular coagulation exists, fibrin proteolysis products may be formed in three ways:

    (a)   By the lysis of the thrombus or intravascular deposit through the actions of the plasminogen-plasmin enzyme system.

(b)   By reticulo-endothelial system action on circulating high molecular weight fibrin polymers formed at the site of local or vascular damage but removed by blood flow before their incorporation into the thrombus or fibrinous deposit.

(c)   By the actions of the blood coagulation system alone or in combination with the plasma fibrinolytic enzyme system on plasma fibrinogen, in the absence of macroscopic fibrin formation (Alkjaersig and Fletcher, 1973).

The products of fibrin proteolysis are released into plasma and become attached to plasma fibrinogen. The complexes produced are of higher molecular weight than fibrinogen (see Figure 4.1.).

Thrombus formation or intravascular fibrin deposition triggers the release of plasminogen activator, either locally or systemically, an action which induces lysis of the thrombus or intravascular fibrinous deposit (Alkjaersig et al., 1959). Activation of the plasminogen-plasmin system also produces mild proteolytic activity in plasma and a proportion of plasma fibrinogen undergoes limited proteolysis to fibrinogen first derivative (267 000 molecular weight); the amount of the latter found is proportional to the degree of activation of the plasminogen-plasmin system. However, with higher levels of plasma thrombolytic activity, fibrinogen first derivative itself may be broken down to fibrinogen second derivative and other derivatives of lower molecular weight; again the proportion of these latter derivatives will also reflect the intensity of plasma thrombolytic activity.

METHOD

Gel exclusion chromatography is a method of fractionating protein mixtures on the basis of molecular weight class. The higher the molecular weight of the protein, or more accurately, the larger the Stokes radius, the higher the degree of its 'exclusion' from the chromatographic matrix, and consequently, the earlier does the protein appear in the chromatographic effluent. Thus, using a chromatographic column, appropriately standardised with proteins of known molecular weight, a plot of effluent protein concentration against chromatographic volume yields a protein molecular weight distribution pattern.

In the chromatography of fibrinogen, plasma is separated on a large-pore agarose gel (Biogel 5M) and the individual chromatographic effluents are assayed (at the rate of 100/hour) for fibrinogen fibrin determinants using a Technicon immunoprecipitator and monospecific antiserum (Fletcher et al., 1972). Quantification of each component in the chromatographic pattern is achieved by analysis of the chromatographic data using chromatographic plate theory and a computer (Alkjaersig *et al.*, 1973). Plasma fibrinogen chromatography has proven to be a highly satisfactory method of quantification of the individual fibrinogen-fibrin reaction end-products found in plasma and characteristic of the pathophysiological states shown in Figure 4.1. However, the method, though simple in principle, is technically complex and is available in only a few laboratories.

INTERPRETATION
It is useful to quantify all the fibrinogen-fibrin derivatives of varying molecular weight underlined in Figure 4.1. However, a simpler classification is adequate for discussion of the venous problem. Figure 4.1 shows that the actions of the coagulation system in plasma, i.e. the direct and indirect results of thrombin release, are to increase the molecular weight of fibrinogen-fibrin derivatives observed. In contrast, the actions of the plasma fibrinolytic enzyme system are characteristically reflected by the presence of fibrinogen derivatives smaller than fibrinogen itself. Consequently, in the discussion that follows, reference will be made to the proportions of three classes of fibrinogen and its derivatives:

1. *Fibrinogen Complexes.* Fibrinogen complexes of higher molecular weight than fibrinogen.
2. *Native Fibrinogen.*
3. Fibrinogen derivatives of smaller molecular weight than fibrinogen itself, referred to collectively as *fibrinogen first derivative.*

1. *Thrombosis or intravascular coagulation.* The formation of fibrin proteolysis products (actions of the plasminogen-plasmin enzyme system on the thrombus or intravascular deposit) results in an increase of fibrinogen-fibrin complexes with an average molecular weight 450-530 000. Normal values for this determination are 8 ± 5 per cent and, consequently, a finding of above 20 per cent complex formation is regarded as pathological (mean ± twice the standard deviation).

2. *Resolution of thrombus* or of intravascular fibrin deposits which occurs as a result of the activity of plasminogen-plasmin system and is characterised by a fall of the proportion of fibrinogen-fibrin complexes present and by an increase in fibrinogen first derivative (267000 MW). The latter reaction occurs because activation of the plasminogen-plasmin enzyme system is not confined to the thrombus and fibrinogen first derivative is derived by proteolysis of plasma fibrinogen. Normal values

for determination of plasma fibrinogen fiirst derivative are 20 ± 9 per cent.

3. *Activation of the plasminogen-plasmin enzyme system* occurs with thrombosis or intravascular coagulation and is charaterised by an increase in fibrinogen first derivative. However, for reasons that will be entered into later (see page 53), if considerable complex formation occurs, this response will not be seen in the chromatogram until the phase of thrombus resolution.

STUDIES IN THE POSTOPERATIVE PATIENT

As a result of the development of the [125] I-fibrinogen test (Hobbs and Davies, 1960; Flanc *et al.*, 1968; Kakkar *et al*,. 1970: Chapter 14) the post-operative patient constitutes an excellent clinical model for test of procedures purported to be of diagnostic value in the detection of clinically silent thrombosis. Accordingly, a cooperative study was arranged with Dr John O'Brien, St. Mary's Hospital, Portsmouth, England, a participant in a British MRC trial of aspirin prophylaxis in postoperative deep venous thrombosis (Report of the Steering Committee of a trial spnsored by the MRC, 1972) and ourselves.

One hundred and seven patients who were operated upon in England, received [125] I-fibrinogen in the postoperative period and their legs were serially scanned for five days thereafter. Deep venous thrombosis was diagnosed by identification of local accumulation of [125] I-fibrin and defined by the location of isotopic 'hot' spots. Preoperative and appropriate postoperative plasma samples were frozen immediately after collection and later air-freighted to St. Louis in a frozen state. Analysis by plasma fibrinogen chromatography was performed under 'blind' conditions; that is, without knowledge of the isotopic findings.

In brief, 31 patients passed through the postoperative period without either isotopic or plasma fibrinogen chromatographic evidence of deep venous thrombosis. Similarly, 41 patients exhibited both isotopic and plasma fibrinogen chromatographic evidence of thrombosis (increase of fibrinogen complexes > 20 per cent. Thus, the results of the methods were wholly concordant in 72 of the 107 patients studied (Fletcher *et al.*, 1972). However, in 22 patients, evidence of deep venous thrombosis was not detected by the ^{125}I-fibrinogen test, but one or more abnormal plasma fibrinogen chromatographic patterns were found postoperatively. In 15 of these 22 patients, abnormal fibrinogen chromatographic patterns had been detected one or two days before operation and the injection of the labelled fibrinogen. We believe that the preoperative findings were the result of thrombosis which occured in a group of ill patients, many suffering from lung carcinoma. Because [125] I-fibrinogen was not administered until the operation we cannot compare the preoperative abnormalities with the postoperative diagnosis. Positive findings could represent either persistent thrombosis in areas other than the legs or thrombi in the legs present before surgery, which had ceased to take up ^{125}I-fibrinogen.

Thus, only seven patients in whom the plasma fibrinogen chromatographic method was positive and the scan negative are relevant to the present inquiry. There were also seven studies in which the isotopic method suggested the presence of leg vein thrombosis, but plasma fibrinogen chromatography was normal. In two instances, it appeared that mislabelling of samples possibly occured and in three of the other five isotopic evidence for the diagnosis of thrombosis appeared to be questionable.

It is noteworthy that clinical signs developed in only 12 of the patients with leg vein thrombosis detected by the ^{125}I-fibrinogen test: thus, the majority of lesions detected by plasma fibrinogen chromatography were clinically silent. Our results have been confirmed by others (Hirsh and Gallus, 1973) who have demonstrated in studies of 103 postoperative patients that the plasma fibrinogen chromatographic method of detecting thrombosis was positive in essentially all patients in whom leg vein thrombus was detected by the ^{125}I-fibrinogen test and confirmed by venography. Hirsh and Gallus also reported that there was a 25 per cent incidence of 'false positive' results with plasma fibrinogen chromatography; that is, that in 25 per cent of postoperative patients, plasma fibrinogen chromatography suggested the presence of a thrombus which was not detected in the legs. These authors remarked that the 'false positive' results were found mainly in patients with carcinoma or with findings which suggested intravascular coagulation. Because they did not examine their patients before operation by plasma fibrinogen chromatography, their results can be regarded as essentially in agreement with our own (Fletcher et al., 1972).

Thus, the presence of greater than 20 per cent fibrinogen complexes in plasma, after operation, indicates that there is an approximately 80 per cent likelihood that deep venous thrombosis is present; The finding of a normal postoperative chromatogram excludes the diagnosis of venous thrombosis.

ORAL CONTRACEPTIVE MEDICATION AND THROMBOEMBOLISM

The predisposition of women receiving oral contraceptive medication to develop thromboembolic vascular disease is now well established and documented (Fletcher et al., 1973; Vessey, 1973). The epidemiological data suggest that the risk of developing thromboembolic vascular complications, usually venous thromboembolism, is increased five- to eleven-fold by the use of oral contraceptives and that the problem has not been solved by reducing the oestrogen content (Boston Collaborative Drug Surveillance Programme, 1973). Moreover, there is evidence that the use of these agents predisposes to the development of stroke (Collaborative Group for the Study of Stroke in Young Women, 1973) and probably also to myocardial infarction. Nevertheless, on a numerical basis, because the prevalence of 'idiopathic' venous thromboembolism is far higher than that of 'idiopathic' arterial disease in the age group affected, the major problem posed by the oral contraceptive agents is predisposition to venous disease and pulmonary embolism.

In the absence of techniques for the detection of clinically-silent thrombosis, all prior estimates of the risk of thromboembolic disease, consequent upon the use of oral contraceptives, have been based either on retrospective epidemiological survey of either hospital admission statistics or the less reliable data provided by national or regional mortality statistics. The best estimates based on hospital admission data suggest that the annual hospital admission rate for 'idiopathic' deep venous thrombosis and pulmonary embolism is approximately 5-6 per 100 000 women at risk for those not receiving oral contraceptives and 45-66 per 100 000 women for those who do.

Our earlier studies on the use of plasma fibrinogen chromatography to measure the degree of thrombogenic risk produced by oral contraceptives have recently been reported (Fletcher et al., 1973). They are based on the principle that the excess clinically-silent thrombotic lesions in the drug group over the control group is a valid measure of thrombogenic risk. Though most of these clinically-silent thrombotic lesions resolve spontaneously, each carries a definite, if small, risk either of extension or of pulmonary embolism.

Our studies demonstrate: (a) that women receiving oral contraceptives experience an approximately 5-fold greater incidence of thrombotic lesions than do controls, a finding in line with the risk established by epidemiological study; (b) that thromboses which develop under these circumstances are characteristically transient, last from 1-4 weeks and show chromatographic patterns of thrombus resolution before return to normality; (c) that the appearance of abnormal chromatographic patterns in patients is significantly ($p < 0.01$) associated with the presence of symptoms suggestive of thromboembolic disease. These observations demonstrate the feasibility of testing oral contraceptive agents for *in vivo* thrombogenicity using comparatively small subject groups (200 subjects) because the incidence of abnormal chromatographic patterns in women receiving oral contraceptive agents is 20 per cent or more.

The use of plasma fibrinogen chromatography in patients on oral contraceptives has practical clinical importance: for instance, in such patients referred to us with clinically suspected, pulmonary embolism or deep venous thrombosis, it has been possible to exclude these diagnoses in over one-third by the finding of a normal plasma fibrinogen chromatogram. Even if initial plasma fibrinogen chromatographic findings are positive for thrombosis, the later findings may be normal providing evidence that the pathological process has regressed.

Findings illustrative of our general study protocol are shown in Figure 4.2.

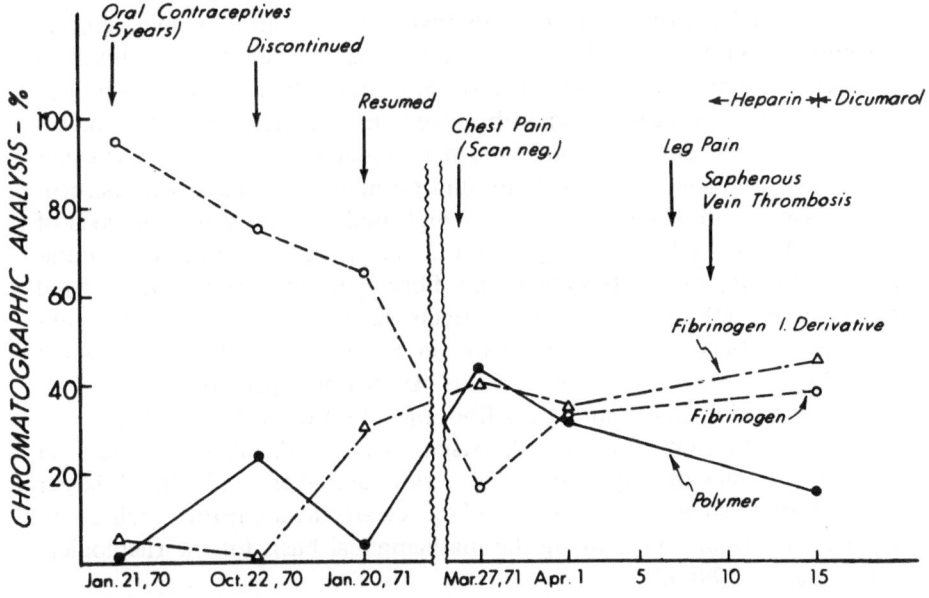

Figure 4.2 Serial fibrinogen chromatographic studies in patients on oral contraceptive medication for five years. Normal chromatographic findings on 1/21/70. When the oral contraceptive was discontinued, findings on 10/22/70 indicate thrombus formation. Normal findings on 1/20/71 when contraceptive medication was restarted. Grossly abnormal chromatographic findings on 3/27/71, when patient was admitted to hospital for suspected pulmonary embolism—a diagnosis not confirmed but contraceptive medication stopped. Persistent grossly abnormal chromatographic findings on 4/1/71. On 4/10/71, patient developed acute iliofemoral and saphenous deep venous thrombosis and received anticoagulant therapy. Note fall on 4/15/71 in polymer and high fibrinogen first derivative—findings characteristic of resolving thrombus. (Reproduced with permission from *Human Reproduction,* Harper and Row, New York, 1973.)

53

BLOOD VISCOSITY

It nas already been stated (Chapter 2) that the rheological behaviour of blood is complex, for at relatively high shear strain rates, usually above $100sec^{-1}$ it exhibits Newtonian behaviour, that is, viscosity independent of shear stress at which it is measured but below this shear strain rate viscosity becomes highly dependent upon the shear rate (see Chapter 6). Attempted mathematical prediction of blood viscosity at low shear rates from the main factors recognised as influencing blood viscosity, the haematocrit and the fibrinogen concentration, has been far from successful. The development of plasma fibrinogen chromatography provide a means by which the influence of the altered biophysical properties of fibrinogen, observed in disease, could be evaluated.

In a recent study (Jacob et al., 1974), involving the analysis of 150 plasma samples from patients with myocardial infarction and cerebral thrombosis, viscosity at low shear rates was measured by a modified capillary viscometer (Benis, 1968), and quantification of fibrinogen derivatives in plasma by plasma fibrinogen chromatography. After correction for blood haematocrit and fibrinogen content, viscosity at low shear rates was shown to be significantly and positively correlated with percentage plasma fibrinogen complexes of high molecular weight. Analysis of the data by multiple linear regression demonstrated that fibrinogen complexes, uncomplexed fibrinogen and fibrinogen first derivative exerted significantly different rheological effects at low shear rates. The approximate ratio of rheological activity in centipoises (100 mg component per 100 ml blood) can be calculated as 10 for fibrinogen complexes, 5 for uncomplexed fibrinogen and 1 for fibrinogen first derivative at shear rates of 0.2 sec^{-1} .In view of the rapidly-rising viscosity displayed by blood at lower shear rates than 0.2 sec^{-1} s, these ratio activities will be much larger at even lower shear rates. These findings clearly account for much of the present uncertainty in defining the mathematical basis for the rheological phenomena of blood.

The pathophysiological significance of a rise in blood viscosity at low shear rates, secondary to the presence of fibrinogen complexes, is reasonably clear in the case of organ infarction, e.g. myocardial infarction and cerebral thrombosis. However, the importance of this phenomenon in deep venous thrombosis, where infarction is not at issue, is less certain. Plasma fibrinogen concentration usually increases in established cases of deep venous thrombosis and the proportion of fibrinogen complexes present invariably rises. As a result of this, blood viscosity at low shear rates increases several fold: such a phenomenon would favour extension of the thrombus, for 'stasis' would appear at higher than normal shear rates.

STUDIES IN OTHER DISEASE STATES

Normal findings in plasma fibrinogen chromatography essentially exclude a clinically suspected diagnosis of pulmonary embolism. Positive chromatographic findings may be due to either thrombosis or pulmonary embolism. They are therefore of little value in confirming the diagnosis of pulmonary embolism in the presence of thrombosis. However, plasma fibrinogen chromatography is a useful method for following patients receiving treatment for pulmonary embolism, because deterioration of chromatographic findings in patients under treatment may be diagnostic of recurrent thromboembolic episodes.

Useful as these methods are in the study of venous disease, their most important uses belong in three different fields: (a) in the study of acute arterial syndromes, e.g., acute myocardial and cerebral infarction; (b) in the study of less-acute syndromes where intravascular coagulation is in question (e.g. in acute renal disease); (c) in the prescription and control of therapeutic agents, where these methods provide information on disease pathophysiology and the effect of therapy upon it obtainable by no other means.

Because positive chromatographic findings occur in many conditions other than venous thrombosis, e.g. cerebral and myocardial infarction, plasma fibrinogen chromatographic results must always be interpreted in terms of the patient's particular clinical problem. Despite this caveat, interpretive difficulties are often less than might be expected.

CONCLUSIONS

It had formerly been thought that the prevalence of clinically-significant pulmonary embolism could be substantially reduced once methods for early diagnosis of deep venous thrombosis had been developed. Unfortunately, now that methods for early diagnosis of the causative venous lesion have been developed (Chapter 14), patient management problems still remain, (Chapter 19), because lower limb thrombosis is now established to be both a common and also a benign disease in the great majority of patients.

Consequently, the problem of preventing pulmonary embolism may be restated either in terms of total prophylaxis, which may be possible in 'high risk' situations such as are seen in the surgically-treated patient, or in terms of differentiating those thrombotic lesions of good prognosis from those likely to embolise—an approach that would be invaluable in the management of less acute situations such as are seen in the case of women receiving oral contraceptive medication. While it is now clear that the anatomical site of thrombosis is of considerable prognostic importance, it is also known that the actual volume of thrombus involved in clinically-severe embolisation is large. Whether the biochemical approach to detection of thrombosis (described in this chapter) may be adapted to quantification of thrombus size is uncertain, but with further refinement of methods, this remains a distinct possibility.

References

Alkjaersig, N. (1967). CPC on Heat Stroke. *Amer. J. Med.,* **43,** 113

Alkjaersig, N. and Fletcher, A. (1974). The proteolysis of fibrin by plasmin and the effect of thrombolysis and of blood hypercoagulability on the biophysical behaviour of plasma fibrinogen. *J. Clin. Invest.* (in press)

Alkjaersig, N., A. and Sherry, S. (1959). The mechanism of clot dissolution by plasmin. *J. Clin. Invest.,* **38,** 1086

Alkjaersig, N., Roy, L., Fletcher, A. and Murphy, E. (1974). Analysis of gel exclusion chromoatographic data by chromatographic plate theory analysis: Application to plasma fibringoen chromatography. *Thromb. Res.* (in press)

Allison, A. and Humphrey, J. (1960). A theoretical and experimental analysis of double diffusion precipitin reaction in gels and its application characterization of antigens. *Immunology,* **3,** 95

Bachmann, F. (1969). Dec. *Disease of the Month* 1, (Chicago, 111: Year Book Publishers, Inc.)

Benis, A. M. (1968). A new simple low-shear capillary viscometer for Blood. *Bio-Rheol.,* **5,** 263

Boston Collaborative Drug Surveillance Program (1973). Oral contraceptives and venous thromboembolic disease, surgically confirmed gallbladder disease and breast tumors. *Lancet,* **i,** 1399

Collaborative Group for the Study of Stroke in Young Women (1973). Oral contraception and increased risk of cerebral ischemia or thrombosis. *New Eng. J. Med.,* **288,** 871

Fisher, S., Fletcher, A., Alkjaersig, N. and Sherry, S. (1967). Immuno-electrophoretic characterization of plasma fibrinogen derivatives in patients with pathological plasma proteolysis. *J. Lab. Clin. Med.,* **70,** 903

Flanc, C., Kakkar, V. and Clarke, M. (1968). The detection of venous thrombosis of the legs using ^{125}I-labelled fibrinogen. *Brit. J. Surg.,* **55,** 742

Fletcher, A., Alkjaersig, N., Fisher, S. and Sherry, S. (1966). The proteolysis of fibringoen by plasmin: The identification of thrombin-clottable fibrinogen derivatives which polymerize abnormally. *J. Lab. Clin. Med.,* **68,** 780

Fletcher, A., Alkjaersig, N. and O'Brien, J. (1972). Blood screening methods for the diagnosis of thromboembolism. *Millbank Memorial Fund Quarterly,* **50,** 1970

Fletcher, A., Alkjaersig, N. and Burstein, R. (1973). Effect of contraceptives on vascular system. In: *Human Reproduction: Conception and Contraception,* Chapter 25, 539 (E. S. Hafez and T. N. Evans, editors) (New York: Harper and Row)

Hirsh, J. and Gallus, A. (1973). Fibrinogen chromatography for the detection of venous thrombosis. *Fourth Int. Cong. Thromb. Haemol. Vienna, Austria* (Abstract), **121,** 155

Hobbs, J. and Davies, J. (1960). Detection of venous thrombosis with ^{131}I-labelled fibrinogen in the rabbit. *Lancet,* **ii,** 134

Jacob, A. Fletcher, A. P. and Alkjaersig, N. In preparation.

Thromboembolism

Kakkar, V., Nicolaides, A., Renney, J., Friend, J. and Clarke, M. (1970). ^{125}I-labelled fibringoen test adapted for routine screening for deep vein thrombosis. **Lancet, i,** 540

Report of the Steering Committee of a trial sponsored by the Medical Research Council. Effect of aspirin on post-operative venous thrombosis (1972). *Lancet,* **ii,** 441

Vessey, M. (1973). The Epidemiology of Venous Thromboembolism. In: *Recent Advances in Thrombosis,* 39-58 (L. Poller, editor) (London: Churchill-Livingstone)

5

Erythrocyte flexibility, blood fibrinogen and surgery

J. A. Sirs

INTRODUCTION

The predisposition of patients undergoing major operation to venous thrombosis is believed to depend upon a complex reaction associated with 'hypercoagulability' and stasis (Chapter 2). The many components involved include changes in blood viscosity, rouleaux formation, aggregation of red cells, platelet stickiness, clotting factors, fibrinogen concentration, cholesterol level and fibrin degradation products. These factors are probably interdependent. It has been suggested, for instance, that the increased rouleaux formation is related to a higher fibrinogen concentration, and it is the dissipation of energy to break down these aggregates at low shear rates that is responsible for non-Newtonian behaviour. However, this is an over-simplification because a similar non-Newtonian characteristic is found whith the blood of ruminants which do not form rouleaux, and with blood of greater than 60 per cent haematocrit, when the cells must always be in contact. An alternative common factor that links the non-Newtonian behaviour of blood, rouleaux formation and fibrinogen concentration, is the flexibility of the red blood cells. It is with the latter aspect that this article is concerned and with recent evidence which suggests that the flexibility of red blood cells changes during surgery and the postoperative period.

Flexibility is identified as the relative force that must be applied to deform a red blood cell. In absolute terms flexibility is dependent on the viscosity of the internal haemoglobin and visco-elastic properties of the cell membrane. This is a complicated problem for which no simple physical and mathematical formulation is available. For this reason the methods used to measure red cell flexibility give a relative index in terms of either shear

59

stress, applied pressure or rate of deformation. Though each technique does not measure exactly the same parameter, there is good correlation between them.

It has been known for some time that red blood cells are deformed during their passage through capillaries (Krogh, 1922). Measurements of the surface tension of red cells indicate that this is less than 0.1 ergs/sq. cm and only very small forces are required to produce deformation (Harvey and Danielli, 1938). Methods of measuring the erythrocyte flexibility have been developed over the last fifteen years. One that has been extensively used is to measure the pressure required to suck a small area of the cell membrane into a micropipette of $1-3\mu$ m diameter. The technique was initially used to study marine eggs (Mitchison and Swann, 1954) and subsequently adapted to investigate the mechanical properties of the red cell membrane (Rand and Burton 1964). It has been demonstrated that deformability is dependent on the metabolism of the red blood cell (Weed et al., 1969) and more recently the technique has been used to study deformation and the rate of volume changes (Jay, 1973). It has been found that distortion of the cell can be produced with pressures as low as 1mm H_2O. Similar studies of erythrocyte flexibility have also been made with larger pipettes (Bayliss, 1952; Bras and Jenett, 1968), comparable to the diameter of capillaries, at flow rates in the physiological range, with haematocrits up to 80 per cent. (Jay et al., 1972). As an alternative to the use of micropipettes the study of flow of cell suspensions through polycarbonate filters has been suggested (Prothero and Burton, 1962), but this particular type of mesh filter does not give reproducible results. A much more satisfactory technique is to use sieves made by irradiating thin plastic sheets with fission fragments, followed by etching (Gregersen et al., 1967; Fleisher et al., 1963; 1965. Such filters are commercially available and have been used to investigate the filterability of red cell suspension in both normal and diseased states (Jandle et al.,1961; Teitel and Nicholau, 1964; Teitel, 1964). At a sufficiently high haematoerit filters with even larger pores can be used, but allowances must be made for aggregation (Swank, 1961).

An indication of erythrocyte flexiblity can also be obtained directly from measurements of blood viscosity. It has been found that when erythrocytes are hardened in acetaldehyde the viscosity increases several fold and becomes Newtonian in character at all haematocrits (Chien et al., 1970). The differences of flexibility occurring *in vivo* are more discernible in studies of blood viscosity at low shear rates, as has been stressed by Dintenfass who has extensively reviewed this field (Dintenfass, 1963; 1971). A more direct method to assess erthrocyte deformability is to measure the viscosity of packed red cells (Jacobs, 1963). However, the disadvantage of this method is that changes in erythrocyte flexibility occur in packing the cells and removing plasma.

Though it is not generally appreciated, the Erythrocyte Sedimentation Rate (ESR) is an index of flexibility, but only to some extent because it is also influenced by rouleaux and aggregation. A centrifuge technique, of measuring the rate of packing at 200-600 g, which overcomes these problems and gives a measure of flexibility has been developed (Sirs,1968). It has the advantages of simplicity, minimum of interference with the blood sample, results available in 15 minutes and only 0.5 ml of blood required. The results discussed in this paper have been obtained with this technique which is explained in detail below.

Using the above methods many factors have been found to alter the erythrocyte flexibility. These may act by producing internal changes in the haemoglobin structure or concentration, in the cell membrane and in the plasma environment. The increase of the viscosity of sickle cells in the deoxygenated state (Harris *et al.*, 1956), is an example of the effect of changes in the internal constituents. Physicochemical factors such as temperature, ionic strength and pH have been shown to affect the cell deformability (Jacobs, 1963; Rand and Burton, 1964; Teitel and Nicolau, 1964). Red cell flexibility is decreased with incubation (Jacobs, 1963) but this can be reversed by the addition of metabolic substrates (Teitel and Nicolau, 1964). The rate of exchange of oxygen and carbon monoxide in erythrocytes is dependent on the cell metabolism and is related to changes in cell flexibility (Sirs,1963; 1964). More recently changes of erythrocyte flexibility have been correlated with ATP concentration (Weed *et al.*, 1969). The flexibility of red blood cells is particularly dependent on the concentration of fibrinogen in the plasma, as is discussed below. Storage of blood in ACD solution for transfusion, can also produce inflexibility (LaCelle, 1969; Sirs 1969). There are variations from one individual to another and in disease but the reasons for some of these variations are not understood.

THE MEASUREMENT OF ERYTHROCYTE FLEXIBILITY WITH A CENTRIFUGE

If red blood cells were rigid and randomly orientated the maximum possible haematocrit would be 35-42 per cent. With the most efficient packed arrangement of erythrocytes the maximum haematocrit obtainable would be 60-65 per cent. The allowance for random orientation was determined by measuring the volume occupied with randomly orientated discs and O-rings (Sirs, 1969). It follows that haematocrits higher than these values can only be obtained by deformation and packing of the erythrocytes. At haematocrits greater than 35 per cent, even flexible cells must be effectively in contact with each other, and the flow of whole blood must involve deformation and interaction between them. Packing of erythrocytes can take place in a centrifuge, or during an ESR test, because they are deformable and flexible. This is not, as commonly assumed, a process of sedimentation (Rampling and Sirs, 1970). Sedimentation only occurs when there is no interaction between the sedimenting particles. When whole blood is centrifuged the packing is brought about by the weight of cells, one on top of the other, squashing themselves together. If the cells were rigid no movement would occur and the plasma could not be separated out. Normal blood packs quickly because the cells are very flexible. The rate of packing is determined by the centrifugal acceleration, the haematocrit, the difference of cell-to-plasma density and the flexibility of the cells (Sirs, 1968). By maintaining the first three factors constant, or by using control samples, the difference of flexibility of the erythrocytes in blood can be assessed. There are two methods of observing the rate of packing. The first, by stopping-and-starting the centrifuge at given time intervals (Sirs, 1968), the second, by automatically recording the length of the red cell column during centrifugation (Sirs, 1970).

Stopping-and-starting procedure: The haematocrit, as indicated by the proportion of the length of the red blood cell column to the total length of plasma plus cells, is measured as a function of the time of spinning. This can simply be obtained by operating a microhaematocrit centrifuge at an acceleration of 600 g, by connecting it to a supply of 80 volts alternating current. The centrifuge is set to run for 2 min, and then the tubes removed and the haematocrit determined. Five consecutive readings are usually made and then the packed cell volume determined by centrifugation at 13 000 g. This method is comparative, in that it is not possible to exactly control the run-up-time, final speed and time-to-stop of the centrifuge, and it is necessary to simultaneously measure a normal blood sample. The advantage of this system is that it is possible on most microhaematocrit centrifuges to run more than twenty samples together. A check should be kept of the cell-to-plasma density difference, but variations in this factor of more than 10 per cent are unusual, and density differences of this magnitude have negligible effect of the packing rate. For direct comparison allowance must also be made for the differences of packed cell haematocrit between samples. To correct for this factor a calibration curve is obtained at different haematocits of the cells diluted in their own plasma (Rampling and Sirs, 1972a; 1972b).

Automatic recording system: The length of the red cell column can be automatically monitored by photographically recording the transmission of light, through the clear layer of plasma above the cells, during centrifugation (Sirs 1970). The apparatus consists of a light source, a rotating disc on which the tube containing the blood sample is held and an optical system, so that a clear image of the tube and its contents is projected onto a moving film each time the sample passes through the light beam. The light beam is automatically switched off for 5 s every minute to provide a series of unexposed calibration lines on the film, one minute apart. The exposure on the film indicates the fall of the top surface of the cells with time, as more clear plasma is formed. Light transmission through the glass seal, at the base of the microhaematocrit capillary tube, similarly indicates the bottom of the cell column. Approximately 0.05 ml of blood is required for each experiment. The blood samples are placed individually into the centrifuge, and after switching on and bringing up to an acceleration of 200g, in 30–40s, they are left to run automatically for 10 min. At the end of each experiment the capillary tube is removed and the sample spun at 13000g for 3 min to determine the packed cell haematocrit. The film is then developed and measurements are made of the packing rates by projection through an enlarger.

This method has the advantage over the stop–start technique that both the time of spinning and speed of rotation can be accurately known and controlled. It is not necessary to run a known standard each time a measurement is made. However, only one sample can be studied at a time, and a series of blood samples are measured by running them sequentially. The reproducibility of this technique is within ± 2 per cent throughout the whole curve, on repeated measurements made on the same blood sample throughout a 5-hour period. This method also confirmed that no significant changes. such as re-expansion, of the cell column occurs during the stopping and starting procedure. There is good agreement, between the results from different blood samples obtained by both methods.

THE EFFECT OF ANTICOAGULANTS ON THE RATE OF PACKING

When the red blood cells are made inflexible (e.g. by fixing them with formaldehyde), the rate at which the cells pack together is slower. Providing a correction is made for the packed cell haematocrit, the packing rate is a relative index of the flexibility of the erythrocytes. All that is involved in making this estimation is to obtain a blood sample, place it in a microhaematocrit centrifuge tube and spin it as described above. A possible difference in flexibility between the *in vitro* sample and the *in vivo* blood may be produced by the method of withdrawing the sample and the anticoagulant used. Differences in packing rate are not observed between blood taken from an artery or vein. The effect of various anticoagulants on the packing rate has been systematically studied (Rampling and Sirs, 1970), and heparin has been found to be the most suitable. Samples are normally collected with 3–6 i.u. of heparin per ml of blood, though no differences of heparin concentration are apparent up to 20 i.u. per ml, but such samples cannot be kept without deterioration longer than 24 hours at 4 °C. ACD and EDTA anticoagulants have a similar effect during the period immediately after collection, though both give significantly slower packing rates than heparin. As the cells are stored, the ACD cells retain their flexibility for a longer period. After five days both the flexibility and efficiency of ACD stored cells to exchange oxygen is considerably reduced (Sirs 1969). Defibrinating blood, with glass beads, leaves the cells relatively inflexible.

ERYTHROCYTE FLEXIBILITY AND BLOOD VISCOSITY

In an extensive study of more than 300 normal subjects (Rampling and Sirs, 1974), it has been found that the packing rates of 90 per cent of these subjects are similar to curve R in Figure 5.1. Outside the scatter of three standard deviations, about curve R, there is a group of approximately 5 per cent of normal healthy subjects whose packing rates are significantly lower, and another group of the remaining 5 per cent who have higher packing rates, such as indicated by curve S in Figure 5.1. What factors are responsible for these differences and what significance can be given to them is not clear. Further detailed investigation of the blood from subjects R and S has not so far revealed what specific factor is responsible for this difference. When the respective red blood cells are separated by centrifugation and resuspended in each other's plasma, the blood groups being identical, the cells from subject S still pack at the faster rate when suspended in the plasma of subject R. Total plasma protein concentrations are normal in both groups but, though both fibrinogen concentrations fall within the normal range, the fibrinogen concentration in the plasma of S group tends to be higher than that of R. However, this has no significant effect on the plasma viscosities, which are 1.6 centipoises at 37°C for both subjects. There are also no differences between the type of haemoglobin, both being HbA. It would appear that the difference in flexibility is due to some structural or functional variation in the red cell membrain. As is reported below, similar differences are found between species of animals.

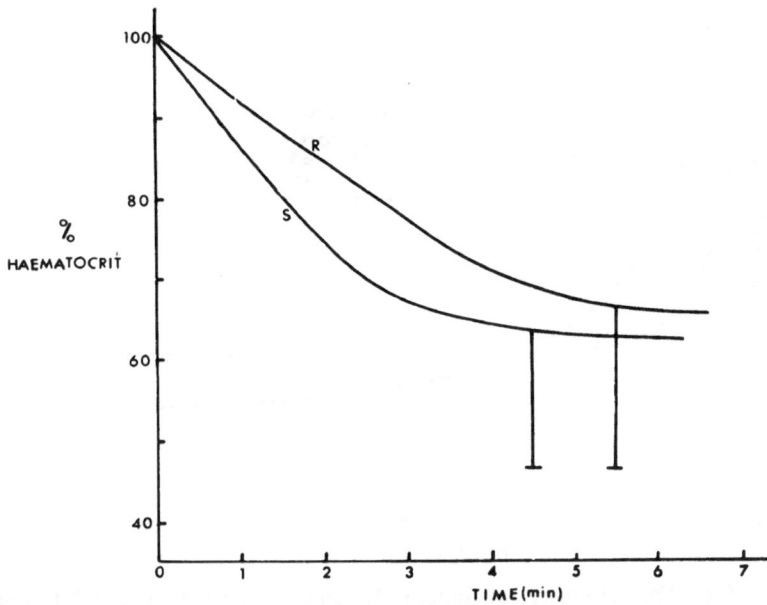

Figure 5.1. The variation of haematocrit with time, for two normal whole blood samples. R is representative of 90 per cent of normal healthy adults and S represents the extreme faster packing rate, found in 5 per cent of normals

When red blood cells are inflexible, the whole blood viscosity is high and independent of shear rate (Chien *et al.,* 1970). The viscosity of normal whole blood is non-Newtonian, with a relatively low value of about 5 centipoise at 37 ^{o}C at high shear rates, which increases several fold at low shear rates. A similar general trend is found between the blood viscosity at the same haematocrits, of subjects R and S, as shown in Figure 5.2. The viscosity values were obtained relative to the flow of isotonic NaCl through a 1 mm bore capillary viscometer. At high shear rates the blood viscosity of a subject S is significantly lower than that of a subject R. At low shear rates the relative difference is reversed. Under normal conditions *in vivo,* when the shear rate is high, subject S would appear to have an advantage over subject R, but under conditions in which stasis may occur subject S is at a disadvantage. The general conclusion may be drawn that whole blood viscosity is related to the deformability of the red blood cells, and when this is altered, keeping other factors constant, the non-Newtonian behaviour is also modified.

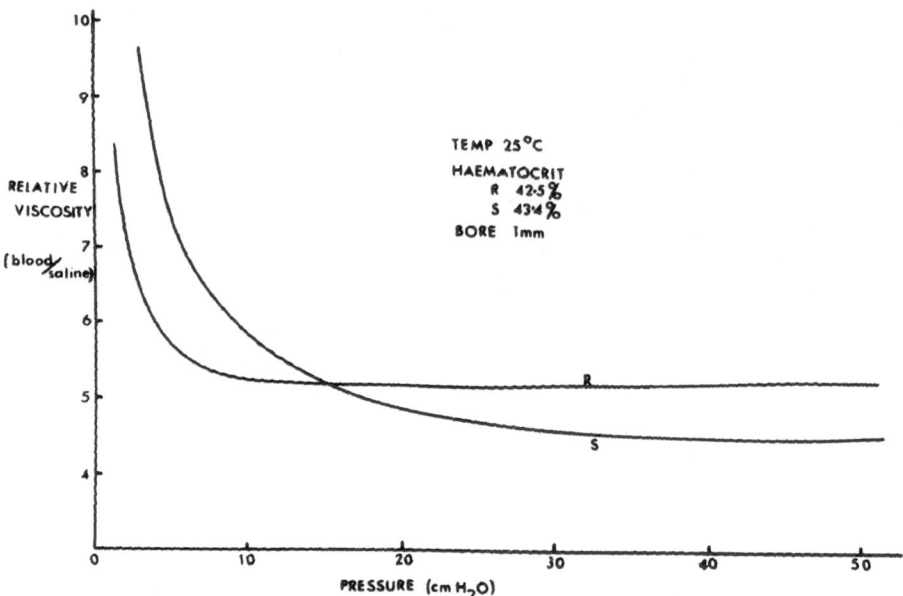

Figure 5.2. The viscosity of bloods R and S (see Figure 5.2.) relative to saline, as measured in a capillary viscometer of 1 mm bore at different pressures

THE ASSOCIATION BETWEEN FIBRINOGEN AND ERYTHROCYTE FLEXIBILITY

It has already been mentioned that when blood is defibrinated by shaking with glass beads, the red blood cells are made relatively inflexible. A similar decrease of erythrocyte flexibility occurs when blood is heated to more than 45°C (Teitel and Nicloau, 1963; Sirs, 1968). In a series of experiments with washed cells and after removal of plasma, it was found that inflexibility and slow packing rates resulted (Sirs, 1971). The following observations were also made:

(a) When whole blood was diluted in its own plasma and in an identical manner with an isotonic Ringer–Locke solution, the packing rates of both samples were the same.

(b) After centrifuging whole blood, or blood diluted by plasma at 600 g for 20 min, and remixing the cells with the supernatant, the flexibility of the cells was the same as the initial untreated control. When blood was mixed with Ringer–Locke solution and centrifuged, the remixed suspension packed at a slower rate.

(c) Blood, diluted with Ringer–Locke solution, was centrifuged and then an equivalent amount of supernatant, to that initially added, was removed. The remixed suspension packed at a slower rate relative to the original whole blood. This effect was found after adding only 1 ml of Ringer–Locke solution to 2 ml of whole blood and could not, therefore, in comparison with (a), be due to simple dilution of the plasma constituents. The degree of change gets progressively more pronounced the greater the initial dilution.

(d) After mixing a 2 ml sample of whole blood with 1 ml of Ringer–Locke, the cells were separated by centrifugation and 1 ml of the supernatant was removed and replaced by 1 ml of Ringer–Locke solution. The cells were then remixed with the supernatant. The packing rate of the remixed suspension was found to be significantly slower than the original diluted sample.

(e) After repeated washing and resuspension of the cells in Ringer–Locke solution, the packing rate fell to one-half that of the original blood sample at the same haematocrit. The washed cells were centrifuged again, the Ringer–Locke removed and replaced by the original plasma. The packing rate of the resuspended cells in plasma was just below that of the original sample.

The only explanation consistent with these experiments would appear to be that some factor is eluted during centrifugation which is necessary to maintain cell flexibility. Providing, however, it is all present when resuspending the cells, the effect is reversible. Preliminary experiments indicate that significant improvement cannot be gained by adding serum albumin, cholesterol or heparin to the Ringer–Locke solution.

The main factor responsible for these changes of flexibility was found to be fibrinogen (Rampling and Sirs, 1972a). If after washing the cells, they were resuspended in Ringer–Locke solutions containing fibrinogen, the flexibility was restored. The degree of restoration was related to the fibrinogen concentration. An equivalent packing curve to that of whole blood cannot be obtained, however, simply by adjusting the concentration of fibrinogen in Ringer–Locke solution. Also the concentration of fibrinogen necessary to obtain an equivalent initial packing rate is some three times greater than in normal plasma. This implies that a subsiduary effect must also be present in normal whole blood because of the presence of other plasma proteins. After adding fibrinogen directly to normal whole blood, and mixing, the packing rate is dramatically increased.

A number of experiments were made to ascertain which particular form of fibrinogen, or its polymers and degradation products, may be associated with this effect (Rampling and Sirs, 1972a). The purified preparation of human fibrinogen used was supplied by the Lister Institute of Preventive Medicine. Of the total protein in the sample 78 per cent was clottable. Warming the fibrinogen— Ringer–Locke solution to 40.5 °C for 1 hour, a procedure known to inactivate the fibrin stabilising factor, had no effect. After the fibrinogen solution was incubated at 52 °C for 1 hour, which denatures fibrinogen, and used to resuspend washed cells, the packing rate was no different from that of the washed cells in Ringer–Locke solution without fibrinogen. The fibrinogen solution was also ineffective after standing at room temperature for one week, because of fibrinolytic decomposition. The above evidence taken together with the inflexibility of erythrocytes after defibrinating blood by thrombin or arvin (see below) suggests that the active component is the uncomplexed fibrinogen (see Chapter 4).Whether the presence of different proportions of uncomplexed fibrinogen, dimer, complexed fibrinogen and degradation products can react in some way has still to be resolved by resuspending cells in plasmas of known fibrinogen composition.

Low molecular weight dextran indirectly reduces the erythrocyte flexibility by interaction with plasma fibrinogen (Rampling and Sirs, 1972a). A fall in the packing rate is observed after adding 0.8 g dextran per 100 ml which corresponds to a reduction of only 10 per cent in the plasma fibrinogen content. Further experiments have shown that when the venom of the malaýan pit viper, arvin, .is used to reduce the plasma fibrinogen concentration, a slower packing rate, indicative of increased erythrocyte rigidity, results (Myers et al., 1972). The addition of arvin to a previously defibrinated blood sample had no additional effect.

How fibrinogen alters the flexibility of red blood cells is not known. The ease by which it can, in part, be removed suggests that it is located in the 'buffy coat' surrounding the cell, in such a way as to utilise its elastic tensile properties, which are similar to myosin and collagen (Bailey et al., 1943). The amount of fibrinogen bound in this way is not simply proportional to the fibrinogen concentration in the plasma (Gramlich, 1963). A practical consequence, of the dependence of flexibility on fibrinogen, is that the individual components which determine the viscosity of whole blood with varying fibrinogen concentration cannot be isolated. As the fibrinogen concentration rises the plasma viscosity increases, but this is compensated by the red blood cells becoming more flexible. If the fibrinogen concentration falls, the reverse compensation applies. The flexibility of normal red blood cells may vary for a number of reasons, and the superimposition of different fibrinogen concentrations on such variability means that it is extremely diffi cult to isolate the decisive factor simply by determining whole blood viscosity.

ROULEAUX FORMATION AND THE ESR

It has been accepted for some time that the erythrocyte sedimentation rate (ESR) under gravity is influenced by the fibrinogen concentration. This, in turn, is considered to be related to the degree of rouleaux formation and aggregation of red cells (Cutler *et al.*, 1938; Dawson, 1960). If the red blood cells in whole blood are effectively in contact, as suggested earlier, then packing cannot be brought about by sedimentation. The formation of rouleaux, which because of their larger size were believed to sediment quicker, would not then directly influence this process. That sedimentation is not the mechanism of packing has already been demonstrated (Sirs, 1968; Rampling and Sirs, 1970).

In order to prove that rouleaux had no effect on the determination of erythrocyte flexibility by centrifugation, the rate of packing under conditions in which the degree of rouleaux formation varied was studied (Rampling and Sirs, 1972a). The simplest method of achieving this is to equally dilute whole blood with plasma, isotonic NaCl or Ringer–Locke solution. Such packing curves serve as a calibration of the effect of packed cell haematocrit on the rate of packing. The amount of rouleaux present in each sample was observed with a microscope and was classified as: 0, no rouleaux; 1, short loose rouleaux, 2, larger more closely packed rouleaux with occasional branching; and 3, very large rouleaux which adhere to form clumps (Engeset *et al.*, 1966).

The results for the rate of packing determined at different haematocrits, measured at 13 000 g, are shown in Figure 5.3. While the degree of rouleaux formation varied with the diluent used, the rate of packing and packed cell haematocrit were the same, for the same dilution. In other experiments it was found that the addition of formalin and dextran lowered the degree of rouleaux formation at the same time as increasing the erythrocyte rigidity. Considerable changes of rouleaux formation occurred after the addition of a dilute concentration of formalin, which was insufficient to significantly alter the packing rate and erythrocyte flexibility.

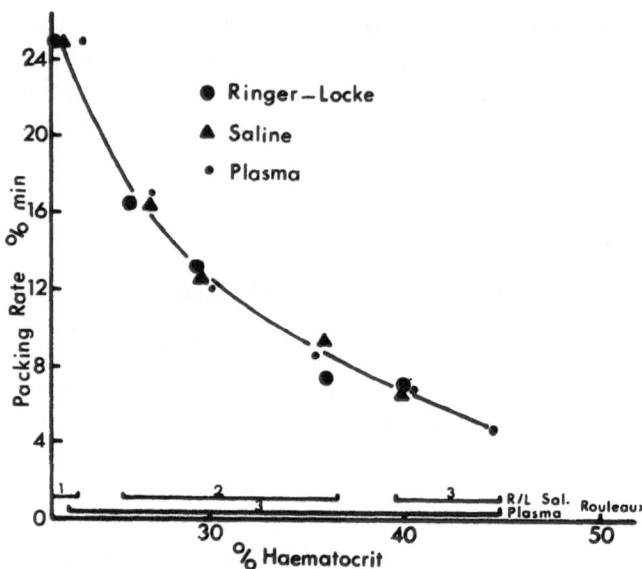

Figure 5.3. The effect of diluting blood in plasma. Ringer–Locke solution and isotonic saline on the rate of packing and rouleaux formation. The rate of packing is the initial slope of curves of haematocrit with time (Figure 5.1).

The formation of rouleaux is a complex interaction depending on many factors. Recent electron microscope studies (Chien *et al.*, 1971 ; Rowlands and Skibo, 1972), indicate that rouleaux are formed by a change of cell shape, the discoidal concavity being replaced by a flat surface which is directly in contact with a similar flat surface of an adjacent cell. There are several requirements for these cells to stick together; they must be able to change shape, have a relatively large area of contact, and some factor or agent must act to provide the adhesion. If the cells are made inflexible then the shape change cannot take place, the area of contact is minimal and rouleaux do not form. This occurs with washed cells, cells made inflexible with dextran or formaldehyde, after defibrination or the addition of any factor that increases the cell rigidity. Conversely, making cells more flexible will help to promote rouleaux formation, such as occurs with high fibrinogen concentrations. The differences of cell aggregation in ruminants and horses can be explained in a similar manner. In this case the fibrinogen concentration is not the determining factor. Horse red blood cells are extremely flexible, with a mean packing rate of approximately 25 per cent/min, compared to 6 per cent/min for man. Sheep and cow red blood cells are not only smaller than those of man, but the respective packing rates are 2.5 per cent/min and 2.35 per cent/min. These differences would appear to be an intrinsic property of the cells. The ESR of horse erythrocytes remains high when mixed with sheep or dog plasma (Osbaldiston, 1971). However, an increase in rouleaux has been observed with patients in which there was no change of flexibility. In these circumstances the surface adhesive factor may be different.

The interpretation of ESR readings is similarly complicated. This is not a process of sedimentation as previously supposed but is brought about by the weight of cells which are in contact with each other, bending and squeezing them together. Under the very small force of gravity it is conceivable that the force of aggregation significantly contributes to the flow properties of the cells during packing. The situation is comparable to studying blood flow in the non-Newtonian region at low shear rates. It was for this reason that the centrifuge method was developed. None the less, though it is more complicated to interpret, the same general considerations must apply to the ESR as to the centrifuge method, and the flexibility of red blood cells must also be a major factor. The association of a faster ESR with increased fibrinogen concentration and aggregate formation (Cutler *et al.*, 1938; Fahraeus, 1939; Dawson, 1960) is also a consequence of the increased flexibility of the erythrocyte. The ESR is lowered by lysolecithin (Fahraeus, 1939) which also decreases the erythrocyte flexibility and the rate of packing in the centrifuge is significantly slower.

The above observations appear to be pertinent to the stickiness of platelets. There has been a tendency to regard venous thrombosis and arterial thrombosis as distinct events. The former is the result of coagulation and the latter of platelet adhesion to collagen at the site of arterial wall damage. A review of factors which affect platelet stickiness, show a remarkable similarity to the agents which alter erythrocyte flexibility. Platelet adhesiveness is reduced by dextran (Cronberg *et al.*, 1966) and lysolecithin. Increased fibrinogen concentration is associated with elevation of platelet stickiness. It is possible that the changes of stickiness of platelets, which must involve deformation of the cells to pack them together, is dependent like rouleaux formation on the flexibility of the cell. In this respect plasma fibrinogen concentration is a factor in both types of thrombosis.

ERYTHROCYTE FLEXIBILITY AND SURGERY

Changes in the flexibility of rabbit's erythrocytes during surgery and the postoperative period have been investigated (Macdonald and Sirs, 1974). It was found that with minor operations, such as insertion of an ear arterial catheter under local anaesthetic, following anaesthesia without surgery,

71

there was no change of erythrocyte flexibility. Changes did occur during and following abdominal incision, removal of one kidney and placing a clip on the remaining renal artery, as is the accepted procedure to induce renal hypertension. Whether hypertension ensued or not it was unrelated to the changes in erythrocyte flexibility observed during surgery. An example of the changes of flexibility during the operation and during the subsequent ten days is shown in Figure 5.4. The initial slope of each packing curve, in per cent per minute, is utilised as an index of flexibility. One ml of blood

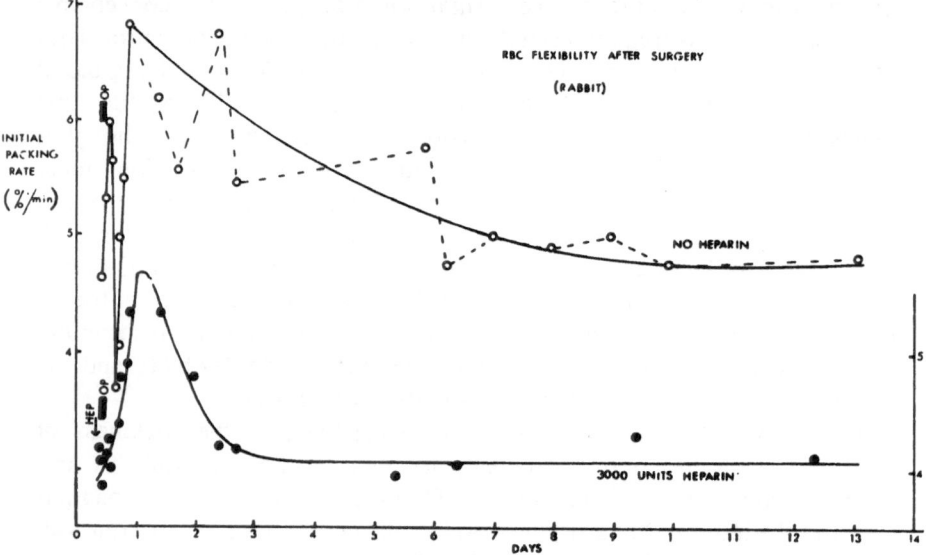

Figure 5.4. The changes in flexibility, as measured by the initial rate of packing, during and following surgery. The upper curve is that obtained without heparin and the lower curve, whose packing rate values are given by the vertical axis of the right-hand side, that obtained after a single intravenous injection of 3000 units of heparin fifteen minutes before the operation

was collected on the day before the operation, using heparin to prevent coagulation. On the day of operation, 1 ml blood samples were drawn at hourly intervals from an arterial catheter, over a 10-hour period, starting before anaesthesia with Nembutal. During the operation the flexibility of the erythrocytes decreased. Three to four hours after the operation, the flexibility started to increase again, at five to six hours was back to normal and then over the subsequent few hours it became significantly more flexible than the preoperative value. This elevated flexibility slowly returned to its original value within ten days. A possible explanation of these changes

72

is an association of the previously indicated relationship of flexibility and fibrinogen concentration with the considerable deposition of fibrin following extensive surgery. To test this hypothesis a single intravenous injection of 3000 units of heparin was given to the anaesthetised rabbit fifteen minutes before the operation. The initial depression of the erythrocyte flexibility did not occur and after operation the flexibility after a sharp rise returned almost to normal in 2–3 days Figure 5.4. This inhibition could also be obtained with a single dose of 200 units of heparin, provided it was given one hour before the operation.

Similar changes have been observed in patients undergoing cholecystectomy (Dupont and Sirs, 1974).

Before attempting to interpret these effects it is necessary to consider the possibility of a direct effect of heparin on red blood cells. There is an interesting difference between the action of high doses of heparin on blood under *in vitro* and *in vivo* conditions. *In vitro* small quantities of heparin, up to 20 i.u. per ml, are without any significant effect. A considerable increase in flexibility was found after adding 250–500 i.u. of heparin to 1 ml of blood (Sirs, 1971). At these concentrations the plasma viscocity was also raised from 1.56 centipoises to 1.72 centipoises. The whole blood viscosity, however, remained unaltered at both high and low shear rates. Only a small and transient change of erythrocyte flexibility was found after an intravenous injection of 5000 units of heparin into a rabbit (Macdonald and Sirs, 1974). The direct effects were negligible in comparison with the changes after operation. No significant changes of blood viscosity occur *in vivo* one hour after infusion of heparin (Meiselman *et al.*, 1971). Although some studies (Zbinden and Tomlin, 1969) indicate that heparin at concentrations above 1 i.u. per ml increases the adhesiveness of platelets *in vitro*, this does not occur to the platelets of patients given heparin (Salzman, 1963).

The effect of the changes of erythrocyte flexibility during and following operation on the rheological properties of blood is uncertain. During the initial phase when erythrocytes are inflexible, the rate of exchange of oxygen is reduced (Sirs, 1964) and to some degree the transport of oxygen is impaired. The more serious effects of introducing inflexible particles into blood occurs in the microcirculation. The injection of starch grains into the jugular vein or right ventricle of goats caused a large portion of the small arteries in the lungs to become occluded (Dunn, 1919). Pulmonary microemboli are found in patients who have received a large blood transfusion. The erythrocytes of ACD stored blood are relatively inflexible Sirs (1969). The perfusion rate of the lung with relatively inflexible cells was found to be decreased, as a result of an increase of the resistance to flow (Greene *et al.*, 1973). The degree of inflexibility during the initial postoperative phase is not as large as that found with ACD stored blood or after defibrination with arvin. It is therefore unlikely that the contribution of this effect to venous thrombosis is great. In a similar manner the increased fibrinogen concentration during the first ten days after operation could involve an increase of the blood viscosity at low shear rates, due to the increased flexibility of the cells. This is not high compared to that found in other diseases, such as rheumatoid arthritis. Though the increased flexibility will predispose to aggregation and stasis, it is unlikely to be a decisive factor in initiating thrombosis.

The most useful aspect of the changes in flexibility following surgery, is to serve as an index of the fibrinogen concentration and as a guide to the coagulation sequence. The initial reaction to surgery is a large deposition of fibrin at the site of the incision, and a fall in the blood fibrinogen level. This is followed in the next few hours by a stimulus to the liver to produce more fibrinogen. The higher fibrinogen levels, and increased erthrocyte flexibility, persist for more than a week. (Wolf *et al.*, 1972; Chapter 4). This reaction is similar to the raised fibrinogen levels found after injections of bacterial products (Ham and Curtis, 1938). That the stimulus to increased fibrinogen production is not simply the fall in fibrinogen concentration is suggested by the postoperative rise of fibrinogen when heparin was used and no significant decrease of flexibility was observed. The observations on the rates of synthesis and breakdown of mammalian fibrinogen (Reeve *et al.*, 1966)., indicate that the stimulus is associated with the breakdown of mammalian fibrinogen and fibrin. This suggests that the decrease of flexibility found in the initial period, without heparin, must be due to fibrinogen and not degradation products, or it would have been found after the addition of heparin as well. The initial phase can thus be explained on the basis of a fall in the fibrinogen concentration as a result of fibrin formation, which must take place even when heparin is present, though to a less degree This is followed by production of more fibrinogen stimulated by the increased degradation products (FDP). The changes and their sequence found in the present study, are the same as those observed after a single injection of typhoid vaccine to a rabbit (Reeve *et al.*, 1968).

The second phase of a change from a high fibrinogen concentration and increased flexibility to the normal level is easier to interpret by considering the heparinised case first. In this situation the flexibility returns to normal in 2–3 days. This is the same as that required for [131] I-fibrinogen, injected into a rabbit, to be cleared from the circulation (Reeve *et al.*, 1966).

The fibrinogen concentration can thus be rapidly increased in a matter of hours, but then takes several days to return to its normal level. The above findings suggest that after heparinisation, there is only a local reaction to surgery with a relatively rapid transient production and decay of degradation products. During the decay phase after heparinisation no degradation products must be present, or they would extend the decay time, and the change of erythrocyte flexibility is simply reflecting the fibrinogen concentration. To explain the longer decay time of the animals following surgery without heparin, some other factors must be involved, and the logical deduction is that degradation products stimulate fibrinogen synthesis. Evidence has been provided that degradation products are present during this phase (Wolf *et al.,* 1972; Chapter 4).

It appears that following surgery, a changing situation exists in which FDP are being continuously produced and fibrinogen concentration and erythrocyte flexibility are increased. In further experiments 200 units of intravenous heparin have been given immediately before operation on a rabbit (Macdonald and Sirs, 1974). Because there was insufficient time for the inhibitory action of heparin to take effect, the initial fall of erythrocyte flexibility occurred, as with the unheparinised animal in Figure 5.4. However, the postoperative increase of fibrinogen concentration and erythrocyte flexibility was only extended a day longer than the increase in the rabbit heparinised with 3000 units. This would suggest that the persistence of degradation products is not associated with excessive deposition and breakdown of fibrin. The heparin is cleared from the circulation with a half-time of 1 hour, and any inhibitory effect on plasminogen (Holemans *et al.,* 1963) during the following days would be negligible. It appears that severe surgical trauma, in the absence of heparin,can initiate intravascular formation and breakdown of fibrin. This results in a sequence of events which persist for more than a week. During this period it is likely that any factor which promotes fibrin formation, such as stasis, high blood viscosity or excessive platelet stickiness, will balance the odds in favour of thrombosis. This risk may be reduced by a low dose of heparin prior to the operation (see Chapter 2).

References

Bailey, K., Astbury, W. T. and Rudall, K. M. (1943). Fibrinogen and fibrin as members of the keratin—myosin group. *Nature (London),* **151,** 716

Bayliss, L. E. (1952). *Deformation and Flow in Biological Systems* (A. Frey-Wyssling, editor) (Amsterdam: North Holland)

Thromboembolism

Braasch, D. and Jemmett, W. (1968). Erythrocyte flexibility, haemoconcentration and friction resistance in glass capillaries with diameters between 6 and 50 /flugers Arch., **302**, 245

Chien, S., Usami, S., Dellenbach, R. and J. and Gregson, M. I. (1970). Shear-sependent deformation of erythrocytes in rheology of human blood. Amer. J. Physiol., **215**, 136

Chien, S., Luse, S. A., Jan, K. M., Usami, S., Miller L. H. and Fremount H. (1971). Effects of macromolecules on the rheology and ultrastructure of red cell suspensions. Proc. Sixth Eur. Conf. Microcirculation, (Basel: Karger)

Cronberg, S., Robertson, B. Nilsson, I. M. and Nilehn, J. E. (1966). Suppressive effect of dextran on platelet adhesiveness. Thromb. Diath. Haemorrh., **16**, 384

Cutler, J. W., Park, F. R. and Herr B. S. (1938). The influences of anaemia on blood sedimentation. Amer. J. Med. Sci., 195, 734

Dawson, J. B. (1960). The E.s.R. in a new dress. Brit. Med. J., **1**, 1697 35

Dintenfass, L. (1963). An application of a cone-in-cone viscometer to study viscosity, thixotropy and clotting of whole blood. Biorheology, **1**, 91

Dintenfass, L. (1971). Blood Microrheology, (London: Butterworth & Co.).

Dunn, J. S. (1919). The effects of multiple embolism of pulmonary arterioles. Quart. J. Med., **13**, 129

Engest, J., Stalker, A. L. and Matheson, N. A. (1966). Effects of Dextran 40 on erythrocyte aggregation. Lancet, **i**, 1124

Fahraeus, R. (1939). The erthrocyte-plasma interface. Lancet, **i**, 630

Fleisher, R. L. and Price, P. B. (1963). Tracks of charged particles in high polymers. Science, 140, 1221

Fleischer, R. L., Price, P. B. and Walker, R. M. (1956). Tracks of charged particles in solids. Science, **149**, 383

Gramlich, F. (1963). Die Bindungsfahigkeit roter Blutkorperchen. Ein Beitrag zur Pathogenese erworbener hamolytischer Zustande. Folia Haemat., Nene Folge, **9**, 15

Greene, R., Hughes, J. M. B., Iliff, I. D. and Pines, G. F. (1973). Red cell flexibility and pressure-flow relations in isolated lungs. J. Appl. Physiol., **34**, 169

Gregersen, M. T., Bryant, C. A., Hammerle, W. E., Usami, S. and Chien S. (1967) Flow characteristics of human erythrocytes through polycarbonate sieves. Science, **157**, 825

Ham, T. H. and Curtiss, F. C. (1938). Plasma fibrinogen response in man: influence of nutritional state, induced hyperpyyrexia, infectious diseases and liver damage. Medicine, **17**, 413

Harris, J. W., Brewster, H. H., Ham, T. H. and Castle, W. R. (1956). The biophysics and sickle-cell disease. Arch. Int. Med., **97**, 145

Harvey, E. N. and Danielli, J. E. (1938). Properties of the cell surface. Biol. Rev., **13**, 319

Holemans, R., Adamis, D. and Horace, J. F. (1963). Interaction of heparin with fibrinolysis. Thromb. Diath. Haemorrh., **9**, 445

Jacobs, H. R. (1963). The viscosity of red cell packs. Biorheology., **1**, 129

Jandle, J. H., Simmons, R. L. and Castle, W. B. (1961). Red cell filtration and the pathogenesis of certain haemolytic anemias. Blood, **18**, 133

Jay, A. W. L., Rowlands, S. and Skibo, L. (1972). The resistance to blood flow in the capillaries. Can. J. Physiol. Pharmacol., **50**, 1007

Thromboembolism

Jay, A. W. L. (1973). Visoelastic properties of the human red blood cell membrane. *Biophys. J., 13*, 1166

Krogh, A. (1962). *The Anatomy and Physiology of Capillaries. (New Haven: University Press, Yale)*

LaCelle, P. L. (1969). *Alteration of deformability of the erythrocyte membrane in stored blood. Transfusion, 9*, 238

Macdonald, G. J. and Sirs, J. A. (1974). (Unpublished data)

Meiselman, H. J., Frasher, W. G. and Wayland, H. (1971). Variable shear rate viscometry of native-dog blood; effect of heparin injection. *Biorheology, 8*, 91

Mitchison, J. M. and Swann, M. M. (1954). The mechanical properties of the cell surface (1) The cell elastimeter. *J. exp. Biol., 31*, 443

Myers, P., Rampling, M. W. and Sirs, J. A. (1972). Interaction of arvin with erythrocyte flexibility. *J. Physiol. 230*, 51P

Osbaldiston, G. W. (1971). Erythrocyte sedimentation rate. Studies in sheep, dog and horse. *Cornell Veterinarian., 61*, 386

Prothero, J. and Burton, A. C. (1962). Physics of blood flow in capillaries. Biophs. J., *2*, 213

Rampling, M. W. and Sirs, J. A. (1970) The effect of haematocrit and anticoagulants on the rate of packing of erythrocytes by a centrifuge. *Phys. Med. Biol., 15*, 15

Rampling, M. W. and Sirs, J. A. (1972a). The interactions of fibrinogen and dextrans with erythrocytes. *J. Physiol. 223*, 199

Rampling, M. W. and Sirs, J. A. (1972b). The measurement of erythrocyte flexibility by centrifugation. *J. Physiol., 230*, 3P

Rampling, M. W. and Sirs, J. A. (1974). (Unpublished data)

Rand, R. P. and Burton, A. C. (1964). Mechanical properties of the red cell membrane (1) Membrane stiffness and intracellular pressure. *Biophys, J., 4*, 115

Reeve, E. B., Takeda, Y. and Atencio, A. C. (1966). Some observation of the mammalian fibrinogen system in non-steady and steady states. *Prot. Biol. Fluid., 14*, 183

Rowlands, S. and Skibo, L. (1972). The morphology of red-cell aggregates. *Thromb. Res., 1*, 47

Salzman, E. W. (1962). Measurement of platelet adhesiveness. *J. Lab Clin. Med., 62* 724

Sirs, J. A. (1963). Metabolic aspects of the uptake of oxygen by haemoglobin in erythrocytes. *Biochim. Biophys. Acta, 66*, 378

Sirs J. A. (1964). The facilitated uptake of nitric oxide by haemoglobin in erythrocytes. *Biochim. Biophs. Acta., 10*, 108

Sirs, J. A. (1968). The measurement of the haematocrit and flexibility of erythrocytes with a centrifuge. *Biorheology, 5*, 1

Sirs, J. A. (1969). The respiratory efficiency and flexibility of erythrocytes stored in Acid-dextrose solution: *J. Physiol., 203*, 93

Sirs, J. A. (1970). Automatic recording of the rate of packing of erythrocytes in blood by a centrifuge. *Phys. Med. Biol., 15*, 9

Sirs, J. A. (1970). Erythrocyte function and aldosterone. Biocheology, *8*, 1

Swank, R. L. (1961). Alteration of Blood on Storage: Measurement of adhesiveness of 'Ageing' platelets and leucocytes, and their removal by filtration. *New Eng. J. Med., 265*, 728

Teitel, P. (1964). Relation of altered plasticity of erythrocytes to their shortened life span. *Sangre, 9*, 421

Thromboembolism

Teitel, P. and Nicolau, C. T. (1963). Chemici, si metabolici care influenteaza reologia eritrocitelor. *Proc. Symp. Molec. Biol. and Pathol* p57; C. Nicolau, editor (Bucharest)

Weed, R. I., LaCelle, B. L. and Merrill, E. W. (1969). Metabolic dependence of red cell deformability. *Clin. Invest.,* **40,** 794

Wolf, P., Farrell, G. W. and Walton, K. W. (1972). The significance of variations in immunoreactive and clottable fibrinogen in health and following thrombosis. *Clin. Pathol.,* **25,** 36

Zbinden, G. and Tomlin, S. (1969). Effect of heparin on platelet adhesivness. *Acta Haematol.,* **41,** 264

6

Abnormal blood viscosity and deep venous thrombosis

J. A. Dormandy

Although the incidence of postoperative deep venous thrombosis has been found to be high by many studies (Atkins and Hawkins, 1965; Kakkar and Flanc, 1968; Flanc *et al.*, 1968; Negus *et al.*, 1968; Kakkar, 1969; Howe, 1970; Chapters 1 and 14) its aetiology is still largely unknown. As can be seen from the reviews in Chapters 2 and 7 the current belief is that in the average patient, deep venous thrombosis is initiated at the time of operation and is facilitated by a number of factors including slowing of the flow of blood (McLachlin *et al.*, 1960; Clark and Cotton, 1968; Chapter 9). This has led to the trial of different techniques designed to reduce perioperative venous stasis (Chapters 9 and 14). The problem is, why in a group of apparently normal patients subjected to similar conditions of reduced venous flow, some develop deep venous thrombosis and others do not. On first principles the velocity of flow of blood along a vessel is dependent on the three primary determinants described by Poiseuille over a century ago (1846). The pressure gradient along the vessel, the size of the vessel lumen and the viscosity of the blood. Of these three, the blood viscosity, or rather the effect of changes in blood viscosity, has been particularly neglected. Poiseuille's original work was carried out using Newtonian fluids in a totally artificial system, but recent work both in animals (Putnam *et al.*, 1967; Dormandy, 1970; Messmer *et al.*, 1972) and in man (Dormandy, 1971) has shown that changes in blood viscosity as measured by current *in vitro* techniques do correlate well with changes in blood flow measured *in vivo*. An increase in blood viscosity raises the peripheral resistance and lowers the cardiac output (almost wholly by an effect on the stroke volume rather than heart rate). For instance a 10 per cent increase in blood viscosity (measured at a shear rate of 230 sec $^{-1}$) is associated with an over 20 per cent decrease in the total circulation through an intact normal human leg (Dormandy, 1971).

Over the past decade, it has been shown that abnormalities of blood viscosity exist in certain clinical conditions and are associated with circulatory disturbances. These conditions include myocardial infarction, (Kellogg and Goodman, 1960; Ditzel *et al.*, 1968); macroglobulinaemia (Fahey *et al.*, 1965); polycythaemia (Burton-Opitz, 1911); sickle-cell disease (Harris *et al.*, 1956; Anderson *et al.*, 1963); spherocytosis (Murphy, 1967); diabetes (Skovborg *et al.*, 1966; Hoare *et al.*, 1973); and some cases of intermittent claudication (Dormandy *et al.*, 1973a ; 1973b). There is therefore considerable circumstantial evidence to suggest that abnormalities in blood viscosity may play a part in the slowing venous blood flow at the time of operation and thus predispose to deep venous thrombosis.

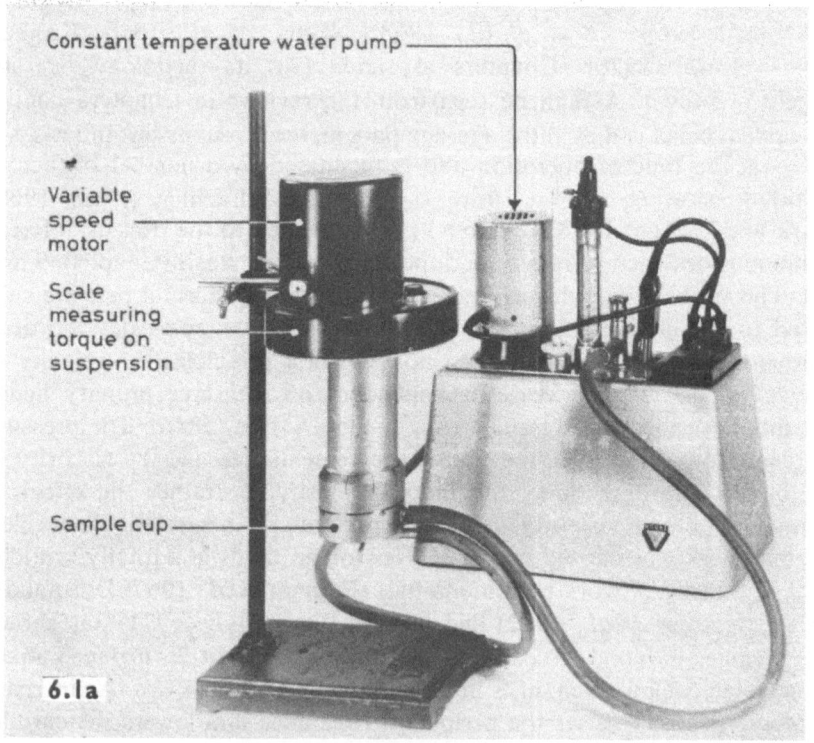

Constant temperature water pump

Variable speed motor

Scale measuring torque on suspension

Sample cup

6.1a

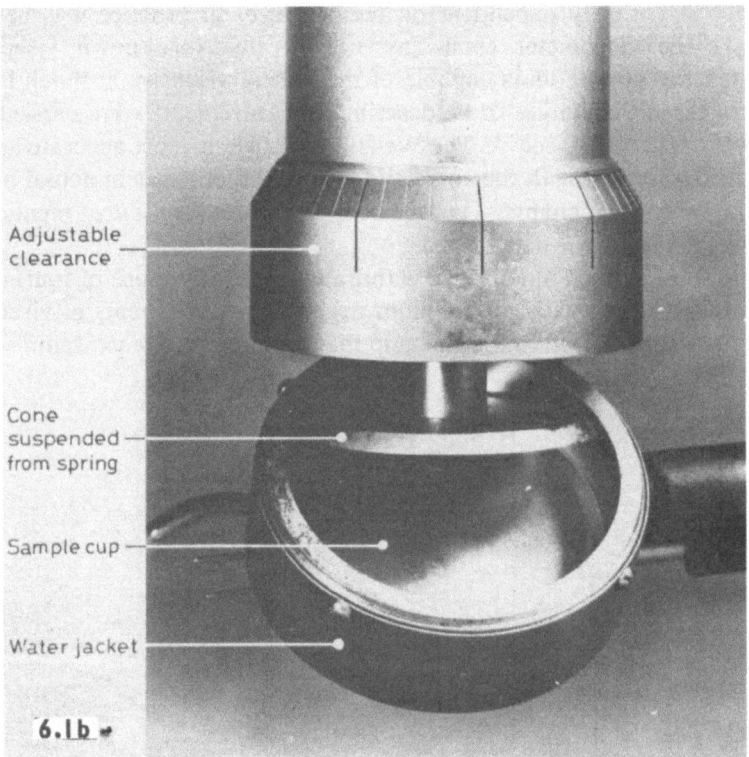

Adjustable
clearance

Cone
suspended
from spring

Sample cup

Water jacket

6.1b

Figure 6.1a and 6.1b The Wells–Brookfield viscometer

The possibility of an abnormal blood viscosity associated with deep
venous thrombosis in the perioperative period was investigated using the
Wells–Brookfield viscometer (Figure 6.1), which is the most commonly
used rotational type viscometer (Wells *et al.*, 1961) and has been adapted from an industrial machine. A conical disk is rotated by a variable
speed motor, through a beryllium copper spring suspension, in a small cup
containing the blood sample. The drag on the rotating cone caused by the
viscosity of the sample can then be measured by the torque on the spring.
Although the difference in velocity between the rotating cone and the cup
increases towards the periphery, the distance between the two surfaces also
increases. Therefore, with a cone of the correct angle, the velocity gradient
or shear rate will be constant throughout the sample. The viscosity in centipoises can be calculated from the dimensions of the chamber, the
rotational speed of the cone and the torque in the spring suspension. The
cup is surrounded by a water-jacket to keep the sample at 37 °C because

viscosity is critically dependent on temperature. In practice it is best to calibrate the viscometer each day with a fluid of known viscosity. Although the apparatus is capable of measuring viscosity at much lower shear rates, in the studies to be described measurements were carried out at a shear rate of 230 sec^{-1}. The Wells–Brookfield is most accurate at this high shear rate at which the correlations between changes in actual blood flow *in vivo* and changes in viscosity measured *in vitro* mentioned previously have been determined.

Samples of venous blood were withdrawn without the use of tourniquet and anticoagulated with solid lithium heparin. Measurements of viscosity were carried out within four hours and the haematocrit of each sample was determined simultaneously.

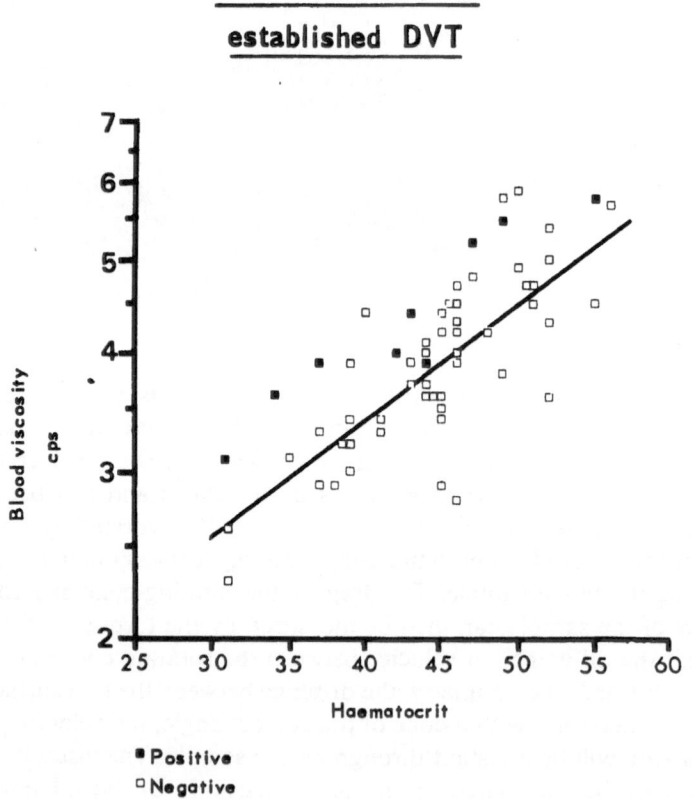

Blood viscosity in
established DVT

■ Positive
□ Negative

Figure 6.2 The relationship between blood viscocity at shear rate of 230 sec^{-1} haematocrit and established deep venous thrombosis

Although it has long been recognised that the red cell concentration is one of the most important determinants of the whole blood viscosity, the nature of the exact relationship has been much debated. The majority of the evidence available suggests that, at least within the physiological range of haematocrit, the relationship is exponential. That is, a linear result is obtained if the logarithm of the viscosity is plotted against the red cell concentration (Gregerson *et al.*, 1963; Begg and Hearns 1966; Meiselman and Merrill, 1966; Weaver *et al.*, 1969; Dormandy, 1970). Figure 6.2 shows the blood viscosity of 50 normal subjects plotted in this way, as well as the regression line defining this relationship. Using the slope of this regression line the 'measured viscosities' can be converted to a 'corrected viscosity' at a constant haematocrit of 45 per cent.

Before embarking on a prospective study of the possible relationship between blood viscosity and postoperative deep venous thrombosis, a pilot investigation was carried out comparing nine patients with established deep venous thrombosis to 50 normal control subjects. None of the patients had an operation in the previous 2 years and the thrombosis appeared to be spontaneous. Three patients had clinical evidence of pulmonary embolism and six were on anticoagulants at the time of the investigation. Figure 6.2 shows the blood viscosities of the patients with established thrombosis plotted against the haematocrit of the samples and the results obtained in 50 normal controls. It can be seen that the patients with established thrombosis had a higher whole blood viscosity than normals with the same haematocrit ($p = 0.001$). This difference may have been the result of venous thrombosis and was not related to its causation; a prospective study was therefore carried out in a general surgical group.

In the prospective study, 72 patients were included who had been admitted for elective general surgical and gynaecological operations. Their average age was 50 years. Patients were excluded if their operation was to be on the legs, groin or thyroid. Table 6.1 shows the operations undergone by the whole group. Patients with a history of previous thrombotic episodes or any known predisposing factor were excluded. The viscosity of the patients' blood was measured immediately before operation using the Wells—Brookfield viscometer. The development of deep venous thrombosis following surgery was detected by the ^{125}I-fibrinogen test (Chapter 14). The legs were scanned before operation and then on the first, third, fifth, seventh and ninth postoperative days. In most cases with a positive scan confirmatory phlebography was performed.

Seventeen of the 72 patients developed deep venous thrombosis. The comparatively low incidence was probably because all patients above 20

Preoperative viscosity

Standard haematocrit of 45 per cent

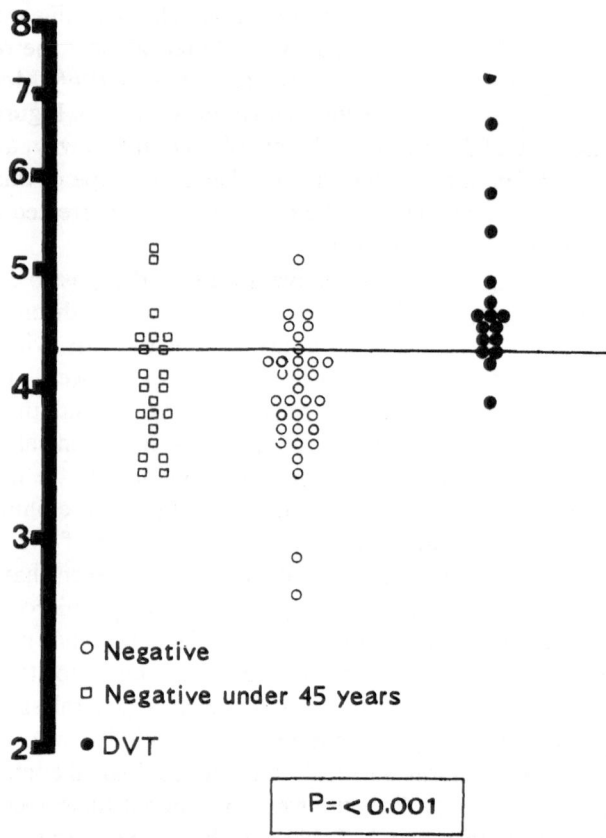

○ Negative

□ Negative under 45 years

● DVT

P= < 0.001

Figure 6.3 Preoperative blood viscosity at shear rate of 230 sec^{-1} corrected to haematocrit of 45 per cent in patients with and without deep venous thrombosis

years of age were included and patients with known factors predisposing to deep venous thrombosis were excluded. The operations performed on the patients who developed thrombosis are also indicated in Table 6.1.

The preoperative blood viscosities of the patients who developed deep venous thrombosis and those who did not are compared in Table 6.2. The measured perioperative mean blood viscosity of the patients who

Table 6.1

Operations performed	Number of patients (with DVT in brackets)
Thoracotomy	3 (1)
Lobectomy	2(1)
Pneumonectomy	1
Major abdominal	
Gastric	9 (2)
Cholecystectomy	10 (4)
Colectomy — Rectal	15 (4)
Splenectomy	1
Aneurysmectomy	1
Renal	1
Major gynaecological	
Hysterectomy	3 (1)
Vaginal ops.	3 (2)
Minor operations	
Haemorrhoidectomy	7 (1)
Appendicetomy	2
Laparotomy	2
Ovarian cystectomy	4 (1)
Hysterotomy	3
Incisional hernia	2
D and C	1
Salpingostomy	1
Excision hydrocele	1

Total 72

developed deep venous thrombosis was higher than the viscosity of the patients who did not ($p<0.001$). This difference was not due to haemoconcentration as, in fact, the patients who developed thrombosis had a lower mean haematocrit. If all the viscosity measurements are corrected to a standard haematocrit of 45 per cent individual variations due to difference in haematocrit are eliminated and the significance of other factors which determine viscosity become more apparent. Figure 6.3 shows the corrected preoperative viscosities and marked difference between the patients who later developed deep venous thrombosis and those who did not ($p<0.001$).

From the above study it would appear that a patient over 45 years of age with no known predisposing factors but who has a corrected

Table 6.2 Preoperative blood viscosity and DVT* in 72 patients

	DVT Negative (55)	DVT Positive (17)	Difference	Significance (_t_ test)
Haematocrit	44.8 per cent (SD – 5.6)	44.1 per cent (SD – 5.3)	0.72 per cent	$p < 0.05$
Measured viscosity	3.99 (SD – 0.76)	4,68 (SD – 0.64)	0.69	$p < .001$
Viscosity corrected for haematocrit	4.00 (SD – 0.50)	4.87 (SD – 0.89)	0.87	$p < 0.001$

*DVT – Deep Venous Thrombosis

preoperative blood viscosity above 4.3 centipoises at a shear rate of 230 sec^{-1} will have a 73 per cent chance of developing post operative deep venous thrombosis. These facts could therefore be used as a screening test to select patients for perioperative scanning with radio active fibrinogen or for the application of any special prophylactic measures which may be available.

Direct treatment of a high blood viscosity is unfortunately not as yet feasible. While haemodilution will lower measured viscosity the present study does not indicate that it will necessarily affect the incidence of thrombosis. Low molecular weight dextran (LMWD) has been suggested as a possible agent with a specific viscosity lowering action by several investigators (Gelin, 1961; Groth and Thorsen, 1965; Ditzel _et al._, 1969). Unfortunately none of them corrected the change in viscosity for the change in haematocrit also produced by LMWD. If this is done then LMWD is found to have no specific effect on viscosity other than by haemodilution (Replogle _et al._, 1965; Meiselmann and Merrill, 1966; Chien _et al._, 1971; Dormandy, 1971).

In the above study only the preoperative blood viscosity was investigated. It is possible that the blood viscosity during or immediately after operation is more critical (Chapter 5). Large changes in viscosity in the postoperative period may be expected because it is known that the plasma fibrinogen is significantly raised following all types of surgery (Langsjoen and Murray, 1971; Kemble and Hickman, 1972). A correlation between plasma fibrinogen and whole blood viscosity is now generally accepted (Eisenberg, 1964; Merrill *et al.*, 1969; Weaver *et al.*, 1969: Chapters 4 and 5) although it is thought to be significant only at low shear rates.

In summary, a high preoperative blood viscosity (measured at a shear rate of 230 sec^{-1}) has been shown to be associated with the development of postoperative deep venous thrombosis in patients with no other known predisposing factors. This could be useful as a predictive screening test. The reason for this association is probably further slowing of venous blood flow in areas of stasis. The high blood viscosity may also reflect an alteration in plasma fibrinogen as a result of a hypercoagulable state in patients predisposed to thrombosis. Unfortunately no specific treatment is as yet available that can correct the abnormally raised blood viscosity. Before such a therapeutic agent is likely to be discovered much more needs to be known about the factors responsible for abnormal blood viscosity.

References

Anderson, R., Cassell, M., Mullinax, G. L. and Chaplin, H. (1963). Effect of Normal Cells on Viscosity of Sickle-Cell Blood. *Arch. Int. Med.* iii, 286

Atkins, P. and Hawkins, L. A. (1965). Detection of Venous Thrombosis in the Legs. *Lancet*, ii, 1217

Begg, T. B. and Hearns, J. B. (1966). Components in Blood Viscosity *Clin. Sci.*, **31**, 87

Burton-Opitz (1911). The Viscosity of the Blood. *J. Amer.* Med. Ass. **57**, 353

Chien, S., Jan, K. and Usami, S. (1971). *Rheological Considerations of Colloid Replacement* (Paris; Les Solutes de Substitution, Librarie Annette)

Clark, C. and Cotton, L. T., (1968). Blood Flow in Deep Veins of Leg, Recording Technique and Evalutation of Methods to Increase Flow during Operation' *Brit. J. Surg.* **55**, 211

Ditzel, J., Bang, H. O. and Thorsen, N. (1968). Myocardial Infarction and Whole Blood Viscosity. *Acta. Med. Scand.*, **183**, 577

Ditzel, J., Bang, H. O. and Thorsen, N. (1969). The Effect of Dextran 40 on Haemorheological Factors during the course of Myocardial Infarction. *Biblio. Anat.* **10**, 132

Dormandy, J. A. (1970). Clinical Significance of Blood Viscosity. *Ann. Roy. Coll. Surg. Eng.*, **47**, 211

Dormandy, J. A. (1971). Influence of Blood Viscosity on Blood Flow and the Effect of Low Molecular Weight Dextran. *Brit. Med. J.*, **4**, 716

Dormandy, J. H. (1973a). Clinical, Haemodynamic Rheological and Biochemical Findings in 126 Patients with Intermittent Claudication. *Brit. Med. J.*, **4**, 576

Dormandy, J. H. (1973b). Prognostic Significance of Rheological and Biochemical Findings in Patients with Intermittent Claudication. *Brit. Med. J.*, **4**, 581

Eisenberg, S. (1964). Changes in Blood Viscosity, Haematocrit and Fibrinogen Concentration in Subjects with Congestive Heart Failure. *Circulation*, **30**, 686

Fahey, J. L., Barth, W. F. and Solomon, A., (1965). Serum Hyperviscosity Syndrome. *J. Amer. Med. Ass.*, **192**, 464

Thromboembolism

Flanc, C., Kakkar, V. V, and Clarke, M. B. (1968). The Detection of Venous Thrombosis of the Legs using 125 I-labelled Fibrinogen. *Brit. J. Surg.* **55**, 742

Gelin, L. E., (1961). Disturbances of the Flow Properties of Blood and its Counteraction in Surgery. *Acta Chirurgca Scand.,* **122**, 287

Gregerson, M, I., Peric, B., Usami, S. and Chien, S., (1963). Relation of Molecular Size of Dextran to its Effect on the Rheological Properties of Blood. *Proc. Soc. Exp. Biol. (n. Y.)* **122**, 325

Groth, C. G., and Thorsen, G. (1965). The Effect of Rheomacrodex and Macrodex on Factors Covering the Flow Properties of Human Blood. *Acta Chirurgia Scand.,* **130**, 507

Harris, J. W., Brewser, H. H., Ham, T. H. and Castle, W. B. (1956). Studies on the Destruction of Red Blood Cells. X. The Biophysics and Biology of Sickle Cell Disease. *Amer. Med. Ass. Arch. Int. Med.,* **97**, 145

Hoare, E., Beckett, A. G., and Dormandy, J. A., (1973). Whole Blood Viscosity in Diabetes. *Excerpta Medica.* (Abstract of Eighth Cong. Int. Diabetic Fed)

Howe, C. T., (1970). Management of Deep Venous Thrombosis. *Brit. J. Hosp. Med.,* **3**, 350

Kakkar, V. V., (1969). The Problems of Thrombosis in the Deep Veins of the Leg. *Ann. Roy. Coll. Surg. Eng.,* **45**, 257

Kakkar, V. V. and Flanc, C., (1968). Role of Phlebography on Deep Vein Thrombosis, *Brit. J. Surg.,* **55**, 384

Kellogg, F. and Goodman, F. R. (1960). Viscosity of Blood: Myocardial Infarction. *Circ. Res.,* **9**, 972

Kemble, J. V. E. and Hickman, J. A. (1972). Post-operative Changes in Blood Viscosity and the Influence of Haematocrit and Plasma Fibrinogen. *Brit. J. Surg.* **59**, 629

Langsjoen, P. H. and Murray, R. A., (1971). Treatment of Post Surgical Thromboembolic Complications. *J. Amer. Med. Ass.,* **218**, 855

McLachlin, A. D., McLachlin, J. A., Jory, T. A. and Rawling, E. G. (1960). Venous Stasis in the Lower Extremities. *Ann. Surg.,* **152**, 678

Meisleman, H. J. and Merrill, E. W., (1966). Haemorheology: the Effect of Haemodilution and L. M. W. D. *Fourth Eur. Conf. Microcirculation*

Merrill, E. W., Cheng, C. S. and Pelletier, G. A., (1969). Yield Stress and Endogenous Fibrinogn. *J. Appl. Physiol.* **26**, 1

Messmer, K., Lewis, D. H., Sunder-Plassman, L., Kloverkorn, W. P., Mendler, N, and Holper, K., (1972). Acute Normovolemic Hemodilution, European Surgical Research, **4**, 55

Murphy, J. R., (1967). The Influence of pH and Temperature on Some Physical Properties of Normal Erythrocytes and Erythocytes from Patients with Hereditary Spherocytosis. *J. Lab. Clin. Med.,* **69**, 758

Negus, D., Pinto, D. J., Le Quesne, L. P., Brown, N. and Chapman, M. (1968). 125 I-Labelled Fibrinogen in the Diagnosis of Deep Vein Thrombosis and its Correlation with Phlebography. *Brit. J. Surg.,* **55**, 835

Poiseuille, J. L. M. (1846). Recherches Experimentales sure le Mouvement des Liquides dans les tubes de tres-petits Diametres. *Comtes Reandes. Academie Sciences Paris,* **9**, 433

Putnam, T. C., Kevy, S. V. and Replogle, R. L. (1967). Factors Influencing the Viscosity of Blood. *Surg. Gynaecol. Obstet.* **124**, 547

Replogle, R. L., Kunder, H. and Gross, R. E. (1965). Studies on the Haemodynamic Importance of Blood Viscosity. *J. Thoracic Cardiovasc. Surg.,* **50**, 658

Thromboembolism

Skovborg et al. (1966). Blood Viscosity in Diabetic Patients. *Lancet,* i, 129

Weaver, J. P. A., Evans, A. and Walder, D., (1969). The Effect of Increased Fibrinogen content on the Viscosity of Blood. *Clin. Sci.,* **36,** 1

Wells, R. E., Denton, R. and Merrill, E. W., (1961). Measurement of Viscosity of Biologic Fluids by Cone Plate Viscometer. *J. Lab. Clin. Med.,* **57,** 646

7

Platelets and venous thrombosis

J. W. Constantine and Irene M. Purcell

Observations on the sequence of events in experimental arterial thrombosis indicate that in the presence of rapid blood flow and vascular injury, coagulation processes are secondary to those of platelet adhesion and aggregation. In an arterial 'white' thrombus, the major component is the platelet 'head', which consists of aggregated platelets attached to a damaged portion of the vessel wall. Strands of fibrin, enmeshing erythrocytes and occasional leukocytes, constitute a 'tail' which streams in the direction of blood flow. The initial phase of thrombus formation involves platelet adhesion to exposed subintimal collagen followed by platelet aggregation; fibrin formation occurs during a later stage which is characterised by consolidation and stabilisation of the platelet mass Poole and French, 1961. Mustard *et al.*, 1962; Mustard *et al.*, 1964; French, 1965, 1969; In contrast, studies on the genesis and morphology of venous thrombi, and clinical experience in the prophylaxis and treatment of venous thromboembolic disease, suggest that reduced blood flow and activation of coagulation mechanisms are more important in the development of venous thrombosis than the processes of platelet adhesion and aggregation. A venous 'red' thrombus consists predominantly of red cells enmeshed in fibrin and layered between fibrin strands and masses of platelets or leukocytes; platelet–fibrin deposits occur at the point of attachment to the vessel wall and at foci throughout the thrombus, but these represent a minor component (Chandler, 1969; Paterson, 1969).

Until recently it was believed that unlike arterial thrombi, venous thrombi were not associated with endothelial lesions. Complete serial sections through early venous thrombi found at necropsy did not reveal endothelial damage in the area of thrombus attachment (Paterson and McLachlin, 1954). In addition, the endothelium in the region of an old deep venous thrombus was similar histologically to the endothelium at the same anatomical location in a vein without a thrombus; no intimal changes were found in the thrombosed vein which could act as a precipitating factor to thrombus formation (McLachlin and Paterson, 1951; Paterson and McLachlin, 1954). Recent studies using scanning electron microscopy suggest that changes and damage to the endothelium may occur as a result of local stasis and tissue, trauma at a distant site. However, the basement membrane remains intact and platelets do not adhere to it. (Chapter 8).

When formed under conditions of stasis a venous thrombus is morphologically similar to a test-tube clot, i.e. it is composed of the formed elements of blood randomly distributed within a fibrin network and it may be referred to as a coagulation thrombus (Deykin, 1967; Wessler, 1962; 1963.). This is not to say, however, that a venous thrombus and a test-tube clot are identical, but rather to emphasise that coagulation mechanisms play a predominant role.

The efficacy of anticoagulant drugs in the prophylaxis and treatment of venous thromboembolic disease further emphasises the difference in the pathogenesis of arterial and venous thrombosis, and provides evidence for the predominance of coagulation processes in the latter. Two principal classes of anticoagulants have been developed for clinical use: heparin which acts both *in vitro* and *in vivo* by potentiating a naturally-occuring inhibitor of activated Factor X (Yin and Wessler, 1970), and by exerting an antithrombin effect (Gurewich *et al.*, 1967); and orally active compounds of the coumarin–indanedione group which suppress synthesis of Factors II, VII, IX and X (Aggeler and O'Reilly, 1966). The effect of anticoagulants of either class is decreased activity of the intrinsic coagulation system and inhibition of fibrin formation.

It is generally accepted that heparin and coumarin analogues have no *direct* effect on platelet behaviour *in vivo* at therapeutic levels (Chan, 1972; Knieriem and Chandler, 1967; Newland and Nordoy, 1967; Poller *et al.*, 1969; O'Brien, 1973). It is therefore not surprising that anticoagulants have only limited effectiveness in the prevention or treatment of coronary artery disease (Arnott, 1969; Borchgrevink, 1966; Brown and MacMillan; 1965; Harvald *et al.*, 1962; Hilden *et al.*, 1961 Pickering, 1964; Seaman *et al.*, 1964), arterial cerebrovascular disease (Hill *et al.*, 1960; Millikan, 1962), or occlusive peripheral arterial disease (Hess, 1966; Lund and Tillgren, 1966). Their benefit in these conditions is, in general, restricted to

Thromboembolism

reducing thrombotic complications such as embolism or further growth of the thrombus, which is in accordance with the concept that the initial phase of arterial thrombogenesis depends more upon platelet adhesion and aggregation than upon coagulation. In contrast, the value of anticoagulants is well established in patients with deep venous thrombosis or where the risk of venous thromboembolic complications is high (Hume *et al.*, 1970). Heparin or oral anticoagulants reduce the incidence of pulmonary embolism in patients with deep venous thrombosis (Barritt and Jordan, 1960; Bauer, 1964; Kernohan and Todd, 1966; Gurewich *et al.*, 1967). They also reduce the incidence of venous thrombosis in bed-ridden patients following surgery, notably orthopedic surgery in the elderly (Sevitt and Gallagher, 1959; Salzman *et al.*, 1966; Sevitt, 1966).

However, the precise role of coagulation mechanisms in venous thromis is not clear. Suggestions about the nature of a hypercoagulable state and its relationship to venous thrombosis have recently been made (Chapters 2 and 4). It is possible that hypercoagulability may occur only locally (e.g. in valve pockets, see below) which, of course, would not be detected by available coagulation tests. In addition to coagulation processes, venous stasis (Chapters 2, 8 and 9) is an important factor in venous thrombogenesis. The majority of venous thrombi are found in the deep veins of the calf, thigh, and pelvis (Paterson, 1969). A reduced rate of blood flow in the legs has been demonstrated during pregnancy and prolonged bed rest, following surgery or trauma, and in a variety of disease states in which there is an increased incidence of deep venous thrombosis (Hume *et al.*, 1970). The sites of origin of venous thrombi—notably valve cusps, bifurcations and solcal veins—are areas where turbulent blood flow or local stasis can develop. Cotton and Clark (1965) perfused vertically-mounted isolated venous segments with a fluid containing India ink; eddy currents were observed at the borders of the valve cusps and fluid stagnated in the valve sinus. Normal laminar blood flow is disturbed producing turbulance and local stasis at bifurcations and in small saccules (Stanton *et al.*,1949; McLachlin *et al.*, 1960; Wells, 1969; Goldsmith, 1970). However, stasis or reduced blood flow alone do not initiate thrombosis (Wessler, 1963; Capter 2).

Ordinarily blood is cleared of activated clotting factors by the reticuloendothelial system (Spaet *et al.*, 1961: Deykin *et al.*, 1966;) so that activated coagulation factors never attain a high enough concentration to cause thrombus formation. Under conditions of stasis, however, this clearance is prevented, and a coagulation thrombus is formed (Wessler *et al.*, 1967; Chapter 2). The importance of clearance mechanisms and blood flow in thrombognesis is further indicated by results of experiments in which Factor XII was activated *in vivo* by ellagic acid injection (Ratnof and Crum, 1964). Thrombosis then occurred only under conditions of stasis in the isolated venous segment (Botti and Ratnoff, 1964; Constantine *et al.*, 1971) and in regions of disturbed blood flow (Nordöy and Chandler, 1967); generalised intravascular coagulation did not —presumably because of rapid clearance of the activated coagulation factors. These experiments also suggest that in regions of turbulent blood flow, there is stasis in that the blood is not truly circulating and hence not cleared of activated coagulation factors; the concentration of procoagulants may thùs increase locally to a level high enough to induce thrombus formation.

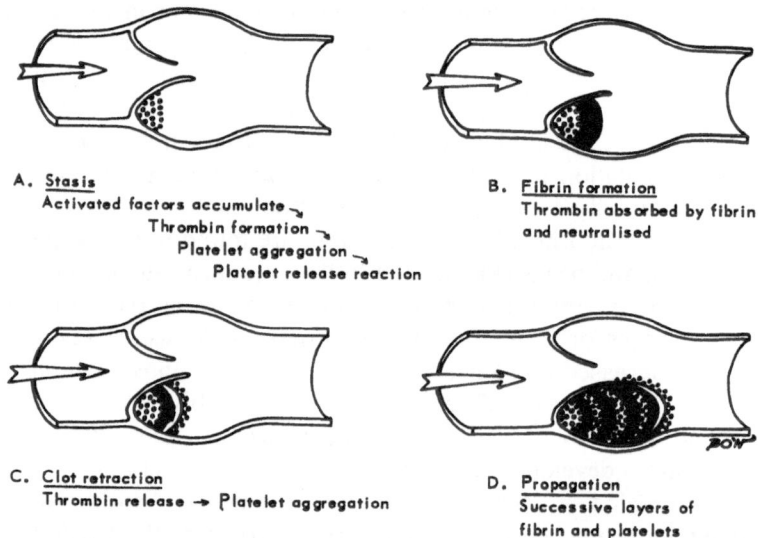

A. <u>Stasis</u>
   Activated factors accumulate
     Thrombin formation
      Platelet aggregation
       Platelet release reaction

B. <u>Fibrin formation</u>
   Thrombin absorbed by fibrin
   and neutralised

C. <u>Clot retraction</u>
   Thrombin release → Platelet aggregation

D. <u>Propagation</u>
   Successive layers of
   fibrin and platelets

Figure. 7.1 Scheme of formation of a valve cusp thrombus. (From Hume *et al.*, 1970, and reproduced by permission of the Harvard University Press, Cambridge, Mass,)

Figure 7.1 illustrates the process of venous thrombosis in a valve pocket as it is presently understood. The valve cusp serves as a nidus for the formation of the thrombus (A) which then propagates in the direction of blood flow by deposition of successive layers composed of formed elements and fibrin (B, C and D). In the earliest venous thrombi in man yet examined, platelet aggregates constitute a minor component and are intermixed with fibrin; it is not possible to say which appeared first (Paterson and McLachlin, 1954). The rheologic properties of blood are such that its viscosity is increased in regions of stasis (Wells, 1969) and platelets may 'silt' into the valve pocket (Cotton and Clark, 1965; Kwaan *et al.*, 1967). Because the concentration of thrombin required to cause platelet aggregation *in vitro* is less than that needed to induce fibrin formation (Zucker and Borelli, 1955), thrombin-induced platelet aggregation may precede fibrin formation within the valve pocket (Figure 7.1). It has been demonstrated that platelet-fibrin thrombi form in regions of slow and turbulent blood flow after activation of the intrinsic coagulation system (Nordoy and Chandler, 1967) and it is possible that activated coagulation factors, brought from another site, or generated locally, may accumulate in the valve pocket eventually causing thrombin formation. However, the fact that aspirin, an inhibitor of platelet aggregation, failed to affect the incidence of deep venous thrombosis in surgical patients (O'Brien *et al.*, 1971; Butterfield, 1972) suggests that the processes of platelet aggregation play a minor role.

Recently there have been improvements in the prophlaxis of venous thrombosis. It has been observed that blood is frequently hypercoagulable during and immediately after major operations as evidenced by an abnormally short coagulation time (Sharnoff *et al.*, 1960). Because the incidence of postoperative venous thrombosis and pulmonary embolism is high in patients undergoing extensive surgical procedures, a study was instituted in which surgical patients at high risk were given low doses of heparin subcutaneously before and after operation, and until they were ambulatory. In contrast to the usual reason for administering anticoagulants, the aim here was to *maintain normal* coagulation time during and after surgery rather than to achieve an anticoagulant effect. At the low dose used, the risk of haemorrhagic complications was reduced, and results in the prevention of fatal pulmonary embolism were encouraging (Sharnoff, 1966; Sharnoff and DeBlasio, 1970; Chapter 15). The efficacy of subcutaneous low dose heparin in the prevention of deep venous thrombosis has, now been established in high risk surgical patients (Kakkar *et al.*, Williams, 1971; Kakkar *et al.*, 1972 Gordon-Smith *et al.*, 1972; Nicolaides *et al.*, 1972; Gellus *et al.*, 1973; Ballard *et al.*, 1973). The antithrombotic effect of beparin in these trials is not related to an inhibitory effect on platelet aggregation because the decrease in the aggregation response of platelets *in vitro* to adenosine diphosphate, which occurs during and after major surgery, is actually reversed by low dose heparin (O'Brien *et al.*, 1972). Recent work, moreover, suggests that heparin may potentiate platelet aggregation (Thomson *et al.*, 1973). The efficacy of low dose subcutaneous heparin may be related to the fact that heparin poten-

Thromboembolism

tiates a naturally occurring inhibitor of activated Factor X at a concentration too low to inhibit the conversion of fibrinogen to fibrin (Yin and Wessler, 1970; Chapter 2). These studies suggest that the immediate future for the successful prophylaxis of venous thrombosis may be in the improved use of presently available anticoagulant drugs rather than in agents which affect those aspects of platelet behaviour (e.g. aggregation) which are of fundamental importance in arterial thrombosis.

References

Aggeler, P. M. and O'Reilly, R. A. (1966). The pharmacological basisi of oral anticoagulant therapy. *Thromb. Diath. Haemorrh.*, **Suppl. 21**, 227

Arnott, W. M. (Chairman) (1969). Report to the Medical Research Council. Assessment of short-term anticoagulant administration after cardiac infarction. *Brit. Med. J.*, **1**, 335

Ballard, R. M., Bradley-Watson, P. J., Johnstone, F. D., Kenney, A., McCarthy, T. J., Campbell, S. and Woston, J. (1973). Low doses of subcutaneous heparin in the prevention of deep vein thrombosis after gynaecological surgery *J. Obstet., Gynaecol.*, **80**, 469

Barritt, D. W. and Jordan, S. C. (1960). Anticoagulant drugs in the treatment of pulmonary embolism. A controlled trial. *Lancet.* **i**, 1309

Bauer, G. (1964). Clinical experiences of a surgeon in the use of heparin. *Amer. J. Cardiol.*, **14**, 29

Borchgrevink, C. R. (1966). Anticoagulant therapy in acute myocardial infarction. *Thromb. Diath. Haemorrh.*, **Suppl. 21**, 311

Botti, R. E. and Ratnoff, O. D. (1964). Studies on the pathogenesis of thrombosis; an experimental (hypercoagulable) state induced by the intravenous injection of ellagic acid. *J. Lab. Clin. Med.*, **4**, 385

Brown K. W. G. and MacMillan, R. L. (1965). Anticoagulant therapy in coronary artery disease; A therapeutic enigma. *Can. Med. Assoc., J.*, **92**, 70

Butterfield, W. J. H. (Chairman) (1972). Report to the Medical Research Council. Effect of aspirin on post-operative venous thrombosis. *Lancet*, **ii**, 441

Chan, K. E. (1972). Relation between the haemorrhagic and anti-thrombotic action of heparin and warfarin in arterial thrombosis. *Cardiovasc. Res.*, **6**, 248

Chandler, A. B. (1969). The anatomy of a thrombus In: S. Sherry., K. M. Brinkhous, E. Genton and J. M. Stengle, editors *Thrombosis*, 279-299 (Washington, D .C: Nat. Acad Sci).

Constantine, J. W., Purcell, I. M. and Gotthelf, M. (1971). Platelets, coagulation and *in vitro* thrombus formation. *J. Pharmacol. Exp. Ther.*, **176**, 76

Cotton, L. T. and Clark, C. (1965). Anatomical localization of venous thrombosis. *Ann. Roy. Coll. Surg. Eng.*, **36**, 214

Deykin, D., Chun, R., Lopez, A. and Silversmith, P. (1966). The role of liver in serum-induced hypercoagulbability. *J. Clin. Invest.*, **45**, 256

Deykin, D. (1967). Thrombogenesis. *New Eng. J. Med.*, **276**, 622

French, J. E. (1965). The structure of natural and experimental thrombi. *Ann Roy. Coll. Sug. Eng.*, **36**, 191

French, J. E. (1969). The fine structure of experimental thrombi. In: Thrombosis, 300-320 S. Sherry, K. M. Brinkhous. E. Genton and J. M. Stengle, editors (Washington. D. C: Nat. Acad. Sci.).

Thromboembolism

Gallus, A. S., Hizsh, J., Tuttle, R. S. Trebilcock, R., O'Brien, S. E., Curroll, J. J., Minder, J.H., Hudecki, S. M. (1973). Small subcutaneous doses of heparin in prevention of venous thrombosis, *New. Eng. J. Med.*, **188**, 545

Goldsmith, H. L. (1970). Motion of particles in a flowing stream. *Thromb. Diath. Haemorrh.*, **Suppl. 40**, 91

Gordon-Smith, I. C., Grundy, D. J., Le Quesne, L.P., Newcombe, J. F. and Bramble, F. J. (1972). Controlled trial of two regiments of subcutaneous if heparin in prevention of post-operative deep-vein thrombosis. *Lancet* **1**, 1933

Gurewich, V., Thomas, D. P. and Stuart, R. K. (1967). Some guidelines for heparin therapy of venous thromboembolic diseases. *J. Amer. Med. Ass.*, **199**, 152

Harvald, B., Hilden, T. and Lund, E. (1962). Long-term anticoagulant therapy after myocardial infarction. *Lancet*, **ii**, 626

Hess, H. (1966). Anticoagulant therapy of peripheral arterial thrombosis. *Thromb. Diath. Haemorrh.*, **Suppl. 21**, 371

Hilden, T. Iveson, K., Raaschou, F. and Schwartz, M. (1961). Anticoagulants in acute myocardial infarction. *Lancet*, **ii**, 326

Hill, A. B., Marshall, J. and Shaw, D. A. (1960). A controlled trial of long-term anticoagulant therapy in cerebrovascular disease. *Quart. J. Med.*, **29**, 597

Hume, M., Sevitt, S. and Thomas, D. P. (1970). *Venous Thrombosis and Pulmonary Embolism.* Cambridge, Mass. Havard University Press

Kakkar, V. V., Field, E. S., Nicolaides, A. N., Flute, P. T., Wessler, S. and Yin, E. T. (1971). Low doses of heparin in prevention of deep-vein thrombosis. *Lancet*, **ii**, 669

Kakkar, V. V., Corrigan, T., Spindler, J., Fossard, D. P., Flute, P. T., Crellin, R. Q., Wessler, S. and Yin, E. T. (1971). Efficacy of low doses of heparin in prevention of deep-vein thrombosis after major surgery. *Lancet*, **ii**, 101

Kernohan, R. J. and Todd, C. (1966). Heparin therapy in thromboembolic disease. *Lancet*, **i**, 621

Knieriem, H. J. and Chandler, A. B. (1967). The effect of warfarin sodium on the duration of platelet aggregation. *Thromb. Diath. Haemorrh.*, **18**, 766

Kwaan, H. C., Harding, F. and Astrup, T. (1967). Platelet befavior in small blood vessels *in vivo. Thromb. Diath. Haemorrh.*, **Suppl. 26**, 207

Lund, F. and Tillgren, C. (1966). Anticoagulant therapty in **occlusive** peripheral arterial disease and its evaluation. *Thromb, Diath. Haemorrh.*, **Suppl. 21**, 385

McLachlin, J. and Paterson, J. C. (1951). Some basic observations on venous thrombosis and pulmonary embolism. *Syrg. Gynaecol. Obstet.*, **93**, 1

McLachlin, A. D., McLachlin, J. A. Jory, T. A. and Rawling, E. G. (1960) Venous stasis in the lower extremities. *Ann. Surg.*, **152**, 678

Millikan, C. H. (1962). Role of anticoagulants in the treatment of cerebrovascular disease. *Amer. J. Med.*, **33**, 731

Mustard, J. F., Murphy, E. A., Rowsell, H. C. and Downie, H. G. (1962). Factors influencing thrombus formation *in vivo. Amer. J. Med.*, **33**, 621

Mustard, J. F., Rowsell, H. C. and Murphy, E. A. (1964). Thrombosis *Amer. J. Med. Sci.*, **248**, 469

Newland, H. and Nordoy, A. (1967). Effect of large doses of warfarin sodium on haemostasis and on ADP-induced platelet aggregation *in vivo* in the rat. *Cardiovasc, Res.*,**1**, 362

Nicolaides, A. N., Dupont, P. A., Desai, S., Lewis J. D., Douglas, J. N., Dodsworth, H., Fourides, G., Luck R. J. and Jamieson, C. W. (1972). Small doses of sodium heparin in preventing deep venous thrombosis after major surgery. *Lancet.* **ii.** 890

Thromboembolism

Nordoy, A. and Chandler, A. B. (1967). Formation of platelet-fibrin thrombi by ellagic acid and adenosine diphosphate in the rat. *Lab. Invest.,* **17,** 3

O'Brien J. R., Etherington. M., Jamieson, S. and Klaber, M. (1972). Platelet function in venous thrombosis and low-dosage heparin. *Lancet,* **i,** 1302

O'Brien, J. R., Tulevski, V. and Etherington, M. (1971).. Two *in vivo* studies comparing high and low aspirin dosage. *Lancet,* **i,** 399

O'Brien, J. R. (1973). Heparin, platelets and venous thrombosis. *Amer. Heart J.,* **85,** 435

Paterson, J. C. and McLachlin, J. (1954). Precipitating factors in venous thrombosis. *Surg. Hynaecol. Obstet.,* **98,** 96

Paterson, J. C. (1969). The pathology of cenous thrombi. In: Thrombosis, S. Sherry, 321-331 K. M. Brinkhous, E. Genton and J. M. Stengle, editors (Washington, D. C. Mat. Acad. Sci).

Pickering, G. (Chairman), (1964). Report to the Medical Research Council Assessment of long-term anticoagulant administration after cardiac infarction. *Brit. Med. J.,* **3,** 837

Poller, L., Thonson, J. M. and Priest, C. M. (1969). Coumarin therapy and platelet aggregation. *Brit. Med. J.,* **I,** 474

Poole, J. C. F. and French, J. E. (1961). Thrombosis. *J. Atheroscler. Res.,* 1, 251

Ratnoff, O. D. and Crum, J. D. (1964). Activation of Hageman Factor by solutions of ellagic acid. *J. Lab. Clin. Med.,* **63,** 359

Salzman, E. W., Harris, W. H. and DeSanctis, R. W. (1966). Anticoagulation for prevention of thromboembolism following fractures of the hip. *New. Eng. J. Med.,* **275,** 122

Seaman, A. J., Griswold, H. F., Reaum R. B. and Ritzman, L. W. (1964). Prophylactic anticoagulant therapy ofr coronary artery disease. *J. Amer. Med. Assoc.,* **189,** 183

Sevitt, S. and Gallagher, N. G. (1959). Prevention of venous thrombosis and pulmonary embolism in injured patients. *Lancet,* ii, 981

Sevitt, S. (1966) Anticoagulant prophylaxis against venous thrombosis and pulmonary embolism after injury. *Thromb. Diath. Haemorrh.,* **Suppl. 21,** 287

Sharnoff, J. G., Bagg, J. F., Breen, S. R., Rogliano, A. G., Walsh, A. R. and Scardino, V. (1960). The possible indication of post-operative thromboembolism by platelet counts anc blood coagulation studies in the patient undergoing extensive surgery. *Surg. Gynaecol. Obstet.,* **111,** 469

Sharnoff, J. G. (1966). Results in the prophylaxis of the post-operative thromboembolism. *Surg. Gynaecol. Obstet.,* **123,** 303

Sharnoff, J. G. and DeBlasio, D. (1970). Prevention of fatal post-operative thromboembolism by heparin prophylaxis. *Lancet,* **ii,** 1006

Spaet, T. H., Horowitz, Zucker-Franklin, D., Cintron, J. and Biezenski. J. J. (1961). Reticuloendothelial clearance of blood thromboplastin. *Blood J. Hematol.,* **17,** 196

Stanton, J, R., Freis, E. D. and Wilkins, R. W. (1949). The accelerarion of linear flow in the deep veins of the lower extremity of man by local compression. *J. Clin. Invest.,* **28,** 553

Thomson, C., Forbes, C. D. and Prentice C. R. M. (19473). The potentiation of platelet aggregation and adhesion by heparin *in vitro* and *in vivo. Clin. Sci. Molec. Med.,* **45,** 485

Wells, R. E. (1969). Rheologic aspects of stasis in thrombus formation In: *Thrombosis* 469-467 S. Sherry, K. M. Brinkhouse, E. Genton and J. M. Stengle, editors (Washigton, D. C.: Nat. Acad. Sci.)

Wessler, S. (1962). Thrombosis in the presence of vascular stasis. *Amer. J. Med.,* **33,** 648

Thromboembolism

Wessler, S. (1963). Stasis hypercoagulability, and thrombosis. *Fed. Proc.,* **22,** 1266

Wessler, S., Yin, E. T., Gatson, L. W.and Nicol, I. (1967). A distinction between the role of precursor and activated forms of clotting factors in the genesis of stasis thrombi. *Thromb. Diath Haemorrh.,* **18,** 12

Williams, H. T. (1971). Prevention of post-operative deep-vein thrombosis with perioperative subcutaneous heparin. *Lancet,* **ii,** 950

Yin, E. T. and Wessler, S. (1970). Heparin-accelerated inhibition of activated Factor X by its natural plasma inhibitor. *Biochim. Biophys Acta,* **201, 387**

Zucker, M. B. and Borelli, J. (1955). Viscous metamorphosis of blood platelets produced by thrombin. *Fed. Proc.,* **14,** 168

8

The role of the vessel wall in deep venous thrombosis

Gwendolyn J. Stewart

The purpose of this chapter is to evaluate the information about the possible mechanisms by which the vessel wall affects the development of venous thrombosis. The role of the vessel wall in deep venous thrombosis will be considered under the headings of initiation, anchoring and fate (i.e. resolution or organisation) of the thrombosis.

THE ROLE OF THE VESSEL WALL IN THE INITIATION OF THROMBOSIS

Different views

There are currently three easily identifiable schools of thought on the role of the vessel wall in deep venous thrombosis. Two of them are opposed while the third occupies an intermediate position. According to one school the initiation of thrombosis is dependent on a lesion of the vessel wall that produces exposure of subendothelial structures on which platelet aggregates form (Spaet and Erichson, 1966; Spaet and Ts'Ao, 1969). This concept is based primarily on experimental thrombosis which is produced by direct injury to the vessel. The investigators who have done extensive postmortem studies of thrombosed veins in man take a more conservative view of the role of endothelial damage in the initiation of venous thrombosis. They believe that there is no damage of the vessel wall before thrombosis and they suggest that the valve pocket serves as a place for nidus formation through the accumulation of platelets and activated clotting intermediates (Hume *et al.*, 1970; Paterson, 1969; Chapter 7). These accumulate behind the valves because of turbulence and local stasis. The third school holds that the vessel wall has no active role in the initiation of thrombosis, that venous thrombosis results entirely from clotting induced by activated factors brought to areas of stasis from other areas of the body (Wessler, 1952; 1955; 1962; Chapter 2).

This diversity of opinion may be because of limitations of experimental design and methods of study. There is as yet no model for experimental thrombosis in which the sequence of events approaches the natural history of deep venous thrombosis in man. To simulate even the commonest clinical situation it is necessary to have a model in which there is considerable to extensive tissue damage to some area of the body well removed from the veins under study. It is also necessary to reduce the flow of blood through the same vessels by some means that does not produce direct mechanical injury to them. The veins must then be studied by some method that will permit examination of most of the luminal surface because vascular damage may be 'patchy' rather than uniform.

Direct injury to small vessels
The concept that a lesion of the vessel wall is an essential factor in the development of thrombosis has been based to a large extent on studies of small blood vessels in thin membranes *in vivo* (Apitz, 1942; Zucker, 1947; Hugues, 1953; Roskam *et al.*, 1959; Berman and Fulton, 1961). In these studies the small blood vessels were severed, partially severed, punctured with microneedles, or ruptured by electrical current applied with micro-electrodes. In every case platelets adhered to the wounded surface and to each other to form a plug that was sufficiently stable to stop bleeding. Platelets were adherent to the cut edges in less than two seconds after arterioles were transected (Roskam, 1961). They did not appear to adhere to the endothelium, but rather to the adventitial side where they were in close contact with collagen (Kjaerheim and Hovig, 1962).

Platelet aggregation and adhesion to the vessel wall was also elicited by more subtle agents that did not produce overt haemorrhage. These included trauma, infection, malignant neoplasia (Lutz *et al.*, 1950), irradiation (Fulton *et al.*, 1953), thrombin (Berman *et al.*, 1954), negative pressure (Shulman *et al.*, 1954) and electrical stimulation (Callahan *et al.*, 1960). At the site of application of the stimulus a platelet thrombus developed. Frequently small portions of the platelet aggregate were broken off and swept away by the circulating blood until eventually a stable platelet mass was formed.

Thromboembolism

Evidence has been presented to indicate that platelets do not adhere to damaged endothelium but only to connective tissue (Bounameaux, 1959; 1961; Roskam, 1961; Hovig, 1962; Hugues, 1962; Zucker and Borelli, 1962; French *et al.*, 1964; Hugues and Lapiere, 1964; Stewart *et al.*, 1974). It is quite possible that platelet aggregation elicited by means that did not produce overt rupture of the vessel was caused by exposure of areas of connective tissue which were too small to be detected in cinemicroscopic studies. This possibility is strongly supported by one study in which micro-electrode technique applied to the hamster cheek pouch produced areas denuded of endothelium (French *et al.*, 1964).

Collagen is the essential substance in connective tissue. Electron microscopy demonstrated that typical collagen fibrils found in 'extract' of tendons produced aggregation of the nearby platelets when added to platelet rich plasma (Hovig, 1963). The incubation of the tendon 'extract' with collagenase completely destroyed its aggregating activity which was independent of calcium ions and heparin and therefore independent of coagulation.

These observations have led to the concept that a vessel wall lesion serves as a point for formulation of platelet aggregates and that the platelet aggregates in turn serve as the trigger mechanism (nidus) for the formation of thrombus. However, observations of the effects of injury to medium and large vessels present a challenge to the uncritical acceptance of this concept.

Direct injury to medium and large vessels

In a number of studies the intima of medium and large size vessels was severely damaged and then exposed to flowing blood without the development of stable platelet aggregates or other thrombotic material. When rat femoral veins were damaged by pinching with fine pointed forceps to produce visible oedema but no bleeding there were areas in which the endothelium became disrupted or even disappeared. In areas denuded of endothelium there was a mesh of fibrin formed in close association with the basement membrane. A few irregularly shaped and degranulated platelets were associated with the fibrin and to some extent with the basement membrane (Ashford and Freiman, 1967). However, there was no dense aggregate of platelets such as was formed when the vessel was disrupted. Although it was not pointed out by the authors, this study suggested that exposure of the basement membrane of medium sized vessels elicited a qualitatively different response from that elicited by damage of small vessels. The loose fibrin net with a moderate number

103

of platelets was decidedly different from the dense aggregates of platelets that form haemostatic plugs.

Insertion of a nylon 'sound' into a marginal ear vein in the rabbit produced uneven damage. The endothelium remained intact in some places while the basement membrane and even deeper layers became exposed in other areas. A layer of platelets was deposited on the basement membrane (1–3 thick). No large platelet aggregates developed and there was not any accumulation of other thrombotic material (Baumgartner *et al.,* 1967).

In a subsequent study the rabbit aorta was denuded of endothelium with a balloon catheter exposing the subendothelium to flowing blood (Baumgartner, 1973). At normal flow, platelets rapidly adhered to the subendothelium to form a near continuous coating. At ten minutes about 18 per cent of this surface was covered by mural platelet thrombi usually in association with leukocytes, especially neutrophiles. However, by twenty minutes this had declined to about 5 per cent and by forty minutes all mural thrombi had disappeared leaving the surface covered with a mono-layer of platelets. No fibrin was observed when the aorta was removed, everted and exposed to flowing citrated blood.

A critical examination of the above studies suggests that platelet aggregation in medium and large vessels (veins and arteries) is limited and does not result in stable, severely obstructing masses such as those which occur in small vessels. Furthermore, the limited accumulations of platelets do not lead to fibrin formation and entrappment of red cells, yet red cells and fibrin certainly comprise the mass of clinical thrombi.

Thrombosis in the absence of detectable vessel injury

In human thrombosis associated with conditions in which there is no *direct* injury to the veins, conventional histological methods have failed to demonstrate evidence of a preceeding inflammatory response in throm-bosed areas or endothelial damage in areas that are not thrombosed in the same or different veins of the same limb (Virchow, 1860; Paterson, 1969; Hume *et al.,* 1970). However, an examination of these studies shows that they were inadequate to exclude either.

The failure to demonstrate an inflammatory response in deep venous thrombosis in man could be the result of the inherent restriction of the experimental design. Veins must be taken as they become available with no clear indication of the time of initiation of the thrombus or the rate or propagation. This, a thrombus which had started at a site which initially displayed certain features of the inflammatory response may have propa-

Thromboembolism

gated slowly so that at the time of examination it displayed characteristics associated with organisation. In the case of occlusive thrombi, leukocytes that had been present on the vessel wall or had migrated into the lumen of the vessel would be expected to die and disintegrate within a few hours. It is also likely that leukocytes would disappear rapidly after death since their normal life span is relatively short (Cartwright *et al.*, 1965). Thus there would be no leukocytes associated with vessels that had been thrombosed for more than a few hours.

The failure to demonstrate endothelial damage in non-thrombosed areas of veins containing thrombi, and in non-thrombosed veins of the same limb can be accounted by the fact that the amount of material examined in histological sections is very limited and that one or a few small foci of damage could be sufficient to initiate thrombosis. The limitations of histological sections was recognised by many investigators (O'Neill, 1947; Samuels and Webster, 1952; McGovern, 1955) who developed and used enface methods for examining blood vessels with the light microscope to demonstrate the 'spotty' nature of vascular lesions.

Stasis (red coagulation) thrombi
Opposition to the concept that a vessel wall lesion is necessary for the initiation of thrombosis has been expressed by Wessler and his associates. Their conclusions were based on observations of stasis (red coagulation) thrombi (Chapter 2). In these studies stasis thrombi were induced experimentally in dogs and rabbits by exposing veins, tying off all tributaries, injecting homologous serum into the systemic circulation and immediately (30–120 sec) tying off segments of the various exposed veins. Unattached thrombi were formed in the isolated segments in 60 sec (Wessler, 1955; Wessler *et al.*, 1959). If the veins were occluded after the clot-promoting effect of the serum had been dissipated (15 min after injection) no clots were formed. From this and from histological studies of veins from 1–43 days following venous narrowing it was suggested that 'significant endothelial injury' was absent (Wessler, 1955).

However, there is evidence which suggests that the negative result was due to the time of sampling and the method of study. In recent studies (Stewart *et al.*, 1974) a combination of scanning and transmission electron microscopy was used to study blood vessels. The entire luminal surface of vessels could be examined with the scanning electron microscope at a resolution of 100–200 A. Thus it was possible to detect and study 'patchy' pathology and assess the overall condition of the vessel wall at higher magnification and greater resolution than was possible by enface techniques with the light

105

microscope. Scanning electron microscopy was also an invaluable guide in interpreting the results of transmission electron microscopy because it provided an estimate of the probability that the small amount of sample examined would contain representative material from apparently normal or abnormal areas (Stewart *et al.*, 1973).

Canine jugular and femoral veins that had been exposed by blunt dissection, and had their tributaries tied off were occluded for 1 or 7 minutes by gentle external pressure applied through the skin proximal to the end of dissection. It was found that large numbers of white cells adhered to the luminal surface, passed through the intercellular junctions and accumulated in pockets between the endothelium and basement membrane. This produced extensive separation of endothelial cells from each other and from the basement membrane, and resulted in frequent desquamation of patches of endothelium. The white cell invasion occurred immediately in response to brief stasis following trauma to tissues adjacent to the veins. Tissue trauma alone or stasis alone did not induce the invasion. Stasis before trauma provoked only sparse, ·patchy white cell invasion (Figures 8.1–8.11) (Stewart *et al.*, 1974).

The white cell invasion and endothelial damage were absent when white cell adhesion and migration were inhibited with lignocaine or the dogs were made neutropenic with vinblastin. The veins in these animals appeared normal when examined with both scanning and transmission electron microscopy. Furthermore, the perfusion of veins exposed to lignocaine or to vinblastin with normal blood resulted in typical white cell invasion. These experiments show that the white cell invasion produced the endothelial damage rather than resulted from it (Figures 8.12–8.21).

The consequences of the white cell invasion were studied at 6, 24 and 72 hours, and at 7, 15 and 28 days (Lynch *et al.*, 1974) after operation. At 6 hours after provocation of the white cell invasion white cells were still abundant on the surface and in pockets under the endothelium. There was also an abundance of amorphous material on the surface (Figures 8.22 and 8.23). One of four veins contained a small mural thrombus composed almost entirely of red cells enmeshed in fibrin. At 24 and 72 hours the white cells had largely disappeared. However, the entire luminal surface of the vein was extensively damaged. Denuded areas and single disintegrating cells were common. Fibro-amorphous material was abundantly scattered over the surface. At 15 and 28 days the vessel had further recovered but even at 28 days amorphous material and giant cells were still present, indicating that recovery was not complete (Figures 8.24–8.28).

Thromboembolism

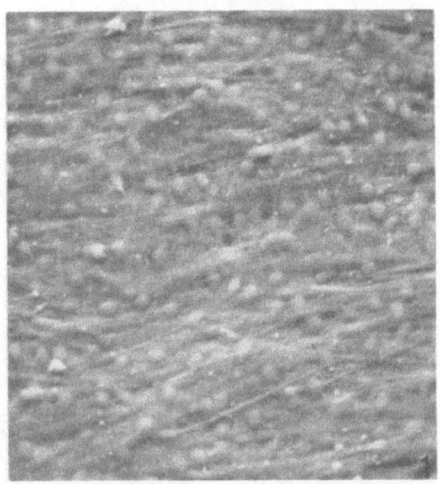

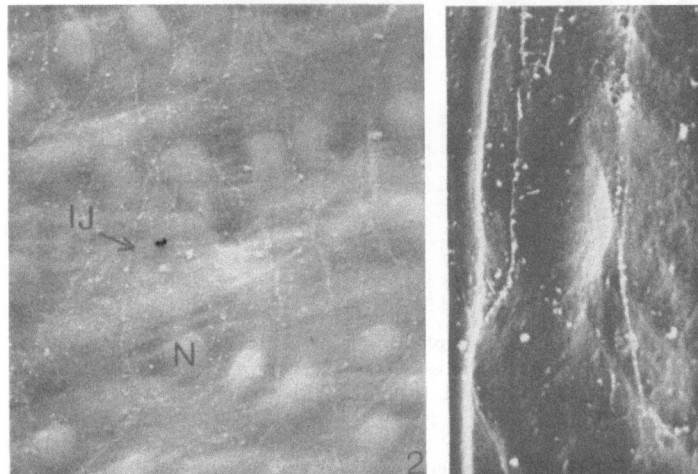

Figures 8.1–8.3 Scanning electron micrographs of typical luminal surface of canine veins that were not occluded. The smooth, intact sheet of elongated endothelial cells with their slightly protruding nuclei and just discernable intercellular junctions was considered normal and used as a basis of comparison for all subsequent treatments. These vessels had of necessity been exposed to the surgical trauma necessary for exposure and perfusion, but care was taken to avoid occlusion of the vessel while it still contained blood.

Figure 8.1 Low magnification showing many cells and underlying cords of fibres and cells in a jugular vein. × 210

Figure 8.2 Intermediate magnification shows the nuclei (N) intercellular junctions (IJ) and mosaic arrangement of the cells. × 700

Figure 8.3 Higher magnification shows the detail of the nuclei and intercellular junctions. The small white dots on the surface are pseudopods (shown by transmission electron microscopy). This is a femoral vein in which the cords of underlying fibres are more prominent than they are in jugulars. × 2100

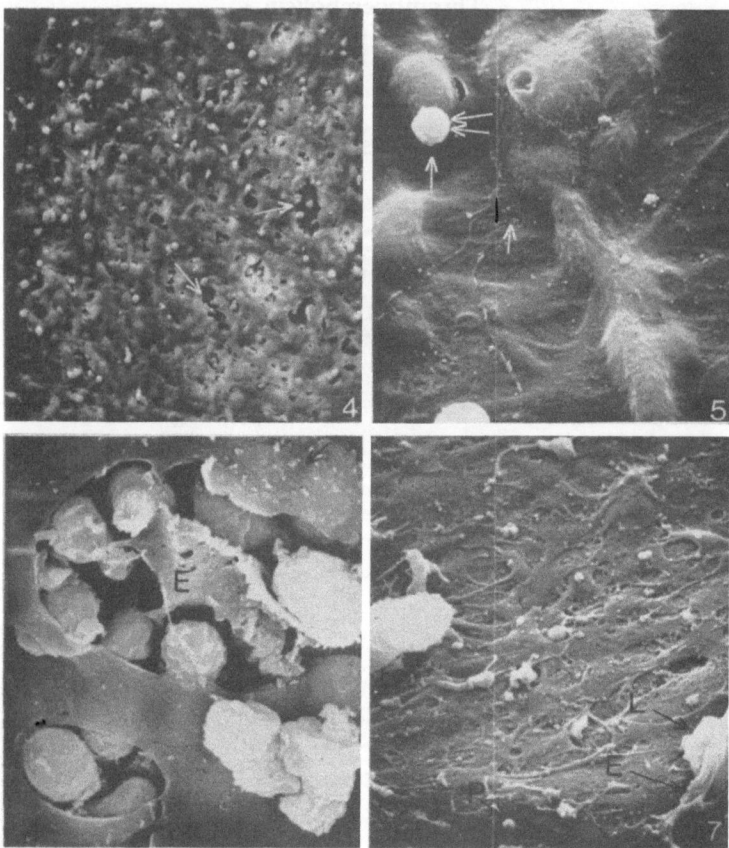

Figures 8.4–8.7 Scanning electron micrographs of the luminal surface of veins that were occluded for seven minutes after surgical exposure so that stasis followed injury to adjacent tissues while the vessel was filled with blood. Leukocyte (L) sticking and emigration were always massive in these veins.

Figure 8.4 Survey of an area about 0·25 mm² in which extensive leukocyte (white spheres) emigration and accumulation led to almost continuous whealing (raised areas) and areas of endothelial desquamation (arrows). × 175

Figure 8.5 Intermediate magnification shows the extent of coalescing of pockets of leukocytes and the frequency of gaps (arrows) between endothelial cells. Leukocytes were caught partially in and partially out in several places (double arrows). × 615

Figure 8.6 A large and a small gap through which leukocytes are visible. A loose, partially degenerated endothelial cell (E) is stretched across part of the larger gap. A loose endothelial cell with pseudopods was still attached to the sheet at the upper right of gap (arrow). × 1750

Figure 8.7 An area of exposed basement membrane with a loose, wrinkled endothelial cell (E) and a white cell (L) at the lower right, and a few platelets (P) are stuck to the exposed membrane. Thin sections show that the flat, spread cells are probably smooth muscle and the fibres are collagen (see Figure 8.10). × 1750

108

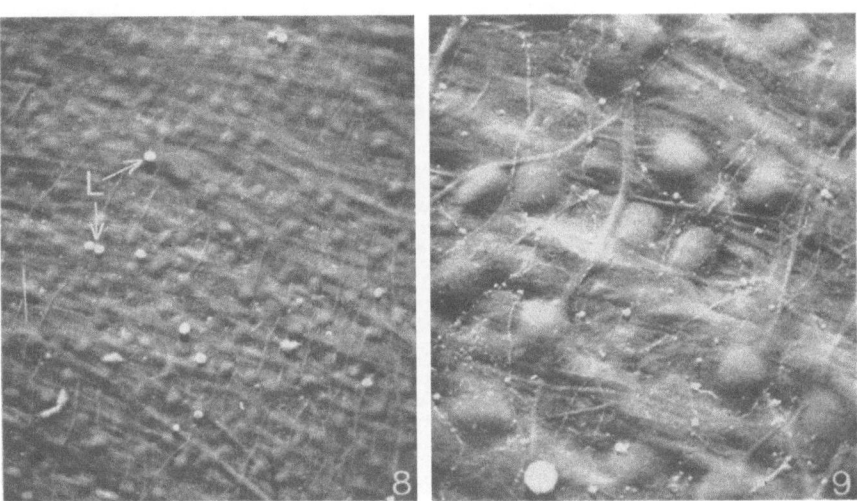

Figures 8.8. and 8.9 Scanning electron micrographs of jugular veins that were occluded for seven minutes prior to surgery, so that stasis occurred when there was no known tissue trauma in the dog's body.

Figure 8.8 Low magnification survey shows scattered, single adhering leukocytes (L) with essentially no migration. · 70

Figure 8.9 Higher magnification shows leukocyte adherent to endothelium. × 700

Figure 8.10 Transmission electron micrograph of section of canine jugular vein. The vein was exposed, perfused *in situ* with Tyrode's solution followed by Tyrode's solution containing 1 per cent glutaraldehyde. The vein was tied off under physiological pressure and submerged in the same fixative for further fixation before being osmicated and further processed for transmission electron microscopy by conventional techniques. All of the structures appear to be well preserved and 'normal'. The endothelium (E) is thin with typical caveolc, rests on a very thin basement membrane (BM) under which is smooth muscle (SM) and collagen (C). The overlap of the endothelial cells was frequently surprisingly great. < 24 640

Figure 8.11 Transmission electron micrograph showing leukocyte invasion of a canine jugular vein. The vein was prepared by exactly the same procedure as the vein in Figure 8.10 except that this vein was occluded by gentle pressure applied externally for one minute before the vessel was perfused with Tyrode's solution. Perfusion was begun almost immediately after occlusion. The leukocytes (L) adhered to the vessel wall and migrated across the endothelium where they accumulated in pockets between the endothelium (E) and basement membrane (BM). The cells, even the endothelium, and fibres of the vessel wall appear to be normal. The short time interval between invasion and fixation combined with the absence of cellular alteration suggests that the separation of endothelial cells from each other and from the basement membrane was a physical phenomenon resulting from the force exerted by the invading leukocytes. × 13 360

109

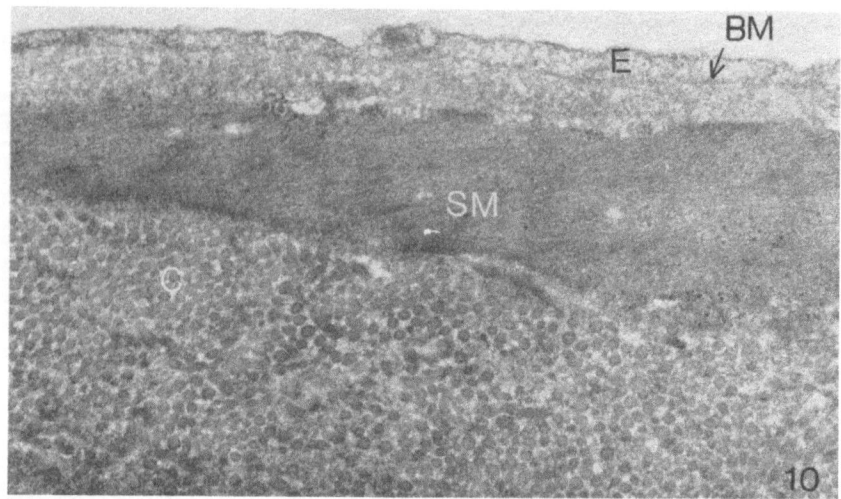

Fig. 8. 10

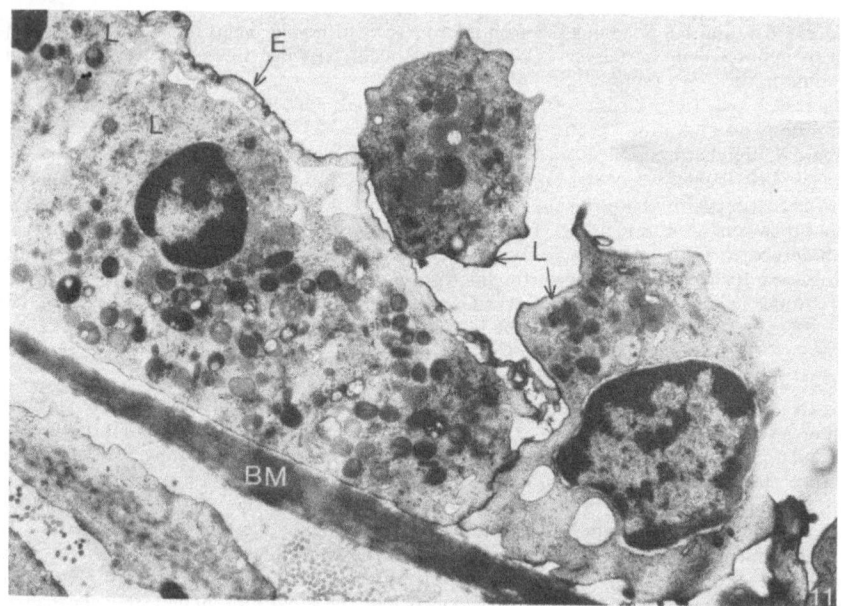

Fig. 8. 11

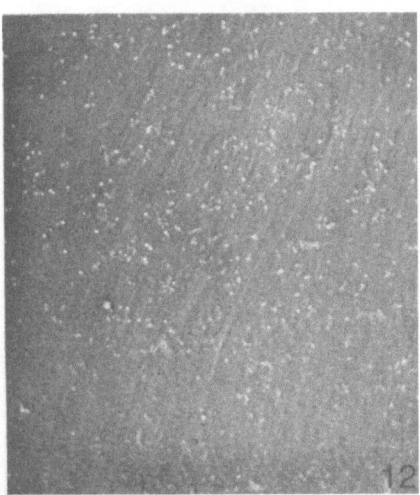

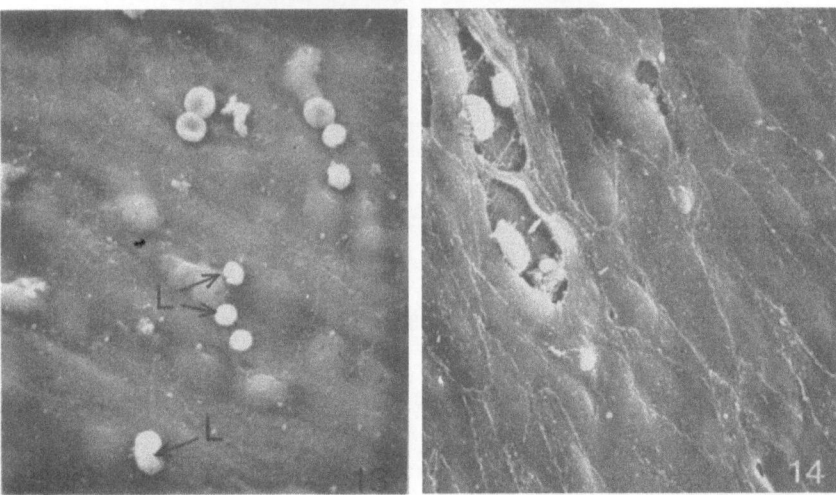

Figures 8.12 and 8.13 Scanning electron micrographs of veins from dog given lignocaine before surgery so that both vessel and blood were treated at the time of surgical trauma and stasis. Lignocaine inhibits leukocyte adhesion and migration. The endothelium is intact and indistinguishable from the controls (Figures 8.1–8.3) as opposed to the extensively invaded vessel shown in Figures 8.4–8.6. There is only scattered leukocyte (L) adhesion and invasion. Figure 8.12 × 70 Figure 8.13 × 700

Figure 8.14 Normal vein perfused with and occluded while containing blood incubated with lignocaine for twenty minutes *ex vivo.* Leukocyte adhesion and migration was minimal with the luminal surface appearing quite normal. An isolated area with limited leukocyte invasion and cell separation is shown in this figure. Normally leukocyte invasion would be massive (see Figures 8.4–8.6)

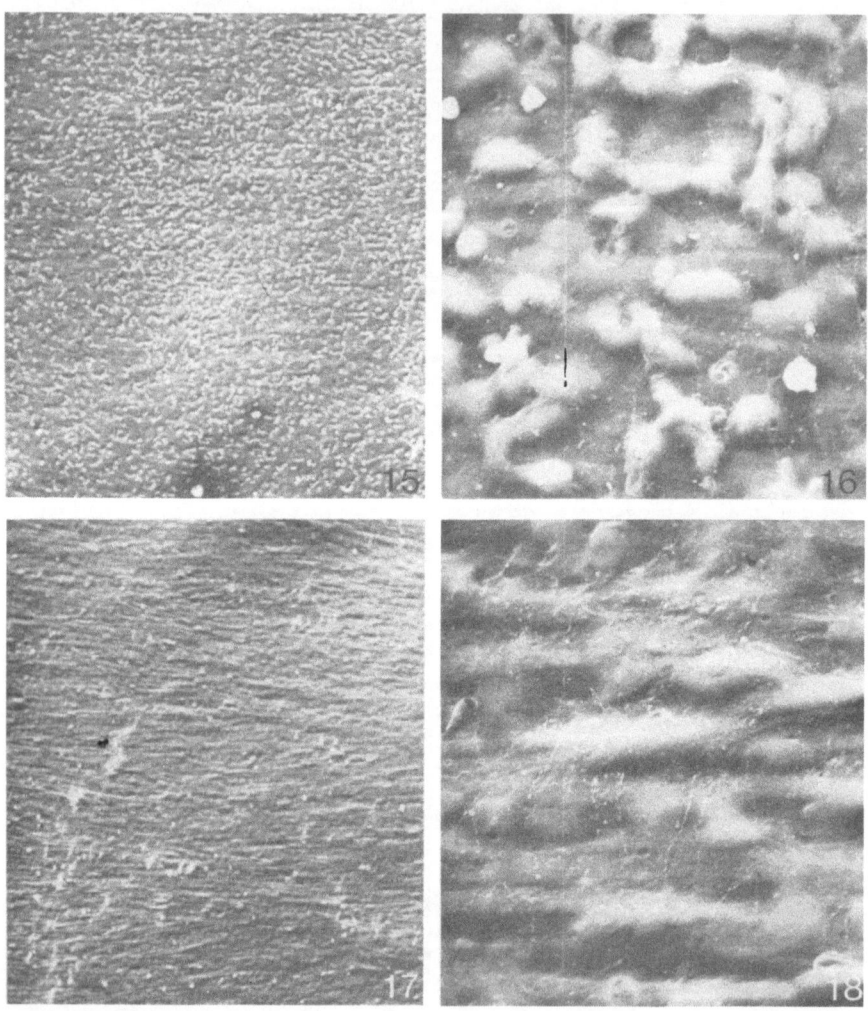

Figures 8.15 and 8.16 Lignocaine treated vessel perfused with and then occluded while containing normal blood. There is extensive leukocyte migration and accumulation between the endothelium and basement membrane as indicated by the coalescing wheals. Figure 8.15 × 70 Figure 8.16 × 700

Figures 8.17 and 8.18 Occluded veins from dogs made neutropenic by treatment with vinblastin. Veins with or without occlusion after surgery were indistinguishable from normal veins (Figures 8.1–8.3). Figure 8.17 × 70 Figure 8.18 × 700

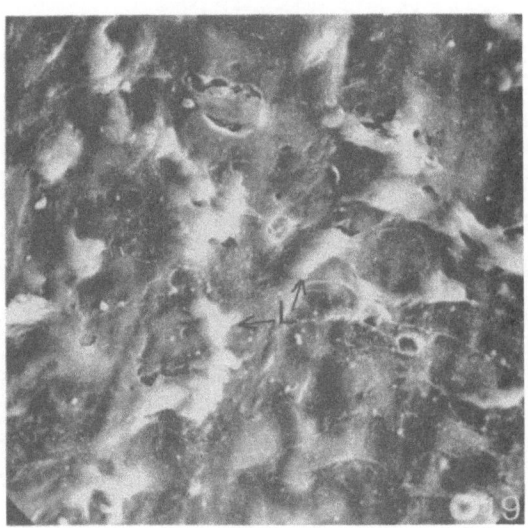

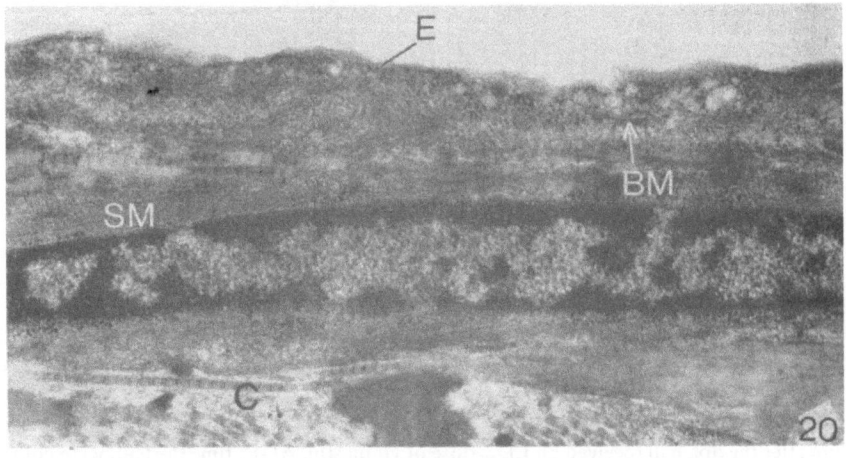

Figures 8.19 Vein from vinblastin-treated dog perfused with and occluded while containing normal blood after surgery. There is fairly extensive leukocyte (L) adhesion with the entrapment of pockets of leukocytes beneath the endothelium. × 700

Figure 8.20 Transmission electron micrograph of non-occluded jugular vein from dog that had received 20 mg of lignocaine intravenously 30 min prior to surgery and an i.v. drip of 2 mg per min during surgery. The ultrastructure of the vein was entirely similar to the control shown in Figure 8.10. ⁄ 25 600

113

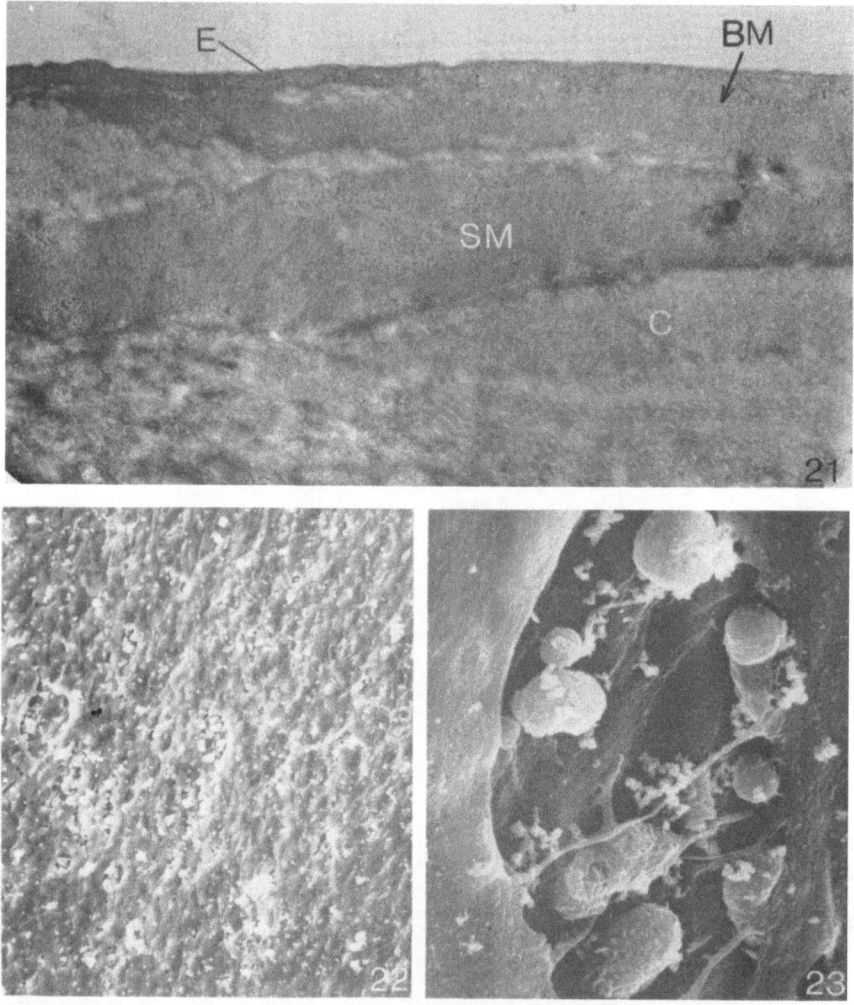

Figure 8.21 Transmission electron micrograph of non-occluded jugular vein removed 24 hours after the dog had received an LD_{50} dose of vinblastin. At the time the leukocyte count was below 1000 and the platelet count above 100 000. The ultrastructure of the vein was entirely similar to the control shown in Figure 8.10. $\times$ 16 200

Figures 8.22 and 8.23 Canine jugular vein perfused and excised six hours after the surgical procedure necessary to expose the vessel and tie the tributaries followed by seven minutes of stasis.

Figure 8.22 shows extensive whealing with frequent spots denuded of endothelium. $\times$ 210

Figure 8.23 shows the details of a damaged area with several missing endothelial cells but with threads of endothelium strung across the exposed basement membrane. The amorphous material has not been identified. Several leukocytes are present. $\times$ 2100

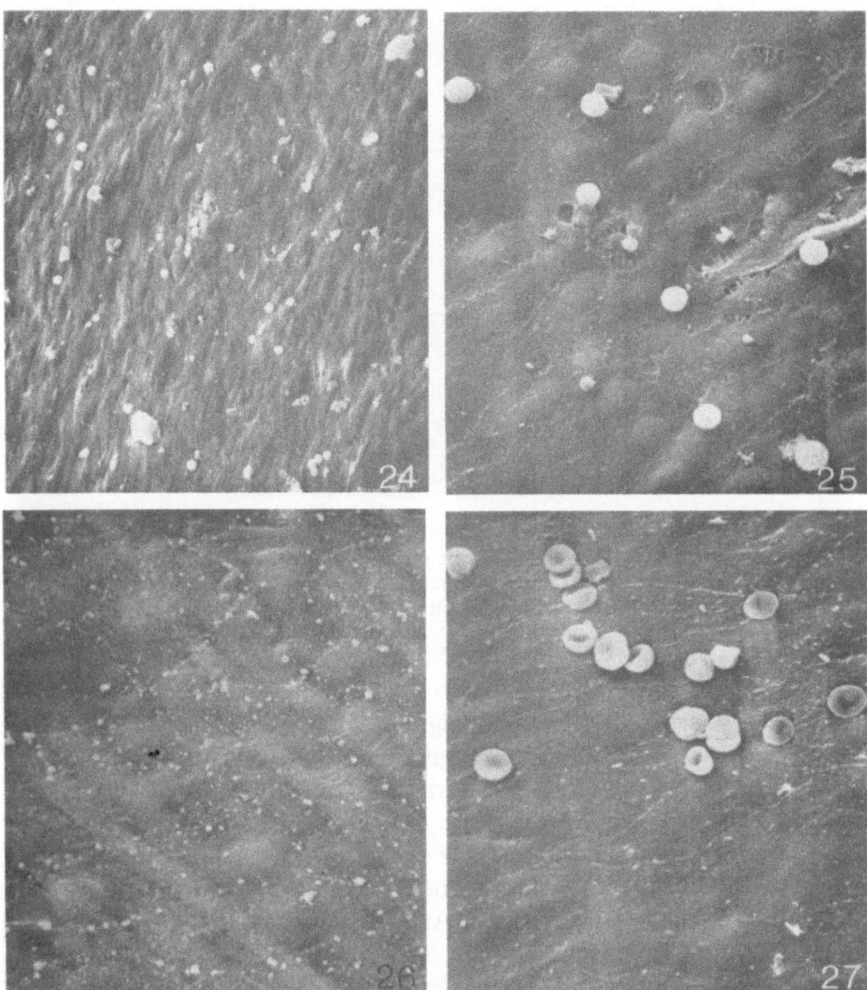

Figure 8.24 Canine jugular vein re-exposed and excised 24 hours after the surgery necessary to expose the vein and tie tributaries. The initial exposure was followed by seven minutes of occlusion by externally applied pressure to induce massive white cell invasion. All surgical procedures were performed under aseptic precautions and the dogs maintained on antibiotics. There was no evidence of infection. There are still scattered leukocytes and foci of damage. × 210

Figure 8.25 Similar treatment as in vein in Figure 8.24. At 72 hours there are still scattered leukocytes and foci of damage that appear to consist of only an occasional damaged or missing cell. × 700

Figure 8.26 Scanning electron micrograph of vessel removed 15 days after the original surgery and temporary occlusion. The endothelial sheet is intact. However, there is still some amorphous material on the surface and an occasional giant cell. × 700

Figure 8.27 At 28 days there were scattered leukocytes, erythrocytes and occasional giant cells on the luminal surface. However, the endothelial sheet was intact. × 700

115

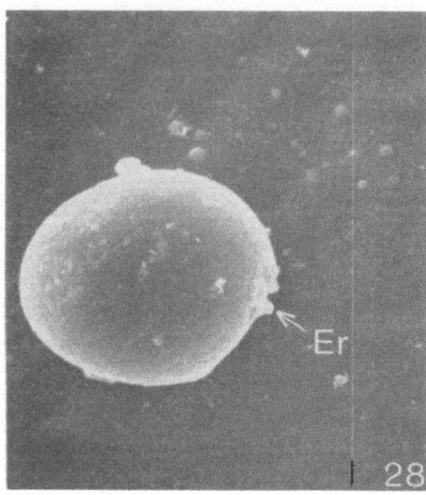

Figure 8.28 Details of a giant cell. There is one and possibly two erythrocytes (Er) adherent to the surface of giant cell. The giant cells may represent macrophages that act as scavengers to remove adherent cells and debris from the luminal surface. They were seldom seen in acute experiments but were frequent in samples obtained from 24 hours to 28 days. × 700

Because the above model (Stewart *et al.*, 1974) iş similar to the model used by Wessler to produce red coagulation thrombi it is suggested that white cell invasion and endothelial damage also occurred in his studies **and that the failure to observe them was due to the time samples were taken** and the method by which they were examined. In the studies with scanning electron microscopy only a few of the invading white cells remained in evidence by the end of 24 hours, the earliest time at which samples were taken by Wessler (Wessler, 1955). At this time endothelial damage was patchy and thus easily missed.

Although the author's observations on the presence of vascular damage disagree with those of Wessler and his associates, they are in agreement with his conclusion that activation of the clotting mechanism is of major importance. In an occasional jugular vein that had been exposed to contrast media (Hypaque 50 or Conray 60) macroscopically visible thrombi that were well enough anchored to withstand perfusion of the vein were found. Similar thrombi were found in one of four veins removed 48 and 72 hours after the original surgery. In all cases these thrombi were composed almost entirely of packed red cells entrapped in fibrin (Ritchie *et al.*, 1974; Lynch *et al.*, 1974). Although an *exogenous* source of activated clotting factors was not added nor was stasis deliberately

116

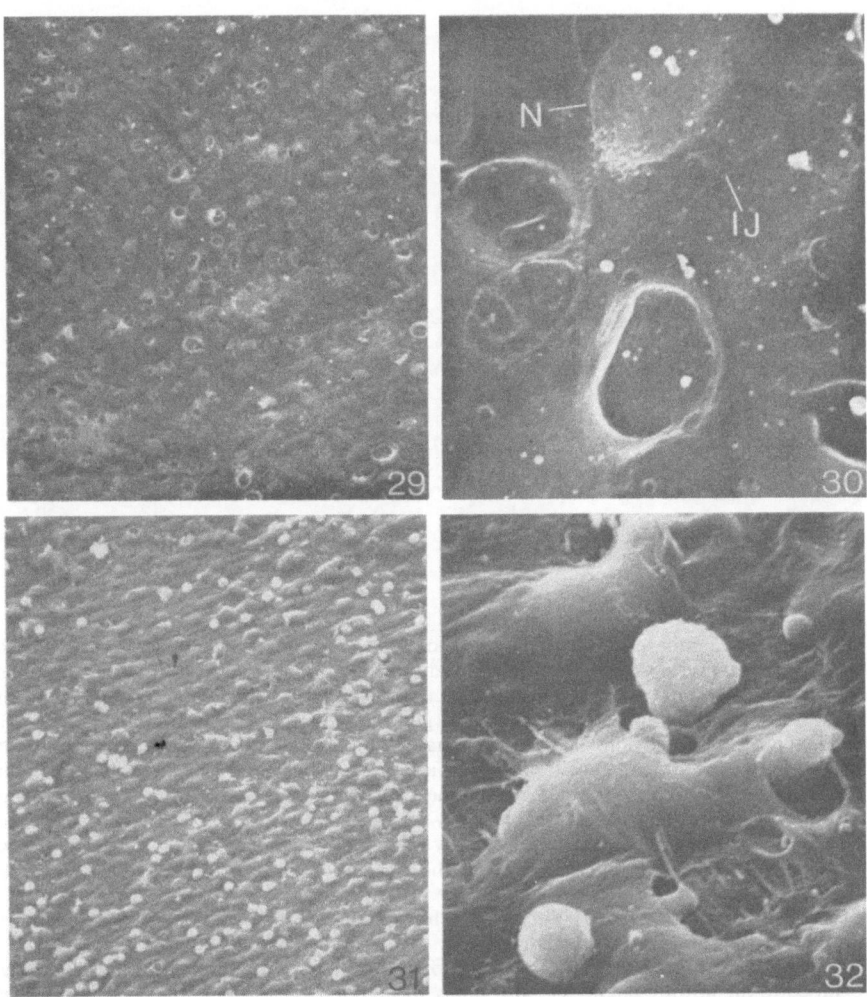

Figure 8.29 This canine jugular vein was exposed and perfused without occlusion one hour after the dog had been subjected to hysterectomy. There was only occasional single leukocyte sticking and migration. However, there were a large number of 'craters', apparently produced from the collapse of vacuoles or blebs. The endothelial sheet remained intact. × 210

Figure 8.30 Details of the endothelial sheet from Figure 8.29 marked with craters are shown here. The nuclei (N) and intercellular junctions (IJ) are still recognisable. × 2100

Figure 8.31 Contralateral jugular to the one in Figure 8.29 and 8.30. It was treated in exactly the same way except that the vein was occluded for seven minutes by externally applied pressure (60 min after hysterectomy) but before any surgery to the neck. Leukocyte adhesion and migration were extensive. This is in sharp contrast to occlusion of the vein for seven minutes in the absence of abdominal surgery (see Figures 8.8 and 8.9)

Figure 8.32 Details of the vessel in Figure 8.31 are shown here. Leukocytes are 'partially in and partially out'. × 2100

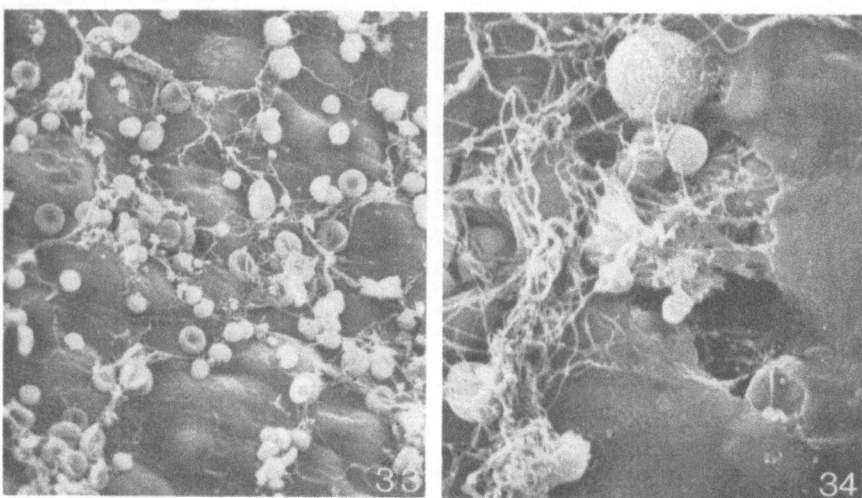

Figure 8.33 Scanning electron micrograph of area of canine jugular vein from which a freshly formed mural thrombus was removed after glutaraldehyde fixation. The thrombus was not over 30 min old, was anchored securely enough to the vessel wall to remain in place during blood flow and perfusion. The glutaraldehyde fixed the components in their original positions relative to each other so that the bulk of the thrombus could be removed and still leave the attachment sites in position. Since there was no valve, it is obvious that the thrombus was attached by some other means. It appears that the means of attachment was through fibrin and leukocytes, possibly by the interaction of polymerising fibrin to leukocytes that had adhered to and partially migrated across the endothelial sheet. × 700
Figure 8.34 Details of Figure 8.33 showing the association of fibrin strands and leukocytes. Platelets are adherent to the fibrin strands. × 2100
Figure 8.35 Luminal surface of blood vessel showing limited deposition of fibrin, leukocytes and erythrocytes on the vessel wall. × 210
Figure 8.36 Scanning electron micrograph of the surface of a mural thrombus that was exposed to the flowing blood. The thrombus was composed almost entirely of a fibrin net that entrapped masses of erythrocytes. An occasional platelet adhered to the fibrin (arrow). × 700
Figure 8.37 Details of the association of fibrin and red cells are shown here. × 7000
Figure 8.38 Internal structure of a thrombus shown by fracture after the thrombus was fixed and dried. The amorphous material on the surface of the erythrocytes is likely bits of broken fibrin strands. What appears to be two platelets (arrows) are also present. × 2100

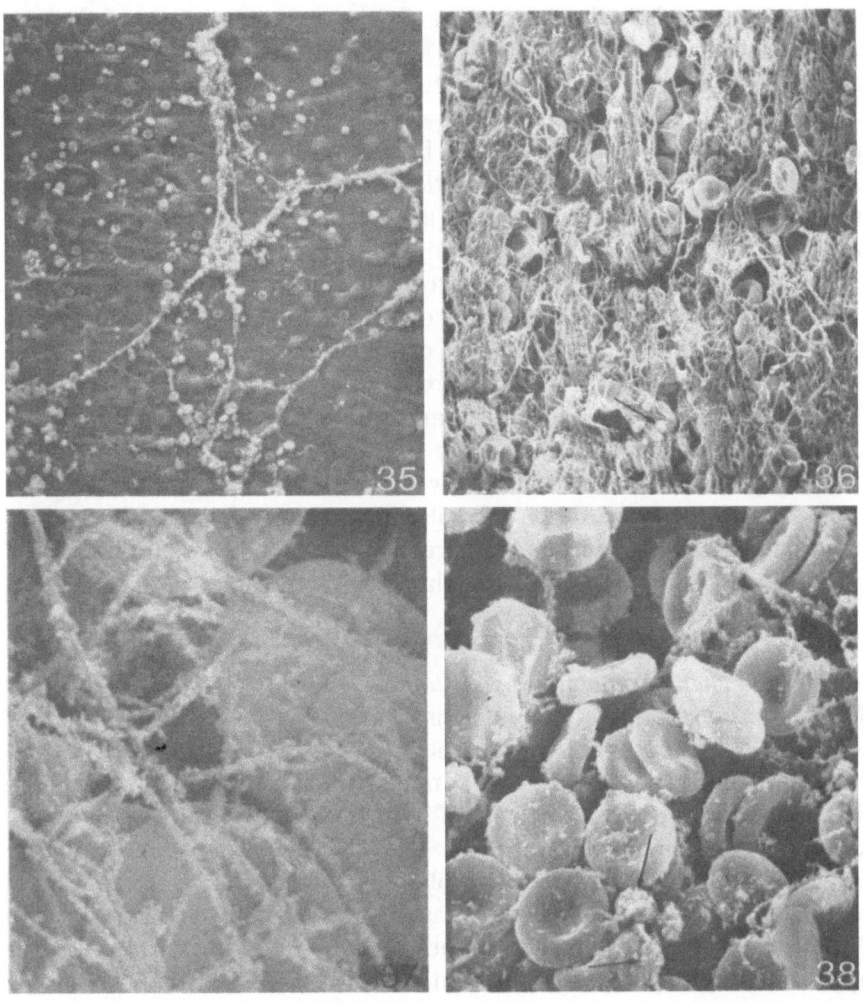

induced, the model did not exclude the presence of a low level of activated endogenous clotting factors in the circulating blood nor the occurrence of stasis due to the position of the animal (Lynch *et al.*, 1974; Ritchie *et al.*, 1974; Stewart *et al.*, 1974). Both could, in fact, be expected. Systemic activation of the coagulation and fibrinolytic systems is observed after dogs are subjected to burns (Guest and Bond, 1968) and patients to surgical trauma (Flute *et al.*, 1972).

119

Response of vessels to the destruction of tissue in a remote part of the body in the presence of stasis

Many of the diverse conditions that predispose to thrombosis have two common characteristics. These are: (1) considerable to extensive cell injury and death in some part of the body remote from the veins that are involved in thrombosis and (2) a period of bed rest. If a combination of injury and death of remote cells and stasis are responsible for the initiation of thrombosis, the following must be considered:

(1) Does the inury and death of cells in one part of the body cause changes in vessels in other parts of the body and if so, what is the mechanism and what form do the changes take?

(2) Does stasis through the lower extremities cause changes in the veins and if so, what is the mechanism and what form do the changes take?

(3) Does a combination of death of distant cells and stasis cause a change in the veins and if so how?

(4) Does injury and death of cells in one part of the body cause a systemic increase in activated intermediates of the coagulation system?

(5) Finally, how do any changes that occur contribute to the initiation of thrombosis?

Generalised changes in blood vessels following localised trauma

The endocrine and metabolic responses to localised cell destruction have been well documented. However, there have been only a few studies on vessels in non-traumatised tissue of animals subjected to localised trauma. Burning the lower legs and backs of hamsters by applying a metal plate at 100 °C for 15 sec was followed in 5–7 minutes by a reduction in corpuscular flow velocity in arterioles and venules accompanied by a reduction in the diameter of the vascular lumen (Branemark *et al.*, 1968). A few minutes after dogs were subjected to third degree burns over approximately 50 per cent of their surface area the microcirculation in the mesentery was hindered by the formation of aggregates of red cells that frequently filled the lumen of small arteries, arterioles and venules (Guest and Bond, 1968). In the rat full-thickness high temperature skin burns over 40 per cent of the body surface produced endothelial swellings and circulating white aggregates or clots in the microcirculation. On the day after the burns there was margination and adhesion of leukocytes in about half of the animals. Occasionally the venous perivascular spaces were larger than normal. The response of larger vessels or their vasa vasorum to trauma in another part of the body has not been reported.

Since the method used by the author for preparing veins (Stewart *et al.*, 1974) has consistently given controls that fulfilled the well established criteria for 'normal' it provided an approach for investigating changes induced by various experimental conditions. In order to simulate the clinical situation it was necessary to cause extensive tissue injury in an area of the dog's body well removed from the jugular veins, to induce stasis in these veins by gentle external pressure (previously shown not to cause leukocyte invasion or other detectable damage in the absence of deliberate tissue destruction in some part of the body) and to look for leukocyte invasion. Tissue destruction was produced by crush injury to the muscular area of both hind legs or by abdominal surgery (hysterectomy on female dogs or removal of the gall bladder on male dogs). Thirty or sixty minutes after the injury one jugular vein was occluded for seven minutes by external pressure. This was done prior to dissection to expose the veins. The contralateral vein was not occluded at any time.

The jugular vein that was not occluded showed variable sticking and migration of single leukocytes (Figures 8.29 and 8.30) while the vein that was occluded showed extensive sticking and accumulation of pockets of leukocytes (Figures 8.31 and 8.32). This resulted in extensive separation and occasional desquamation of endothelial cells. These results suggested that extensive tissue damage to any area of the body influenced the medium sized veins in non-traumatised areas and that the influence was enhanced by local stasis.

Leukotaxis
It is established that white cells migrate only in response to an increasing gradient of chemotactic agent *in vitro* (Sorkin *et al.*, 1970) and most likely *in vivo* (Buckley, 1963; Hurley, 1964). Therefore, it follows that some change has occurred in the vessel wall external to the endothelium or in the adjacent tissues and that the change has resulted in the formation of a chemotactic substance. This substance must then diffuse across the wall to the lumen of the vein to establish a concentration gradient so that white cells would migrate from the lumen into the wall. The identity of the chemotactic substances has been indicated by studies of complement induced chemotaxis. Antigen–antibody complexes incubated in a medium containing fresh, normal rabbit serum exerted a strong chemotactic response on rabbit polymorphonuclear leukocytes. This phenomenon suggested that the active substance could be a component of complement (Boyden, 1962). Since then rapid strides have been made in elucidating the mechanism of complement induced leukocyte migration. It has now been established that the serum complement system provides substrates for the

enzymatic generation of at least three different chemotactic factors for neutrophiles. There is a high molecular weight C567 complex and two low molecular weight fragments derived by the cleavage of C3 and C5. Each of these chemotactic factors can be generated by the action of enzymes which are either intrinsic or extrinsic to the complement systems (Ward, 1972). Of particular interest is the formation of C3a by plasmin (Taylor and Ward, 1967; Ward, 1967; Bokisch and Muller-Eberhard, 1970). There are also several chemotactic factors independent of complement such as kallikrein (Kaplan et al., 1972) which may cause white cell adhesion and migration in veins. Certain products of cells infected with viruses (Ward et al., 1972) and bacteria (Keller and Sorkin, 1967; Ward et al., 1968; Walker et al., 1969) may be of significance in thrombosis in patients with various infectious diseases.

A generalised increase in vascular permeability could set in motion a series of complex interactions that would result in the generation of chemotactic complement fragments (C3a and C5a, anaphylotoxins). This could happen if considerably higher than 'normal' levels of plasma proteins including components of the clotting, fibrinolytic and complement systems escaped from the vessels, especially the vasa vasorum, and came into contact with the mass of collagen in the vessel wall. Factor XII could then become activated by collagen and lead to the generation of plasmin, thrombin and kallikrein.

The above discussion appears to provide a partial answer to the question, 'Does the death of cells in a distant part of the body cause changes in vessel walls and if so, what is the mechanism and what form do the changes take?' In crush injuries and surgical trauma there is extensive endothelial cell separation and desquamation induced by the migration and accumulation of leukocytes between the endothelium and the basement membrane.

A similar response could be expected in patients suffering from other forms of trauma. However, in the case of septicaemia the invading organisms may produce endothelial damage directly or through products such as endotoxin (McGrath and Stewart, 1969; Stewart and Anderson, 1971; Gaynor, 1973). There are indications (oedema) that pregnancy and oral contraceptives as well as immune reactions (histamine release) lead to increased vascular permeability which would allow the escape of plasma proteins into the vessel wall where collagen would activate the fibrinolytic system and generate plasmin. This in turn could form chemotactic complement fragments C3a and C5a kallikrein and plasminogen activator.

Thromboembolism

Stasis and the vessel wall

It is now accepted that reduced blood flow through the lower extremities is a contributing factor in the initiation of thrombosis (Chapter 2). Vessel wall damage, accumulation of activated clotting factors and silting out of platelets have all been mentioned as possible consequences of reduced flow (Chapters 2 and 7). Several studies have purported to demonstrate endothelial damage produced by ischaemia of the vessel wall resulting from interruption of the blood flow to the vasa vasorum (O'Neill, 1947; Samuels and Webster, 1952; McGovern, 1955). Although these studies have contributed to the development of methods for investigating the luminal surface of blood vessels (see page   ) they do not demonstrate the effects of ischaemia *per se* on the vessel intima. In all of them trauma to tissue adjacent to the vein was a factor that could have contributed to the observed endothelial damage.

In an extensive study of the effect of complete ischaemia on small blood vessels in skin (Williams-Kretschmer and Majno, 1969) no significant changes were found with the light microscope when the duration of complete ischaemia was 2 hours or less. In rats ischaemia for periods of 4–6 hours with 0–2 hours reflow produced loss of the smooth muscle fibres in the wall accompanied by considerable polymorphonuclear infiltration, oedema and necrosis. With 8 hours of ischaemia there was almost complete loss of muscle (even with no reflow), blebbing of the vascular wall and intense polymorphonuclear diapedesis and infiltration. Tissue damage was considerably less in the rabbit; there was blebbing of the vascular wall, but polymorphonuclear infiltration was rarely seen.

At the ultrastructural level these investigators found that one of the characteristic features of ischaemic damage was the focal nature of the lesions. Severely damaged vessels were often adjacent to vessels that appeared normal. In general the proportion of damaged vessels increased with increasing times of ischaemia. The earliest evidence of endothelial damage was a diffuse swelling either of individual or of all the cells of some small venules and capillaries. Swelling was accompanied by blebs which become detached in many cases. Swelling of the perinuclear space was another type of early endothelial change. After 6 hours or more of complete ischaemia, condensation and margination of nuclear chromatin was a constant feature of endothelial cells. The pericytes most frequently exhibited swelling of endoplasmic reticulum and perinuclear spaces.

Reduction of the flow rate in the inferior vena cava of the rabbit by a restricting but not occluding ligature for periods ranging from 1 to 21 days caused changes in the endothelium and smooth muscle, but no deposition of thrombotic material (Tedder and Shorey, 1966). The effects of partial ligation for periods ranging up to 24 hours (Ts'Ao and Spaet, 1967) caused endothelial desquamation and limited platelet aggregation at the site of ligation.

These studies suggest that reduced flow through the deep veins of the legs of patients at bedrest does not result in sufficient ischaemic damage to cause the accumulation of platelets and fibrin on the vessel walls. However, the significance of the accumulation of platelets or activated clotting factors in valve pockets is uncertain. Most of the thrombi in valve cusps in one study were 'white thrombi' (Paterson, 1969), and most thrombi near the apex of the valve pocket in another were composed largely of red cells and fibrin (Hume *et al.*, 1970). Histological examination of valve pockets without visible thrombi in the femoral vein revealed some small condensed clumps of fibrin on a valve leaf with granular material (possibly platelets) nearby. However, isolated and packed islets of red cells were observed in other pockets. It should be pointed out that there is no evidence that these aggregates of material serve as nidi for developing thrombi. It may well be that there is some accumulation of material in most valve pockets normally and that these have nothing to do with initiation of thrombosis.

If reduced blood flow through the legs does not produce ischaemic damage or silting of platelets, what then is its role in the production of thrombosis? Our studies suggest that venous stasis helps in establishing a chemotactic gradient which induces extensive leukocyte migration. The leukocytes that leave the lumen of the vessel become trapped, either singly or in pockets, between the endothelium and the basement membrane. This results in endothelial cell separation and desquamation. Since this does not occur in the absence of tissue destruction at some site in the body it would explain the observation that chronic paralysed patients who must have considerable to severe stasis but not tissue destruction do not have frequent episodes of thrombosis (Lockhart-Mummery, 1924; Tribe, 1963; and Wolman, 1965). Stasis may also play a role in spontaneous thrombosis by reducing the clearance rate of activated clotting factors arriving in normal veins from traumatised areas or produced locally (Wessler *et al.*, 1959; 1967; Spaet, 1962; Guest and Bond, 1968; Flute, *et al.*, 1972); Chapters 2 and 7).

Vascular damage and reduced flow in the initiation of thrombosis
Evidence has been presented that extensive cell death in one part of the

body causes leukocyte adhesion and migration in another part of the body and that these are increased by local stasis (Stewart *et al.*, 1974). The relevance of these observations depends on their ability to contribute to the initiation of thrombosis. Extensive disruption of the endothelial lining provides an opportunity for plasma proteins including fibrinogen and clotting factors to come into contact with collagen that composes a large part of the vessel wall. Since Factor XII is activated by collagen (Niewiarowski *et al.*, 1965) this provides a means of setting in motion the intrinsic clotting process with the ultimate conversion of fibrinogen to fibrin. It is also possible that the extrinsic coagulation mechanism is activated if the white cells were sufficiently modified during their migration. It has been shown that leukocytes exposed to endotoxin exhibit thromboplastic activity (Niemetz and Fani, 1973), and that polymerising fibrin adheres to white cells *in vitro* (Niewiarowski *et al.*, 1972a). The attachment of fibrin to leukocytes that are in the process of migrating across the endothelial sheet (Figures 8.33–8.35) has been observed on several occasions (Stewart *et al.*, 1974). Thus, the leukocytes may produce endothelial damage and anchor fibrin to the vessel wall.

Surprisingly few platelets adhering to the exposed subendothelial structure on the venous side have been observed (Stewart *et al.*, 1974). This is in agreement with the observation that venous thrombi contain very few platelets and in some cases do not have demonstrable platelet nidi (Hume *et al.*, 1970). Platelet adhesion and aggregation were frequently observed on damaged arterial walls and woven Dacron grafts immediately after insertion into the canine thoracic aorta (Reichle *et al.*, 1973). Other investigators have reported that the extent of platelet adhesion and aggregation is dependent on the flow rate with few platelets accumulating at low flow rates (Begent and Born, 1970; Friedman *et al.*, 1970; Friedman and Leonard, 1971). It may be that the relatively low flow of blood in the venous circulation contributes to the scarcity of platelet aggregates on the venous wall and in venous thrombi.

Doubtless platelets play a significant role in deep venous thrombosis through their participation in the intrinsic coagulation mechanism (Biggs, 1972) and through the recently discovered platelet coagulation properties that are independent of platelet factor three (Walsh, 1972a; 1972b; Walsh and Biggs, 1972). It appears that platelets may also accumulate to a limited extent in propagating thrombi by adhering to polymerising fibrin (Figures 8.34, 8.36 and 8.37). The adherence of platelets to *polymerising* fibrin but not to fully polymerised fibrin has been well documented *in vitro* (Niewiarowski *et al.*, 1972b). This may be the mechanism of formation of the lines of Zahn so commonly observed in clinical thrombi (Hume et al., 1970).

In an extensive study (Borgstrom and Gelin, 1959) ligation of the femoral veins of rabbits in the absence of trauma caused a low incidence of thrombosis (1 of 20). However, muscle contusion inflicted immediately after vein ligation greatly increased the incidence of thrombosis with the increase depending on the degree of trauma. In the groups with contusion of one hind limb by 50, 100, 150 and 200 blows, 5, 14, 17 and 19 thrombi were found out of 20 possible in each case. The number of thrombi was the same on contused and non-contused sides. Focal vessel damage by point cauterisation did not increase the incidence of thrombosis. The veins were dissected free and examined for thrombi at 6–7 days after the trauma. The influence of increasing stasis on thrombus formation in animals subjected to various degrees of trauma was also investigated by ligating both the femoral vein and the first tributary below the femoral ligature. In the group with no contusion the additional stasis increased the incidence of thrombosis from 1/20 to 14/20. With 50 blows the rate increased from 5/20 to 17/20 while with 100 blows it increased from 14/20 to 19/20.

These studies showed that a combination of trauma and stasis caused thrombosis and that the incidence of thrombosis increased as the degree of stasis or the degree of trauma was increased. When the degree of stasis and trauma were increased simultaneously, the incidence of thrombosis increased even faster.

ATTACHMENT OF VENOUS THROMBI TO THE VESSEL WALL

There are apparently no studies specifically on the means by which fresh venous thrombi are attached to the vessel wall. According to some authors (Paterson, 1969; Hume et al., 1970) thrombi are attached only at valve cusps, bifurcations or small saccules. This means that the attachment is largely physical although it has been suggested that the initial attachment is 'probably fibrinous' (Hume et al., 1970). However, no mechanism by which fibrin could attach to the vessel wall has been suggested. As the thrombus becomes organised, i.e. converted into vascular connective tissue, it becomes part of the vessel wall.

The concept that thrombi are always attached by anchoring behind valves is not supported by clinical venographic studies (Nicolaides et al., 1971a). By using the ^{125}I-fibrinogen test it has been shown that practically all thrombi start in the calf and extend proximally (Flanc et al., 1968; Negus et al., 1968; Murray et al., 1970; Nicolaides et al., 1971b). Further investigations with venography have shown that about 46 per cent of venous thrombi are confined to the calf, and 42 per cent had extended into the popliteal and more proximal veins. In only 12 per cent of the cases were thrombi found in the popliteal, femoral, common and external iliac veins in the presence of normal distal veins. The majority of thrombi that start in the calf start in the soleal veins (Nicolaides *et al.*, 1971a; Chapter 11). On the basis of these observations it was stated that in the majority of patients venous thrombi started in the calf and particularly the soleal veins. The soleal veins were always valveless (Nicolaides *et al.*, 1971a; Tragardh, 1973; Chapter 11). Therefore, it seems unlikely that the growing thrombus is retained in a soleal vein by mere physical lodging since during venography there is considerable filling of the vessel with contrast medium around the thrombus whose diameter is no larger than the diameter of the vein immediately proximal ot it. If the thrombus were not attached to the vessel wall by some means, it would be carried along until it reached a narow place in the vein where it would then lodge, totally occluding the vessel distal to the thrombus.

A possible mechanism for the attachment of fresh thrombi to the venous wall has been shown by scanning electron microscopy of canine jugular veins (Stewart *et al.*, 1973). Following white cell induced injury to the endothelium thrombi as much as 3–5 cm in length and covering about one fourth of the circumference were formed in some veins. These were not associated with valves or bifurcations yet were anchored firmly enough to withstand perfusion at pressures of 10–20 cmH$_2$O. After initial fixation to preserve structures in their original relationships, the thrombi were gently lifted off the vessel wall and oriented so that the attached side of the thrombus as well as the vessel wall could be examined. It appeared that the thrombi had been anchored to the wall by the attachment of fibrin strands to white cells that were partially or completely beneath the endothelium (Figures 8.33–8.35). The structure of the thrombi is shown in Figures 8.36–8.38.

FATE OF THROMBI

Resolution of thrombi

Thrombi, produced by stasis and subsequently released as emboli, underwent a rapid reduction in size, presumably due to lysis. The emboli were detectably smaller after only 24 hours; after five days only a few residual emboli remained and after six weeks only small organised nubbins were found (Wessler *et al.*, 1961). Red coagulation thrombi, induced by.

thrombin in occluded veins or the rabbit's ear, showed evidence of extensive lysis after 18 hours and lysis of more than half the mass was complete at 48 hours (Scott, 1968). It has also been observed that lysis of the periphery of venous thrombi induced by stasis occurs shortly after the thrombi are formed (Kwaan and Astrup, 1965) and depends on the production of plasminogen activator by the vessel wall.

The ability of tissues to induce the lysis of plasma clots has been studied extensively (Fleisher and Loeb, 1915). Small pieces of various tissues were either embedded in or placed on the top of plasma clots and observed for zones of clot lysis. It was concluded that organs had a 'certain dissolving effect' on the coagulum. Later, it was discovered that the fibrinolytic activity induced by tissues is due to a substance (activator) which brings about the activation of a proenzyme (plasminogen) which is present in plasma in an inactive form (Fischer, 1946; Astrup and Permin, 1947).

The activator content of organs of a given species varies considerably as does the content of the same organ in different species (Albrechtsen, 1957; Ende and Auditore, 1961). The tissue activator was shown to be associated with vasa vasorum in normal arteries. However, activity has been reported in the endothelium of aortic grafts from dogs sacrificed six weeks after operation and to some extent from the aortic wall (Warren and Brock, 1964). The activator is released from the endothelium to become the blood or plasma activator and the trigger mechanism responsible for its release appears to be abrupt changes in vascular tone (Rahn and Von Kaulla, 1964). The relationship between vascular plasminogen activator and urokinase is uncertain. Although some workers had suggested that the two were identical (Bernik and Kwaan, 1969), others found that the two activators were different imunologically, biochemically and enzymatically (Kucinski et al., 1968; Aoki and Von Kaulla, 1971). Fibrinolytic activity has also been shown to exist in reparative connective tissue (Kwaan and Astrup, 1964; Glas and Astrup, 1970) and in fibroblasts in tissue culture (Niewiarowski and Goldstein, 1973).

Organisation of venous thrombi

According to French and MacFarlane, 'At the same time as the thrombus is undergoing partial resolution, reactive changes occur in the vessel wall and gradually transform the mass, in whole or in part, into vascular connective tissue' (French and MacFarlane, 1970). The organisation of a thrombus resembles wound healing in which fibrin and tissue debris are gradually replaced by organised connective tissue.

Although there is some disagreement about the area of the vessel from which cells migrate and about the type of cells involved, most investigators believe that the vessel wall is the source of cells involved in the organisation of venous thrombi (Weiner and Spiro, 1962; Stirling, 1966; Scott, 1968; Sevitt, 1970). Others have suggested that blood-born monocytes (macrophages) are the progenitors of the fibroblast (Paul, 1958; Ross and Benditt, 1961). In organising venous thrombi the most prominent cells are fibroblasts, histiocytes, macrophages and **endothelial.** Smooth muscle cells may be found after some time. So far, it has not been established whether the vessel wall or the blood is exclusively the source of cells. Cells from both sources have opportunity and potential for invading the thrombus and may well do so.

SUMMARY AND CONCLUSIONS

Most of the diverse clinical conditions which predispose to deep venous thrombosis have two characteristics in common: considerable tissue destruction in some part of the body well removed from the veins in which thrombosis occurs and a period of bed rest. Localised tissue destruction causes systemic responses in addition to the local responses in the damaged area. One aspect of the localised response (i.e. the inflammatory process) is increased vascular permeability that results in swelling. While a systemic increase in vascular permeability has not been shown directly, some increase has been indicated by reversible haemoconcentration. The return of normal flow has been attributed to the return of normal permeability. The generalised increase in vascular permeability could result from the localised release of histamine and formation of plasma kinins that are taken up by the blood and circulated to other parts of the body during the brief interval before their inactivation.

Such an increase in the vascular permeability provides an opportunity for the passage of plasma proteins including Factor XII into extravascular areas. Plasma proteins may escape into the collagen matrix of the medium and large veins from the lumen and from the small vessels composing the vasa vasorum. Contact with collagen can act as a trigger mechanism for the activation of the clotting, fibrinolytic, plasma kinin and complement systems. The products that are formed by the activation of these systems must diffuse in all directions and may reach the lumen of the vessel, especially if the junctions between the endothelial cells are 'opened' by histamine.

Thromboembolism

There is no evidence that increased vascular permeability *per se* can serve as a stimulus for thrombus formation. However it may do so indirectly by contributing to leukocyte invasion of the vessel wall. Massive migration of leukocytes across the endothelial sheet and their accumulation in pockets between the endothelium and basement membrane results in extensive endothelial cell separation and desquamation. In a small percentage of cases, even without stasis induced deliberately, thrombi formed in these vessels, invaded by leukocytes.

The invasion of the vessel wall by leukocytes almost certainly results from the formation of a chemotactic substance or substances at some place external to the endothelium since leukocytes migrate only from an area of low concentration to an area of high concentration of such an agent.

In the 'remote trauma' studies abdominal surgery 'primed' the animal so that stasis in the jugular veins resulted in leukocyte invasion. This can best be explained by assuming substances from the damaged site, carried throughout the body, caused alterations of the vessel wall or surrounding tissue which resulted in the generation of one or more chemotactic agents. The chemotactic agents would diffuse in every direction, eventually reaching the lumen of the vessel, especially if it were formed in the wall of the vessel (external to the endothelium). This would result in a chemotactic gradient with a higher concentration in the outer aspect of the vessel wall than at the luminal surface. If a similar sequence of events occurs in man, it could explain how trauma to one part of the body (abdominal surgery for instance) 'primes' the patient for deep venous thrombosis when stasis is added as a necessary, accessory condition.

During infection it is possible that the infectious agents or their products not only damage or destroy their target tissues but also cause direct injury to blood vessel walls. The predisposition to thrombosis associated with pregnancy and the use of oral contraceptives are major exceptions to the presence of known tissue destruction and bed rest but the chronic low level oedema usually associated with both indicate some increase in vascular permeability over prolonged periods.

Stasis in the deep veins may be also involved in establishing a chemotactic gradient. As long as blood flow is adequate, chemotactic agents that diffuse across the wall and reach the luminal surface will be washed away so that no gradient could be established. However, in complete stasis and even in greatly reduced flow the chemotactic substance reaching the lumen could accumulate and produce leukocyte migration.

The endothelial damage caused by the white cell invasion combined

Thromboembolism

with the accumulation of activated clotting intermediates in the stagnant blood provide a possible means of initiation of thrombosis with platelets participating through their role in coagulation. Platelet factor three and the other recently discovered clotting activities of platelets probably serve to promote fibrin formation. Platelets have been observed to be attached to fibrin strands suggesting that they adhere to polymerising fibrin *in vivo* as well as *in vitro*.

References

Albrechtsen, O. K. (1957). The fibrinolytic activity of human tissues. *Brit. J. Haematol.*, **3**, 284

Aoki, W. and Von Kaulla, K. N. (1971). Dissimilarity of human vascular plasminogen activator and human urokinase. *J. Lab. Clin. Med.*, **78**, 354

Apitz, K. and Der, E. (1942). Influss Experimenteller gerinnungs-ktorugen auf die blutsxilling. *Virchow Arch.*, **308**, 590

Ashford, T. P. and Freiman, D. G. (1967). The role of the endothelium in the initial phases of thrombosis. *Amer. J. Pathol.*, **50**, 257

Astrup, T. and Permin, P. M. (1947). Fibrinolysis in the animal organism. *Nature (London)*, **159**, 681

Baumgartner, H. P., Tranzer, J. P. and Studer, A. (1967). An electron microscopic study of platelet thrombus formation in the rabbit with particular regard to 5-hydroxytryptamine release. *Thromb. Haemorrh. Diath.*, **18**, .592

Baumgartner, H. P. (1973). The role of blood flow in platelet adhesion, fibrin deposition and formation of mural thrombi. *Microvasc. Res.*, **5**, 167

Begent, N. and Born, G. V. R. (1970). Growth rate *in vivo* of platelet thrombi, produced by iontophoresis of ADP, as a function of mean blood flow velocity. *Nature (London)*, **227**, 926

Berman, H. J., Fulton, G. P., Lutz, B. R. and Pierce, D. L. (1954). Effect of irradiation, cortisone, heparin and aging on susceptibility to thrombosis in hamsters. *Anat. Rec.*, **120**, 802

Berman, H. J. and Fulton, G. P. (1961). Platelets in the peripheral circulation. In: *The Henry Ford Hospital Symposium on Blood Platelets*, 7–22 (S. A. Johnson, editor) (Boston, Mass.: Little, Brown and Co.)

Bernik, M. B. and Kwann, H. C. (1969). Plasminogen activator activity in cultures from human tissue: An immunological and histochemical study. *J. Clin. Invest.*, **48**, 1740

Biggs, R. (1972). Intrinsic prothrombin activation. In: *Human Blood Coagulation, Haemostasis and Thrombosis*, Chap. 5, 64–78. (Oxford, London, Edinburgh and Melbourne: Blackwell Scientific Publications)

Bokisch, V. A. and Muller-Eberhard, H. J. (1970). Anaphylatoxin inactivator of human plasma: its isolation and characterisation as a carboxypeptidase. *J. Clin. Invest.*, **49**, 2427

Borgstrom, S. and Gelin, E. (1959). The formation of vein thrombin following tissue injury. An experimental study in rabbits. *Acta Chir. Scand.*, **Suppl. 247**

Bounameaux, Y. (1959). The coupling of platelets with subendothelial fibers. *C.R. Soc. Biol.*, **153**, 865

Bounameaux, Y. (1961). The adherence of blood platelets to subendothelial fibers. *Thromb. Diath. Haemorrh.*, **6**, 504

Thromboembolism

Boyden, S. (1962). The chemotactic effect of mixtures of antibody and antigen on poly-morphonuclear leucocytes. *J. Exp. Med.,* 453

Branemark, P. I., Breine, U., Joshi, M. and Urbaschek, B. (1968). Microvascular patho-physiology of burned tissue. *Ann. N.Y. Acad. Sci.,* **150,** 474

Buckley, I. K. (1963). Delayed secondary damage and leucocyte chemotaxis following focal aseptic heat injury *in vivo. Exp. Molec. Pathol.,* **2,** 402

Callahan, A. B., Lutz, B. R., Fulton, G. P. and Degelman, J. (1960). Smooth muscle and thrombus threshold to unipolar stimulation of small blood vessels. *Angiology,* **11,** 35

Cartwright, G. E., Athens, J. W., Boggs, D. R. and Wintrobe, M. M. (1965). The kinetics of granulopiesis in normal man. *Series Haematol.,* **1,** 1

Ende, N. and Auditore, J. V. (1961). Mast cells and fibrinolysin. *Nature (London),* **189,** 593

Fischer, A. (1946). Mechanism of the proteolytic activity of malignant tissue cells. *Nature (London),* **157,** 442

Flanc, C., Kakkar, V. V. and Clarke, M. B. (1968). The detection of venous thrombosis of the legs using ^{125}I-labelled fibrinogen. *Brit. J. Surg.,* **55,** 742

Fleisher, M. and Loeb, L. (1915). On tissue fibrinolysis. *J. Biol. Chem.,* **21,** 477

Flute, P. T., Kakkar, V. V., Renney, J. T. G. and Nicolaides, A. N. (1972). The blood and venous thromboembolism. In: *Thromboembolism: Diagnosis and Treatment,* 2–12 (V. V. Kakkar and A. J. Jouchar, editors) (Baltimore, Maryland: The Williams and Wilkins Co.)

French, J. E., Macfarlane, R. G. and Sanders, A. G. (1964). The structure of haemostatic plugs and experimental thrombi in small arteries. *Brit. J. Pathol.,* **45,** 467

French, J. E. and Macfarlane, R. G. (1970). Haemostasis and thrombosis. In: *General Pathology,* 305 (Philadelphia and London: W. B. Saunders Co.)

Friedman, L. I., Liem, H., Grabowski, E. F., Leonard, E. F. and McCord, C. W. (1970). Inconsequentiality of surface properties for initial platelet adhesion. *Trans. Amer. Soc. Artif. Infern. Organs.,* **16,** 63

Friedman, L. I. and Leonard, E. F. (1971). Platelet adhesion to artificial surfaces: Consequences of flow, exposure time, blood condition and surface nature. *Fed. Proc.,* **30,** 1641

Fulton, G. P., Lutz, B. R., Joftes, D. L. and Maynard, F. W. (1953). Vascular effects in the hamster cheek pouch after irradiation. *Anat. Rec.,* **115,** 446

Gaynor, E. (1973). The role of granulocytes in endotoxin-induced vascular injury. *Blood,* **41,** 797

Glas, P. and Astrup, T. (1970). Thromboplastin and plasminogen activator in tissues of the rabbit. *Amer. J. Physiol.,* **219,** 1140

Guest, M. M. and Bond, T. P. (1968). Release of thromboplastin after thermal injury. *Ann. N.Y. Acad. Sci.,* **150,** 528

Hovig, T. (1962). The ultrastructure of rabbit blood platelet aggregates. *Thromb. Diath. Haemorrh.,* **8,** 455

Hovig, T. (1963). The effect of calcium and magnesium on rabbit blood platelet aggregation *in vitro. Thromb. Diath. Haemorrh.,* **12,** 179

Hugues, J. (1953). Contribution a l'etude des facteurs vasculares et sanguins dans l'hemostase spontanee. *Arch. Int. Physiol.,* **61,** 565

Hugues, J. (1962). Accolement des plaquettes aux structures conlonctives perivasculaires. *Thromb. Diath. Haemorrh.,* **8,** 241

Hugues, J. and Lapiere, M. (1964). Nouvelles researches sur l'accolment des plaquettes aux fiberes de collagere. *Thromb. Diath. Haemorrh.,* **11,** 327

Thromboembolism

Hume, M., Sevitt, S. and Thomas, D. P. (1970). In: *Venous Thrombosis and Pulmonary Embolism*, 32–35 (Cambridge, Mass.: Harvard University Press)

Hurley, J. V. Substances promoting leukocyte emigration. *Ann. N.Y. Acad. Sci.*, 116, 918

Kaplan, A. P., Kay, B. A. and Austen, K. F. (1972). A prealbumin activator of prekallikrein. III. Appearance of chemotactic activity for human neutrophils by the conversion of human prekallikrein to kallikrein. *J. Exp. Med.*, 135, 81

Keller, H. N. and Sorkin, E. (1967). Studies on chemotaxis. V. On the chemotactic effect of bacteria. *Int. Arch. Allerg.*, 31, 505

Keller, H. N. and Sorkin, E. (1968). Chemotaxis of leucocytes. *Experientia*, 24, 641

Kjaerheim, A. and Hovig, T. (1962). The ultrastructure of hemostatic blood platelet plugs in rabbit mesenterium. *Thromb. Diath. Haemorrh.*, 7, 1

Kucinski, C. S., Fletcher, A. P. and Sherry, S. (1968). Effect of urokinase antiserum on plasminogen activators. Demonstration of immunologic dissimilarity between plasma plasminogen activator and urokinase. *J. Clin. Invest.*, 47, 1238

Kwaan, H. C. and Astrup, T. (1964). Fibrinolytic activity of reparative connective tissue. *J. Pathol. Bacteriol.*, 87, 409

Kwaan, H. C. and Astrup, T. (1965). Fibrinolytic activity in thrombosed veins. *Circ. Res.*, 17, 477

Lockhart-Mummery, P. (1924). Pulmonary embolism. *Brit. Med. J.*; 2, 850

Lutz, B. R., Fulton, G. P. and Akers, R. P. (1950). White thromboembolism in the transiluminated cheek pouch of the hamster following trauma, anticoagulant therapy, infection and malignant neoplasia. *Ant. Rec.*, 108, 544

Lynch, P. R., Stewart, G. J. and Ritchie, W. G. M. (1974). (Unpublished data)

McGovern, V. J. (1955). Reactions to injury of vascular endothelium with special reference to problems of thrombosis. *J. Pathol. Bacteriol.*, 69, 283

McGrath, J. M. and Stewart, G. J. (1969). The effects of endotoxin on vascular endothelium. *J. Exp. Med.*, 129, 833

Murray, T. S., Lorimer, A. R., Cox, F. C. and Lawrie, T. D. V. (1970). Leg-vein thrombosis following myocardial infarction. *Lancet*, ii, 792

Negus, D., Pinto, D. J., LeQuesne, L. P., Brown, N. and Chapman, M. (1968). 125I-labelled fibrinogen in the diagnosis of deep vein thrombosis and its correlation with phlebography. *Brit. J. Surg.*, 55, 835

Nicolaides, A. N. Kakkar, V. V., Field, E. S. and Renney, J. T. G. (1971a). The origin of deep vein thrombosis: a venographic study. *Brit. J. Radiol.*, 44, 653

Nicolaides, A. N., Kakkar, V. V., Renney, J. T. G., Kinder, P. H., Hutchison, D. C. S. and Clarke, M. B.(1971b). Myocardial infarction and deep vein thrombosis. *Brit. Med. J.*, 1, 432

Niemetz, J. and Fani, K. (1973). Thrombogenic activities of leukocytes. *Blood*, 42, 47

Niewiarowski, S., Bankowski, E. and Rogowicka, I. (1965). Studies on the absorption and activation of the Hageman factor (factor XII) by collagen and elastin. *Thromb. Diath. Haemorrh.*, 14, 398

Niewiarowski, S., Regoeczi, E. and Mustard, J. F. (1972a). Platelet interaction with fibrinogen and fibrin: comparison of the interaction of platelets with that of fibroblasts, leukocytes and erythrocytes. *Ann. N.Y. Acad. Sci.*, 201, 72

Niewiarowski, S., Regoeczi, E., Stewart, G. J., Senyi, A. F. and Mustard, J. F. (1972b). Platelet interaction with polymerising fibrin. *J. Clin. Invest.*, 665

Niewiarowski, S. and Goldstein, S. (1973). Interaction of cultured human fibroblasts with fibrin: Modification by drugs and aging *in vitro*. *J. Lab. Clin. Med.*, 605

Thromboembolism

Paterson, J. C. (1969). The pathology of venous thrombi. In: *Thrombosis*, 329 (S. Sherry, K. M. Brinkhouse, E. Genton and J. M. Stengle, editors) Washington D.C.: Nat. Acad. Sci.)

Paul, J. (1958). Establishment of permanent cell strains from human adult peripheral blood. *Nature (London)*, **182**, 808

Rahn, B. and Von Kaulla, K. N. (1964). Pharmacological induction of fibrinolytic activity in the dog. *Proc. Soc. Exp. Biol. Med.*, **115**, 359

Reichle, F. A., Stewart, G. J. and Essa, N. (1974). A transmission and scanning electron microscopic study of luminal surfaces in Dacron and autogenous vein by-passes in man and dog. *Surgery* (in press)

Ritchie, W. G. M., Lynch, P. R. and Stewart, G. J. (1973). (Unpublished data)

Roskam, J., Hughes, J., Bounameux, Y. and Salmon, J. (1959). The part played by platelets in the formation of an efficient hemostatic plug. *Thromb. Diath. Haemorrh.*, **3**, 510

Roskam, J. (1961). Role of platelets in the formation of a hemostatic plug. In: *Blood Platelets*, Henry Ford Hospital International Symposium on Blood Platelets, 153 (S. A. Johnson, editor) (Boston, Mass.: Little, Brown and Co.)

Samuels, P. B. and Webster, D. R. (1952). The role of venous endothelium in the inception of thrombosis. *Ann. Surg.*, **136**, 422

Scott, G. B. D. (1968). A quantitative study of the fate of occlusive red venous thrombi. *Brit. J. Exp. Pathol.*, **49**, 544

Sevitt, S. (1970). (Unpublished data. 1967–1969) Cited in: *Venous Thrombosis and Pulmonary Embolism*, 34–43 (M. Hume, S. Sevitt and D. P. Thomas, editors) (Mass.: Harvard University Press, Cambridge)

Shulman, M. H., Mode, R. K.; Kagen, R. and Fulton, G. P. (1954). Petechial susceptibility of the hamster cheek pouch subjected to negative pressure. *Anat. Rec.*, **118**, 408

Sorkin, E., Stecker, V. J. and Borel, J. F. (1970). Chemotaxis of leucocytes and inflammation. *Ser. Haematol.*, **III**, 131

Spaet, T. H. (1962). Studies on the *in vivo* behaviour of blood coagulation product I in rats. *Thromb. Diath. Haemorrh.*, **8**, 276

Spaet, T. H. and Erichson, R. B. (1966). The vascular wall in the pathogenesis of thrombosis. *Thromb. Diath. Haemorrh.*, **Suppl. 21**, 67

Spaet, T. D. and Ts'Ao, C. H. (1969). Vascular endothelium and thrombogenesis. In: *Thrombosis*, 416–436 (S. Sherry, K. M. Brinkhous, E. Genton and J. M. Stengle, editors) (Washington, D.C.: Nat. Acad. Sci.)

Stewart, G. J. and Anderson, M. J. (1971). An ultrastructural study of endotoxin induced changes in mesenteric arteries. *Brit. J. Exp. Pathol.*, **52**, 75

Stewart, G. J., Ritchie, W. G. M. and Lynch, P. R. (1973). A scanning and transmission electron microscopic study of canine jugular veins. Scanning electron microscopy (Part III). *Proceeding of the Workshop on Scanning Electron Microscopy in Pathology, IIT Research Institute, Chicago, Ill.*, April, 25

Stewart, G. J., Ritchie, W. G. M. and Lynch, P. R. (1974). (Unpublished data)

Stirling, G. A., Isapagos, M. T. and Girolami, P. L. (1966). Organisation of thrombi. *Brit. J. Surg.*, **53**, 232

Taylor, F. B. and Ward, P. A. (1967). Generation of chemotactic activity in rabbit serum by plasminogen–streptokinase mixtures. *J. Exp. Med.*, **126**, 149

Tedder, E. and Shorey, C. D. (1965). The fine structure of rabbit inferior vena cava. *Aust. J. Exp. Biol. Med. Sci.*, **43**, 99

Thromboembolism

Tragardh, B. (1973). (Personal communication)

Tribe, C. R. (1963). Causes of death in the early and late stages of paraplegia. *Paraplegia*, **1**, 19

Ts'Ao, C. H. and Spaet, T. D. (1967). Ultramicroscopic changes in the rabbit inferior vena cava following partial constriction. *Amer. J. Pathol.*, **51**, 789

Virchow, R. (1860). Metastatical dyscrasiae. *Lectures in Cellular Pathology*, 196–229 (Churchill)

Walker, W. S., Barlet, R. . and Kurtz, H. M. (1969). Isolation and partial characterization of a staphylococcal leukocyte cytotoxin. *J. Bacteriol.*, **97**, 1005

Walsh, P. N. (1972a). The role of platelets in the contact phase of blood coagulation. *Brit. J. Haematol.*, **22**, 237

Walsh, P. N. (1972b). The effects of collagen and kaolin on the intrinsic coagulant activity of platelets. Evidence for an alternative pathway in intrinsic coagulation not requiring factor XII. *Brit. J. Haematol.*, **22**, 393

Walsh, P. N. and Biggs, P. (1972). The role of patients in intrinsic factor-Xa formation. *Brit. J. Haematol.*, **22**, 743

Ward, P. A. (1967). A plasmin-split fragment of C`3 as a new chemotactic factor. *J. Exp. Med.*, **126**, 189

Ward, P. A., Lepow, I. H. and Newman, L. J. (1968). Bacterial factors chemotactic for polymorphonuclear leukocytes. *Amer. J. Pathol.*, **52**, 725

Ward, P. A. (1972). Natural and synthetic inhibitors of leukotaxis. In: *Inflammation Mechanisms and Control*, 301–310 (Lepow and Ward, editors) (New York and London: Academic Press)

Ward, P. A., Cohen, S. and Flanagan, T. D. (1972). Leukotactic factors elaborated by virus-infected tissues. *J. Exp. Med.*, **135**, 1095

Warren, B. A. and Brock, L. J. (1964). The electron microscopic features and fibrinolytic properties of neointima. *Brit. J. Exp. Pathol.*, **45**, 612

Weiner, J. and Spiro, D. (1962). Electron microscope studies in experimental thrombosis. *Exp. Molec. Pathol.*, **1**, 554

Wessler, S. (1952). Studies in intravascular coagulation. I. Coagulation changes in isolated venous segments. *J. Clin. Invest.*, **31**, 1011

Wessler, S. (1955). Studies in intravascular coagulation. III. The pathogenesis of serum-induced venous thrombosis. *J. Clin. Invest.*, **34**, 647

Wessler, S., Reimer, S. M. and Sheps, M. C. (1959). Biologic assay of a thrombosis inducing activity in human serum. *J. Appl. Physiol.*, **14**, 943

Wessler, S. (1962). Thrombosis in the presence of vascular stasis. *Amer. J. Med.*, **33**, 648

Wessler, S., Freiman, D. G., Ballon, J. D., Katz, J. H., Wolff, R. and Wolf, E. (1967). Experimental pulmonary embolism with serum-induced thrombi. *Amer. J. Pathol.*, **38**, 89

Williams-Kretschmer, K. and Majno, G. (1969). Ischemia of the skin. An electron microscopic study of vascular injury. *Amer. J. Pathol.*, **54**, 327

Wolman, L. (1965). The disturbance of circulation in traumatic paraplegia in acute and late stages: A pathological study. *Paraplegia*, **2**, 213

Zucker, M. B. (1947). Platelet agglutination and vasoconstriction as factors in spontaneous hemostasis in normal, thrombocytopenic and heparinized. *Amer. J. Physiol.*, **148**, 275

Zucker, M. B. and Borelli (1962). Platelet clumping produced by connective tissue suspensions and by collagen. *Proc. Soc. Exp. Biol. Med.*, **109**, 779

9

Venous stasis* in the lower limb

A. N. Nicolaides

Evidence has been presented in previous chapters (2, 7 and 8) that stasis predisposes and facilitates deep venous thrombosis though it cannot initiate it on its own. This is because stasis prevents the clearance of activated clotting factors arriving from a distance or produced locally (Chapters 2 and 7) and induces endothelial damage by white cells when tissue trauma is present at a distant site (Chapter 8).

The purpose of this chapter is to discuss the factors responsible for stasis in the lower limb, the sites it occurs and the efficacy of various methods which are believed to prevent it.

FACTORS PRODUCING VENOUS STASIS

Venous stasis may be produced by diminished limb perfusion, venous dilatation, failure of the action of the peripheral pump, gravity and obstruction of the veins. In most patients in hospital several of these factors are present simultaneously and it is not surprising that venous stasis is considerable in their limbs.

Diminished limb perfusion may be the result of a fall in the cardiac output, occlusive arterial disease or an increase in the peripheral resistance. A fall in the cardiac output may occur during operation or in clinical conditions such as myocardial infarction and hypovolaemia. An increase in the peripheral resistance occurs with age (Allwood, 1958) and in patients with high blood viscosity. A 10 per cent increase in blood viscosity is associated with an over 20 per cent decrease in limb perfusion (Dormandy, 1971;

*The term 'stasis' is used in this chapter to mean reduced velocity.

137

Chapter 6). Retarded flow increases blood viscosity (Wells, 1969) which causes further increase in the peripheral resistance. A high concentration of fibrinogen and particularly high molecular weight fibrinogen complexes which occur in 'hypercoagulable' states and after operation (Chapter 4), a high haematocrit and polycythaemia (Chapters 5 and 6) are factors responsible for elevated blood viscocity. Occlusive arterial disease will reduce the arterial perfusion of a limb and therefore the venous return. *Venous dilatation* may occur as a result of drugs such as halothane and pethidine; it may also occur passively during recumbency (Lundbrook and Loughlin, 1964) or in patients with cardiac failure as a result of

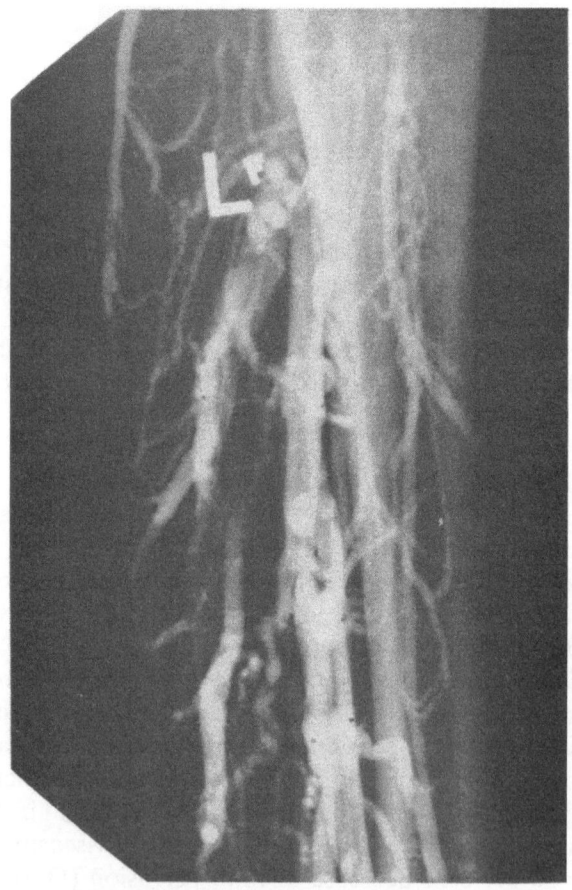

Figure 9.1 Long and spindle-shaped soleal veins

increased intraluminar pressure.

The peripheral pump consists of the soleus muscle and its veins. Cinephlebographic studies (Almen and Nylander, 1962) have demonstrated that the soleal veins fill during relaxation and empty during contraction. Because of the valves present in the axial veins, the soleal veins are filled with blood from the tibial veins and the blood expelled is directed proximally. The action of the peripheral pump is abolished during anaesthesia, in paralysed and in inactive limbs. It is ineffective when the valves of the axial veins are damaged.

The effect of gravity on the flow of blood in the veins depends on posture. Venous velocity in the axial veins of the lower limb, measured by an injection of ^{24}NaCl (Wright and Osborn, 1952) is halved when the subject stands or sits when compared with that in the supine position. Venous

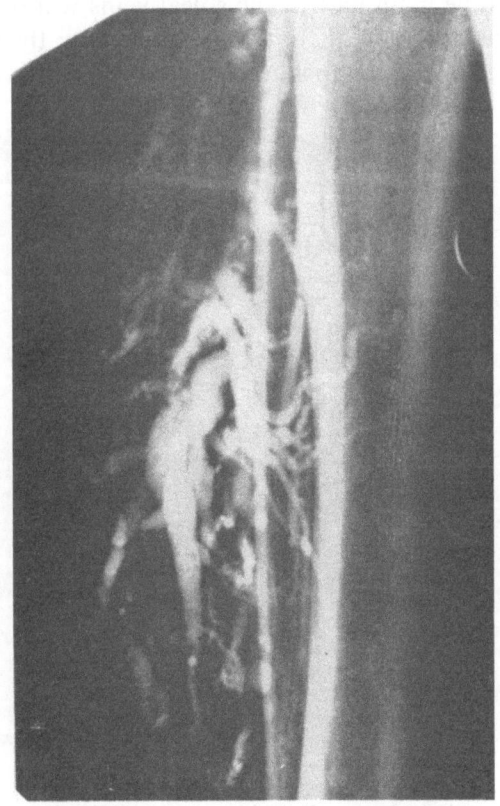

Figure 9.2 Short and bag-like soleal veins

velocity is doubled when the subject is tipped head downwards or after vigorous repeated plantar-flexion of the foot. The anatomical arrangement of the soleal veins is such that marked stasis occurs in them also when the patient is supine and immobile. The soleal veins are either long and spindle-shaped (Figure 9.1) or short and bag-like (Figure 9.2). They may be over one centimetre in diameter. They are usually arranged in two groups, the smaller in the upper part and the larger in the lower part of the soleus muscle; often they are double, one for each belly of the muscle and very rarely contain valves. They are connected proximally and distally to the posterior tibial veins, thus forming arcades (Figure 9.3). In some venograms (this is more obvious in stereoscopic views) the distal part of the soleal veins has been seen to be connected to the superficial system (Figure 9.4). Such **anastomotic** veins are rare but have been described in the past (Le Dentu, 1867; Limborgh, 1961, 1961a; Andel, 1967). When the leg is horizontal the main part of the soleal veins will be dependent and unless the soleus contracts there will be little flow through them. The efficacy of the peripheral pump is at its highest when the venous valves are

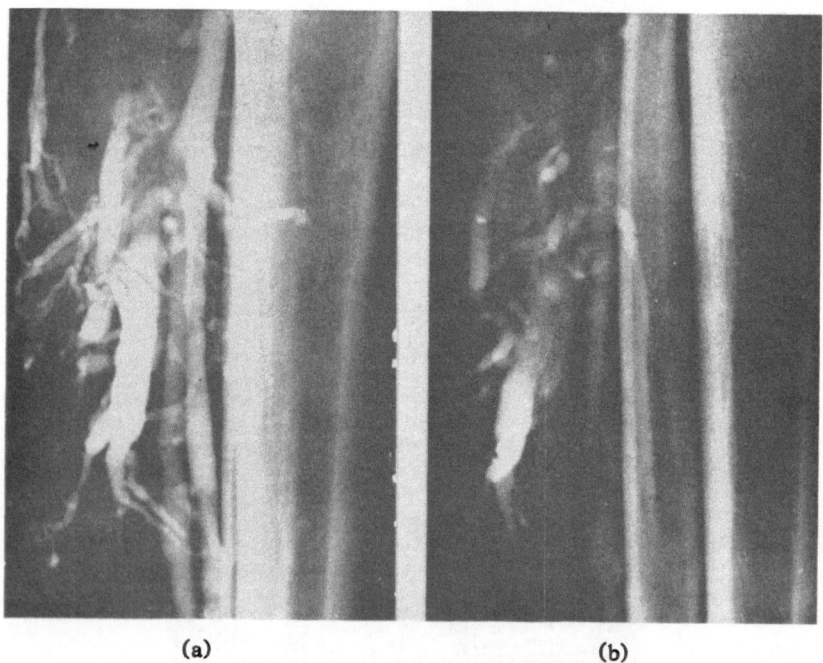

(a) (b)

Figure 9.3 (a) Soleal and tibial veins filled with contrast medium just before releasing the mid-thigh cuff. (b) One minute after the mid-thigh cuff has been released

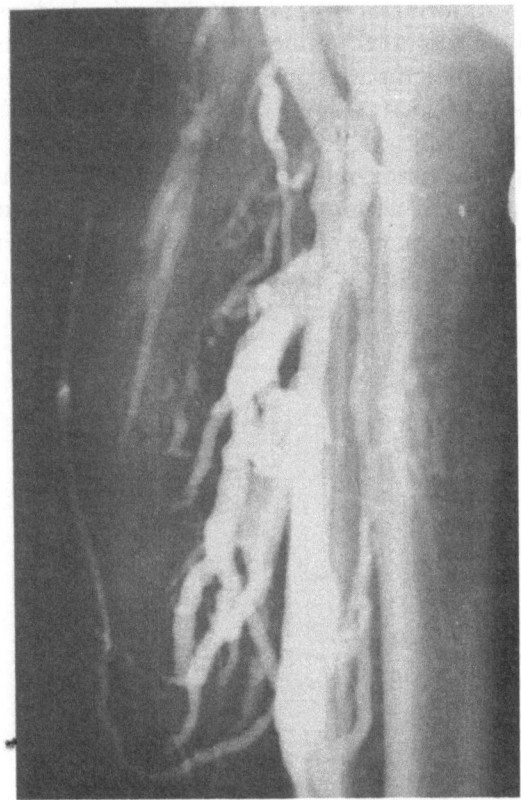

Figure 9.4 Direct communication between soleal and superficial veins

competent, the limbs are dependent and plantar flexion of the foot is against resistance (Nicolaides *et al.*, 1971; Nicolaides, 1972; Nicolaides *et al.*, 1972a). When the limbs are dependent maximum filling of the soleal veins will occur and muscle contraction will result in a maximum stroke volume.

Obstruction of veins will produce stasis distally. Obstruction may be the result of thrombosis or of extra-mural compression by haematoma, pelvic tumours, lymph nodes involved by malignant disease, retroperitoneal fibrosis and lymphocyst. Compression of the left common iliac vein by the right common iliac artery is not uncommon.

VENOUS STASIS IN CLINICAL SITUATIONS

Axial velocity is greatly reduced when the limbs are horizontal and still (Wright *et al.*, 1951; Dodd and Cocket, 1956; McLachlin *et al.*, 1960) and at the end of operation (Doran *et al.*, 1964). During bed rest axial velocity progressively falls reaching a minimum at 7–14 days. This fall does not occur in ambulant patients after operation (Wright *et al.*, 1951). Reduction in the resting arterial perfusion of the calf also occurs after surgery and any increase due to physical activity is transient (Browse, 1962a; 1962b).

The changes in the blood velocity of the femoral vein during operation have been investigated with an ultrasonic doppler blood flow detector (Doptone) (Nicolaides, 1974) in 10 patients undergoing simple mastectomy. The flat probe of this instrument was fixed to the skin over

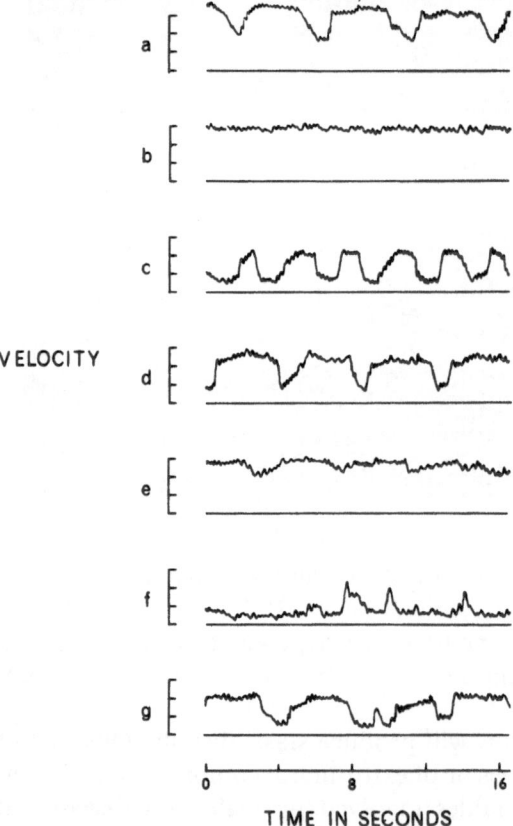

VELOCITY

TIME IN SECONDS

Figure 9.5 Changes in the femoral vein velocity (in arbitrary units) during simple mastectomy. The tracings have been obtained at different stages during the operation. (a) Just before induction of anaesthesia (b) During the application of sterile drapes; spontaneous breathing (c) Patient paralysed; hand-ventilated by anaesthetist (d) On positive pressure ventilator; tidal volume 500 ml (e) As in (d) but with negative phase (f) Patient waking up at the end of the operation; breath holding (g) Patient conscious in the recovery room; spontaneous breathing

the femoral vein in the groin. A continuous recording of mean blood velocity was obtained via a pen recorder. The response of this instrument to blood velocity has been shown to be linear (Sampson *et al.*, 1970) and although blood velocity cannot be measured in absolute units, changes in blood velocity can be measured with an experimental error not greater than ± 10 per cent. The changes in the mean blood velocity in the femoral vein before the induction of anaesthesia and during operation are demonstrated in Figure 9.5. The effect of spontaneous breathing and positive pressure ventilation with and without a negative phase is also illustrated. The results indicate that blood velocity in the femoral vein is phasic with respiration. There is also a progressive fall in the mean blood velocity during the operation with marked variation according to type of ventilation.

The clearance time of contrast medium in the deep veins of the leg was prolonged when the limb was horizontal in concious patients undergoing pyelography and during operation (McLachlin *et al.*, 1960; Hodgson, 1964). Leg elevation and vigorous voluntary contractions of the thigh and calf muscles reduced the clearance time to less than one third.

Necropsy studies have demonstrated a direct relationship between deep venous thrombosis and the length of bed rest (Gibbs, 1957; Sevitt and Gallagher, 1961; Roberts, 1963). They have also suggested that thrombi begin at valve pockets, vein junctions and sinuses (Sevitt and Gallagher, 1959; Diener, 1971; Chapter 10). Diminished flow in the axial veins will increase the amount of stasis and turbulance in valve pockets (McLachlin *et al.*, 1960; Cotton and Clarke, 1965).

STASIS IN SOLEAL VEINS AND ITS PREVENTION
Recent studies using the ^{125}I-fibrinogen test during the first week after operation and venography have demonstrated that most thrombi start in the calf (Flanc *et al.*, 1968; Negus *et al.*, *1968; Nicolaides, 1972; Chapter* 11) and particularly the soleal veins (Nicolaides *et al.*, 1970; Nicolaides *et al.*, 1971a; Nicolaides, 1972; Chapter 11). Therefore, it seemed appropriate to investigate stasis in this region. The greatest difficulty in the past has been the lack of a venographic technique which demonstrated the soleal veins consistently. A technique has been developed which has overcome this difficulty (Nicolaides, 1972; Nicolaides *et al.*, 1972a; 1972b). Briefly, the patient lies horizontal on the X-ray table. A scalp-vein infusion needle is introduced into a vein on the dorsum of the foot. A 5 cm wide pneumatic cuff is placed at the ankle to prevent any filling of the superficial leg veins and a similar cuff is placed on the mid-thigh to occlude the

femoral vein. The veins of the leg are first partially emptied by a lightly applied elastocrepe bandage. The ankle cuff is then inflated to 120 mmHg and the mid-thigh cuff to 200 mmHg. This does not occlude the arterial blood flow because of the narrowness of the cuff. The injection of 45 per cent sodium diatrizoate is commenced and the bandage is removed. The contrast medium is seen on the image intensifier to ascend in the tibial veins and to fill the soleal veins in a retrograde fashion. After injecting 30 ml to fill the soleal and tibial veins the injection is stopped, the mid-thigh cuff is removed, and the clearance time of contrast medium is measured using a stopwatch.

This technique was used in 46 conscious patients who had normal veins. Venography was performed in these patients in order to prove or disprove the clinical diagnosis of deep venous thrombosis. Patients with thrombi, oedema or cellulitis were excluded. When the leg was horizontal and immobile the tibial veins emptied first, while contrast medium remained in the soleal veins on an average for 10 min (Figure 9.6). The marked degree of stasis in the soleal veins may explain why the majority of thrombi start in the soleal and not in the tibial veins; This study has also demonstrated that there is no correlation between age and the rate of emptying of the soleal veins (Figure 9.7) as previously suggested (McLachlin *et al.*, 1960). Therefore the higher incidence of deep venous thrombosis associated with elderly patients may be related to factors

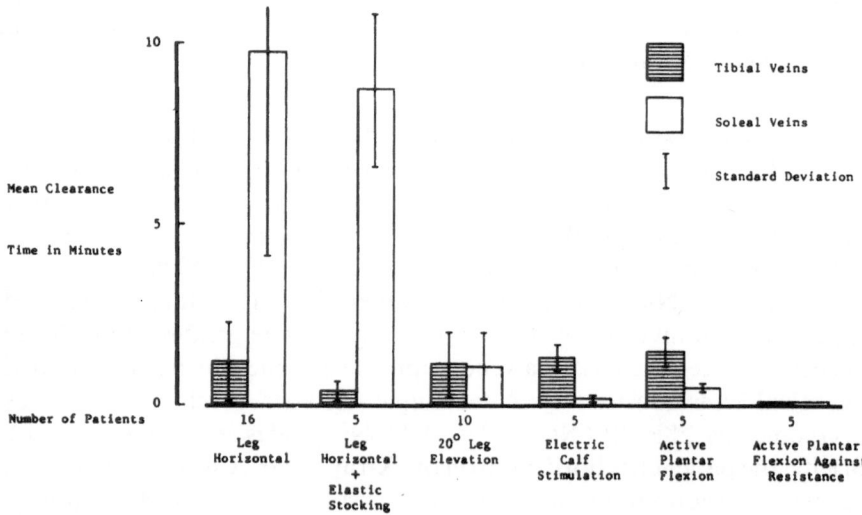

Figure 9.6 The effect of methods believed to prevent stasis on the clearance of sodium diatrizoate from tibial and soleal veins

144

Thromboembolism

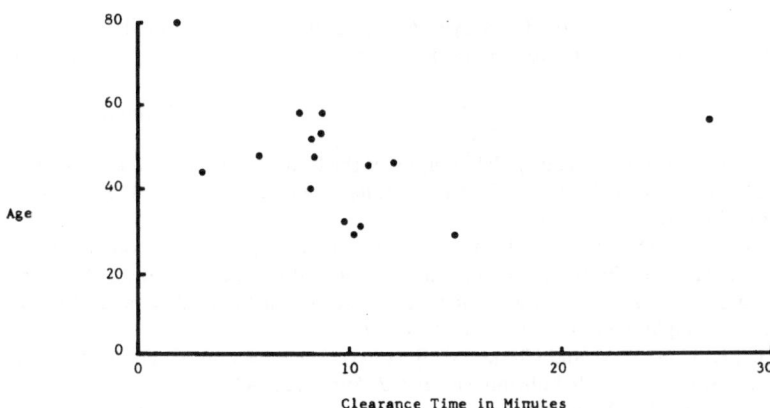

Figure 9.7 Lack of correlation between age and clearance time of contrast medium from the soleal veins

other than stasis. Elastic stockings had a small effect in hastening the clearance of contrast medium from the tibial veins and had no effect on the emptying of the soleal veins. These results would be compatible with the work of Makin and his colleagues who showed that 'Tubigrip' increases the velocity of venous return in the legs (Makin *et al.*, 1969) and would also explain why elastic stockings had no effect on the incidence of deep venous thrombosis (Rosengarten *et al.*, 1970; Browse *et al.*, 1974). Stasis in the soleal veins, however, was prevented by 20 degree leg elevation, active plantar flexion of the foot and electrical calf stimulation. It appears that active plantar flexion is more effective than leg elevation in preventing stasis in the soleal veins. From the methods studied the best ones to prevent stasis in the soleal veins are active plantar flexion against resistance in the conscious patient and electrical calf muscle stimulation in the unconcious patient (Figure 9.6). These findings provide some guidance to the worth of physical methods used by physiotherapists before and after operation. Their value in preventing deep venous thrombosis will be discussed in Chapter 14.

References

Allwood, M. J. (1958). Blood flow in the foot and calf in the elderly; a comparison with that in young adults. *Clin. Science*, **17**, 331

Almen and Nylander (1962). Serial phlebography of the normal lower leg during muscular contraction and relaxation. *Acta Radiol.*, **57**, 264

Andel, Z. (1967). Scheme anatomo-clinique de la localisation des veines communicantes insuffisante de l'extremite inferieure. *Societe Francaise de Phlebologie*, **1**, 19

Browse, N. L. (1962a). Effect of bedrest on resting calf blood flow of healthy adult males. *Brit. Med. J.*, **1**, 721

Browse, N. L. (1962b). Effect of surgery on resting calf blood flow. *Brit. Med. J.*, **1**, 1714

Thromboembolism

Browse, N. L., Jackson, B. T., Mayo, M. E. and Negus, D. (1974). The value of mechanical methods of preventing postoperative calf vein thrombosis. *Brit. J. Surg.*, **61**, 219

Cotton, L. T. and Clarke, C. (1965). Anatomical localisation of venous thrombosis. *Ann. Roy. Coll. Surg. Engl.*, **36**, 214

Diener, L. (1971). Intraosseous phlebography of the lower limb. *Acta Radiol.*, **Suppl. 304**

Dodd, H. and Cockett, F. B. (1956). *The Pathology and Surgery of the Veins of the Lower Limb* (Edinburgh and London: Livingstone)

Doran, F. S. A., Drury, M. and Sivyer, A. (1964). A simple way to combat the venous stasis which occurs in the lower limbs during surgical operations. *Brit. J. Surg.*, **51**, 486

Dormandy, J. A. (1971). Influence of blood viscosity on blood flow and effect of low molecular weight dextran. *Brit. Med. J.*, **4**, 716

Flanc, C., Kakkar, V. V. and Clarke, M. B. (1968). The detection of venous thrombosis of the legs using 125I-labelled fibrinogen. *Brit. J. Surg.*, **55**, 742

Gibbs, N. M. (1957). Venous thrombosis of the lower limbs with particular reference to bedrest. *Brit. J. Surg.*, **45**, 209

Hodgson, D. C. (1964). Venous stasis during surgery. *Anaesthesia*, **19**, 96

Le Dentu, A. (1867). *Circulation Veineuse du Pied el la Jambe* (Thesis No. 276, Paris)

Limborgh, J. van (1961). Demonstration d'un modele anatomique des veines du membre inferieur. *Bull. Soc. Sc. Med. Luxemb.*, **98**, 247

Limborgh, J. van (1961a). L'anatomie due systeme veineux de l'extremite inferieure en relation avec la pathologie variqueuse. *Fol. Angiol.*, **8**, 240

Lundbrook, J. and Loughlin, J. (1964). Regulation of volume in postarteriolar vessels of the lower limb. *Amer. Heart J.*, **67**, 493

Makin, G. S., Mayes, F. B. and Holroyd, A. M. (1969). Clinical and experimental studies on the effects of calf compression on deep venous flow-rates and thrombosis. *Brit. J. Surg.*, **56**, 369

McLachlin, A. D., McLachlin, J. A., Jory, T. and Rawlings, E. G. (1960). Venous stasis in the lower extremities. *Ann. Surg.*, **152**, 678

Negus, D., Pinto, D. J., Le Quesne, L. P., Brown, N. and Chapman, M. (1968). 125I-labelled fibrinogen in the diagnosis of deep-vein thrombosis and its correlation with phlebography. *Brit. J. Surg.*, **55**, 835

Nicolaides, A. N., Kakkar, V. V. and Renney, J. T. G. (1970). The soleal sinuses. Origin of deep-vein thrombosis. *Brit. J. Surg.*, **57**, 860

Nicolaides, A. N., Kakkar, V. V. and Renney, J. T. G. (1971). Soleal sinuses and stasis. *Brit. J. Surg.*, **58**, 307

Nicolaides, A. N., Kakkar, V. V., Field, E. S. and Renney, J. T. G. (1971a). The origin of deep-vein thrombosis: a venographic study. *Brit. J. Radiol.*, **44**, 653

Nicolaides, A. N. (1972). *The Prevention of Postoperative Deep Venous Thrombosis* (Jacksonian Prize Essay)

Nicolaides, A. N., Kakkar, V. V., Field, E. S. and Fish, P. (1972a). Venous stasis and deep-vein thrombosis. *Brit. J. Surg.*, **59**, 714

Nicolaides, A. N., Kakkar, V. V., Field, E. S. and Fish, P. (1972b). Soleal veins, stasis and prevention of deep-vein thrombosis. Chapter in Kabi: *Thromboembolism*, (V. V. Kakkar and J. Juhar editors) (Churchill – Livingstone)

Nicolaides, A. N. (1974). Unpublished data

Roberts, G. H. (1963). Venous thrombosis in hospital patients: A post-mortem study. *Scot. Med. J.*, **8**, 11

Thromboembolism

Rosengarten, D. S., Laird, J., Jeyasingh, K. and Martin, P. C. (1970). The failure of compression stockings (Tubigrip) to prevent deep venous thrombosis after operation. *Brit. J. Surg.*, **57**, 296

Sampson, D., Papadimitriou, M., Kulatilake, A. E. (1970). Ultrasonic blood flow measurement in haemodialysis. *Brit. Med. J.*, **1**, 340

Sevitt, S. and Gallagher, N. G. (1959). Prevention of venous thrombosis and pulmonary embolism in injured patients: A trial of anticoagulant prophylaxis with phenindione in middle-aged and elderly patients with fractured necks of femur. *Lancet*, **ii**, 981

Sevitt, S. and Gallagher, N. G. (1961). Venous thrombosis and pulmonary embolism: A clinico-pathological study in injured and burned patients. *Brit. J. Surg.*, **48**, 495

Wells, R. E. (1969). Rheological aspects of stasis in thrombus formation. In: *Thrombosis*, 469 (S. Sherry *et al.*, editors) (Washington, D.C.: National Academy of Sciences)

Wright, H. P., Osborn, S. B. and Edmunds, D. G. (1951). Effects of postoperative bedrest and early ambulation on the rate of venous blood flow. *Lancet*, **i**, 222

Wright, P. A. and Osborn, S. B. (1952). Effect of posture on venous velocity, measured with ^{24}Na Cl. *Brit. Heart J.*, **14**, 325

10

Origin and distribution of venous thrombi studied by postmortem intraosseous phlebography

L. Diener

INTRODUCTION

Pulmonary embolism is a major cause of death in geriatric patients, especially when they are submitted to operation. Most emboli originate in the deep veins of the lower limbs.

In clinical practice venography is accepted as the best method for exact anatomical localisation of thrombi (Chapters 11 and 19). However, for more extensive investigations of the frequency and morphology of venous thromboembolism, autopsy studies with complete venous dissection of the lower extremities are desirable. In order to facilitate the exploration of the veins of the lower limbs, intraosseous venography (Drassner, 1946; Arnoldi and Bauer, 1960) was adopted at Stureby Sjukhus Geriatric Unit as a new procedure for postmortem studies (Lund *et al.*, 1969). The purpose of this chapter is to present the distribution and extent of venous thrombi and pulmonary emboli found at postmortem examination in geriatric patients and discuss their significance.

METHOD

The postmortem technique of intraosseous venography has been described in detail elsewhere (Diener, 1971). Briefly the method is as follows: The cadaver is placed on a tilting table and fixed with a belt across the thorax. The table is tipped legs down to form an angle of 60 degrees to horizontal to avoid layering of contrast medium (Lindblom, 1941; Greitz, 1954). A tourniquet is placed at the ankle to prevent filling of the superficial venous system. Barium sulphate suspension (300–400 ml) containing 0·1 g barium sulphate per ml is injected into each calcaneum (Figure 10.1). Anteroposterior and lateral films are taken with an exposure between 50 mA by 60 kV and 10 mA by 85 kV at a constant film distance of 1 metre.

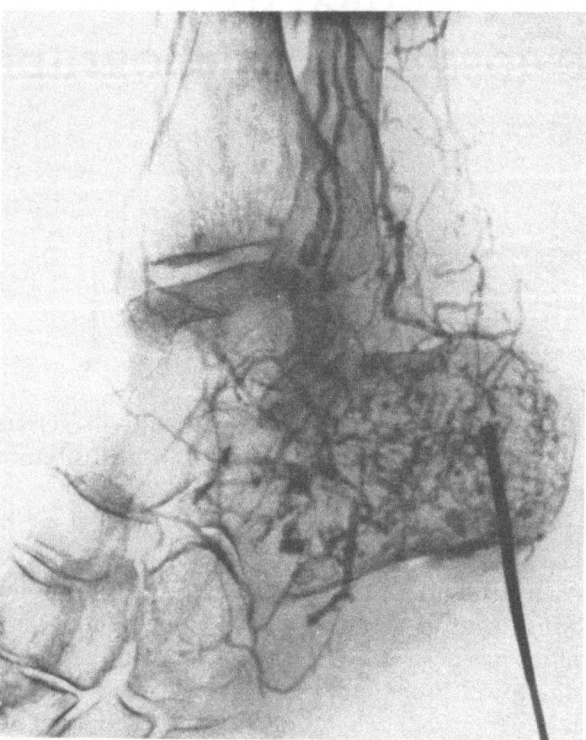

Figure 10.1 Contrast medium injected into the calcaneum. It is seen in the sinusoids of cancellous bone from which it passes directly into deep veins of the leg

During the development of the method the veins of the legs were dissected down to the ankles to compare venographic and autopsy findings. Venography provided comprehensive and accurate information on the site and size of venous thrombi (Diener, 1971). Figure 10.2 shows an example of this comparison.

Two anatomical regions of the lower limb present special problems in detecting thrombi by intraosseous venography. The first consists of the muscular veins of the lower leg and the second of the deep femoral vein, both of which are not often demonstrated. They are filled inconsistently, even during clinical venography (Rogoff and De Weese, 1960; Arroldi,

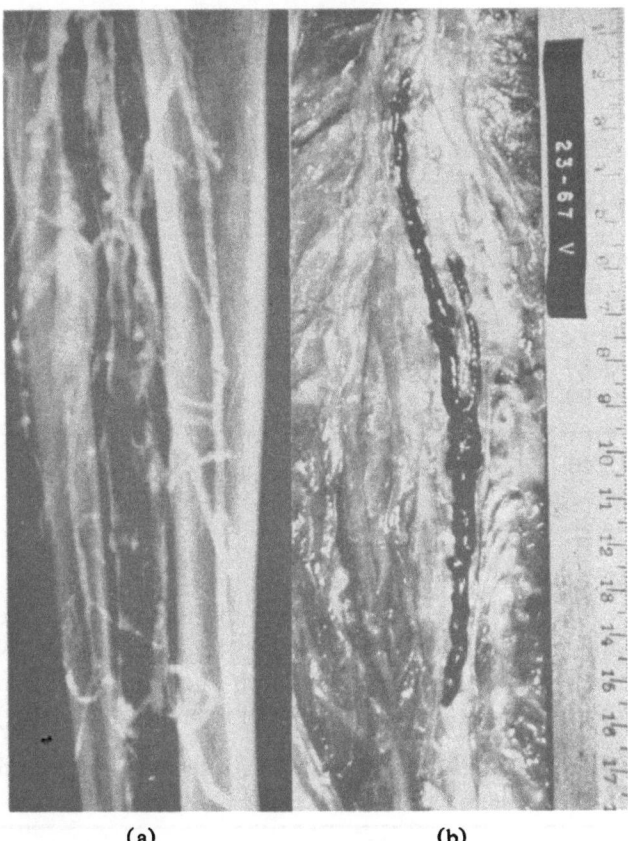

(a)   (b)

Figure 10.2 Striking correspondence between (a) venographic and (b) pathological demonstration of a 14 cm long thrombus in peroneal vein branched in its proximal portion

1961; Britton, 1964; Cotton and Clark, 1965). In the present series the muscular veins of the lower leg often were not filled with contrast medium. Although a better filling could be obtained with the cadaver horizontal, the semivertical position was used to avoid layering, and the muscular veins were explored by sectioning the calf at short intervals (1–2 cm). However, failure to detect small thrombi in the muscular veins in a few cadavers could not be definitely excluded.

The branches of the pulmonary artery were also dissected down to a diameter of approximately 2 mm in search of pulmonary emboli.

MATERIAL
The reported findings are based on 400 autopsies. Intraosseous venography

of the lower limbs was performed prior to dissection. In 5 cases one of the legs had been amputated. The distribution of the material according to age and sex is shown in Table 10.1.

Table 10.1 The distribution of the 400 cases studied according to age and sex

Age group	Men	Women	Total
50–59	2	2	4
60–69	10	5	15
70–79	59	44	103
80–89	75	147	222
90–99	24	32	56
Total	170	230	400
Mean age	81·0	83·3	82·3

RESULTS

Frequency of thrombi. Thrombosis was found in 187 (47 per cent) of 400 autopsies and in 286 (36 per cent) of 795 limbs examined. Ninety-nine patients (25 per cent) had bilateral thrombi. There was no difference in the incidence of thrombosis between men and women (Table 10.2).

Table 10.2 The distribution of the cases with thrombosis according to age and sex (number of legs within brackets)

Age group	Men	Women	Total
50–59	0	0	0
60–69	2 (4)	4 (6)	6 (10)
70–79	23 (36)	22 (31)	45 (67)
80–89	36 (54)	73 (114)	109 (168)
90–99	11 (17)	16 (24)	27 (41)
Total	72 (111)	115 (175)	187 (286)

Localisation and distribution of thrombi. The localisation and distribution of thrombi in the lower limbs is shown in Figures 10.3–10.5. Figure 10.3 denotes continuous and Figure 10.4 discontinuous thrombi.

Of the 53 limbs which had continuous thrombi confined to the calf

152

(Figure 10.3), 6 had additional distinct thrombi in some other deep vein of the lower leg. As the continuous thrombi were predominant, they were all presented as one group.

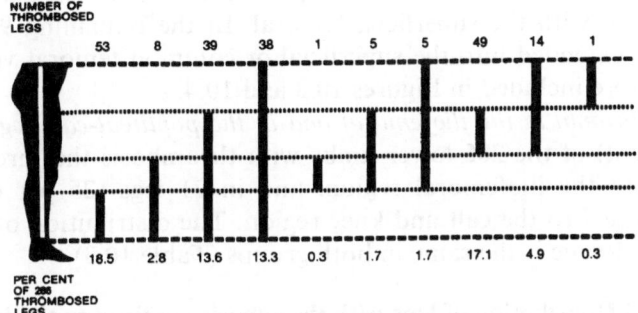

Figure 10.3 Localisation and distribution of continuous thrombi in 213 legs. The horizontal fields represent iliac, femoral, popliteal and calf regions

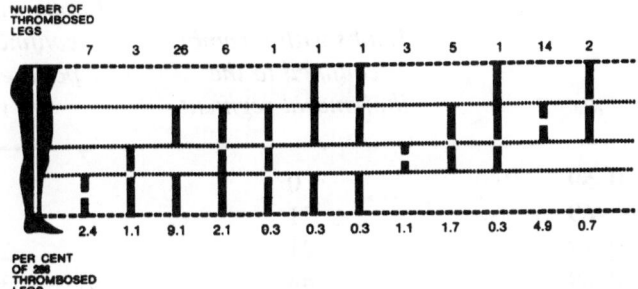

Figure 10.4 Localisation and distribution of discontinuous thrombi in 70 legs. The horizontal fields represent iliac, femoral, popliteal and calf regions.

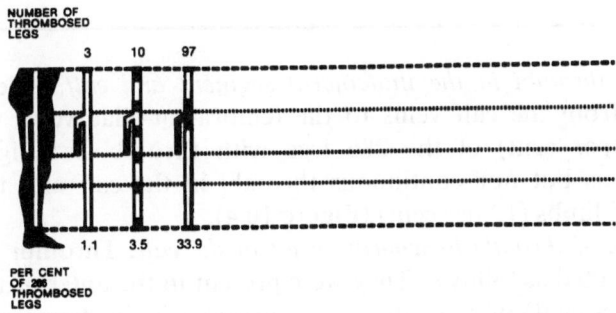

Figure 10.5 Localisation and distribution of thrombi in deep femoral vein and coexisting thrombi in other deep veins in 110 legs. The horizontal fields represent iliac, femoral, popliteal and calf regions.

153

Thrombi in the deep femoral vein. Of 286 legs with thrombosis 110 (38 per cent) had a thrombus in the deep femoral vein (Figure 10.5). Only 3 of these 110 legs had an isolated thrombus in this region. In 10 legs there was a thrombus in the deep femoral vein which did not reach the junction with the superficial femoral. In the remaining 97 legs the thrombus extended into the superficial or common femoral vein. These 107 legs were included in Figures 10.3 and 10.4.

Isolated thrombi in the iliofemoral and in the popliteal-calf region. In 80 (29 per cent) of the 286 lower limbs with thrombosis the thrombi were localised to the iliofemoral region, and in 71 legs (25 per cent) they were confined to the calf and knee region. The distribution of the cases according to age is the same in both groups (Table 10.3).

Table 10.3 Distribution of legs with thrombosis confined to the iliofemoral, and the popliteal-lower leg region

Age group	Limbs with thrombi confined to the iliofemoral segment	Limbs with thrombi confined to the popliteal-lower leg region
50–59	0	0
60–69	1	1
70–79	21	24
80–89	46	39
90–99	12	7
Total	80	71

Coexisting thrombi in the iliofemoral segment and calf. A continuous thrombus from the calf veins to the femoral or iliac veins was found in 77 (27 per cent) of the 286 legs with thrombosis (Figure 10.3). Simultaneous but non-continuous thrombi in the calf and thigh were found in 35 limbs (12 per cent) (Figure 10.4).

Distribution of thrombi in separate veins of the calf. Thrombi in the calf were distributed as follows: They were present in the anterior tibial veins in 47 (26 per cent) of 183 calves with thrombosis, in the peroneal veins in 148 legs (81 per cent) and in the posterior tibial veins in 108 legs (59 per cent). Thrombi in the muscular veins were found in 35 lower legs (19 per

154

cent). Isolated thrombi solely localised to the muscular veins of the calf were noted in 12 legs (4·1 per cent), 5 on the right and 7 on the left.

Multiple thrombi. Many of the legs had two or more separate thrombi. To this group belong the 70 limbs with discontinuous thrombi shown in Figure 10.4 and also the 6 legs, mentioned earlier, which had both continuous and simultaneous but non-continuous thrombi in the calf.

Thrombi in valve pockets. In the early stages of this study attention was not directed to the very small thrombi often located in valve pockets. It is therefore possible that some may not have been detected at autopsy. Only the X-ray films remain for re-examination. However, some incipient thrombi could have been masked by contrast medium or misinterpreted

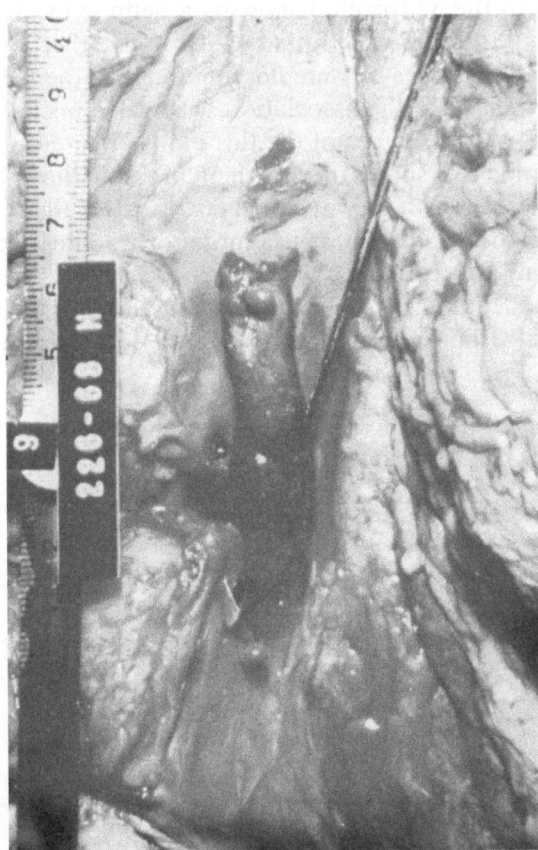

Figure 10.6 Remnant of a thrombus presumed to have formed in a valve pocket in the femoral vein. A probe is inserted into the pocket. Note the fractured edge of the thrombus. Needle-heads have been placed immediately under the valve pocket and at the fractured end of the thrombus.

as postmortem clots. Because of these sources of error, only thrombi demonstrated to be localised in venous valve pockets by dissection in the last 300 cases are presented here. In these cases the total incidence of thrombosis in the deep veins of the leg was 146 (48 per cent). Out of the 596 legs examined venous thrombi were found in 229 (38 per cent). In 32 of the latter (5·4 per cent), a definite thrombus related to a valve pocket was noted. Altogether, 37 such thrombi were encountered, which were either confined to the pocket or had their distal end in a pocket. None of the thrombi ending in valve pockets occluded the lumen completely, but some of them had a rugged, 'fractured' proximal end (Figure 10.6) and in these cases pulmonary emboli were found.

In addition to the 37 thrombi showing a definite localisation to valve pockets, 9 small thrombi were found which were either localised but not adherent to valve pockets or were floating freely in the lumen just above a pocket. In some cases the association with valve pockets was revealed by impressions on the surface of the thrombus apparently caused by the valve cusps. Table 10.4 shows the length of all the 46 thrombi with definite or presumed localisation to valve pockets. Most of them were found in the veins having the widest lumen (femoral or popliteal). Small thrombi (less than 2 cm) not associated with valve pockets were extremely rare. It should be added that in the lower leg veins the possible association of thrombi to valve pockets was more difficult to establish for technical reasons.

Table 10.4 Length of 46 thrombi located within or having their distal end in valve pockets

Length of thrombi	2 cm or less	2 to 5 cm	5 cm or more
Number	33	9	5
Per cent	71·7	19·7	10·9

Distribution of thrombi in right and left leg. The distribution of thrombi in the right and left leg is shown in Table 10.5. In men, the incidence of thrombosis was the same on both sides. In women there was a higher incidence on the left side but this difference was not statistically significant.

156

Table 10.5 Case distribution according to side of thrombosis

Legs involved	Right only	Left only	Bilateral	Total
Men	16	17	39	72
Women	24	31	60	115
Total	40	48	99	187

Pulmonary embolism. Pulmonary emboli were recorded in 83 (22 per cent) of the 400 cases. There was no significant difference in the frequency of pulmonary embolism in various age groups or between men and women. The diameter of the emboli was classified as large in 50 cases (60 per cent) and small in 33 cases (40 per cent). By definition, 'large' pulmonary emboli were those·with a diameter equal to or larger than the lumen of the superficial femoral vein of the same patient (Figure 10.7).

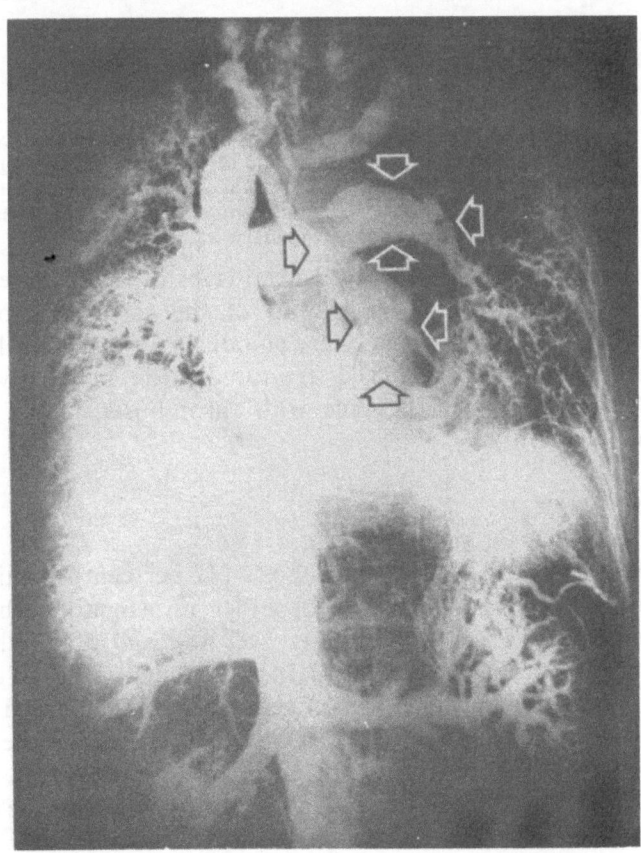

10.7 (a)

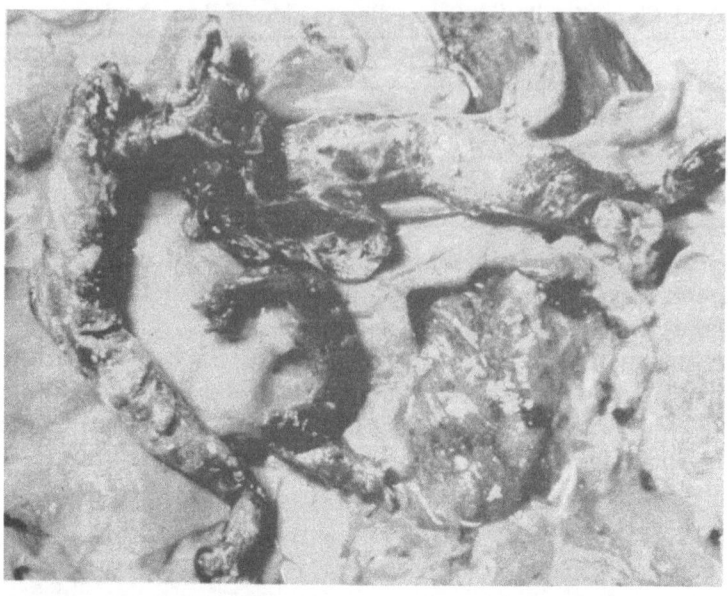

(b)

Figure 10.7 (a) Venogram of abdomen and thorax. Contrast medium has entered the inferior vena cava, hepatic and splenic veins, the right side of the heart and pulmonary arteries. Multiple filling defects are present (arrows) in the pulmonary artery and its left main trunk caused by an embolus. (In this case 1,500 ml of contrast medium were injected into the calcaneum.) (b) The embolus *in situ* in the pulmonary artery

The presence of thrombosis in the deep veins of the lower extremities was demonstrated in 70 (84 per cent) of the cases with pulmonary emboli. In some cases with pulmonary embolism a remaining iliofemoral thrombus remnant with a rugged 'fractured' proximal end was found (Figure 10.6). Of the 186 patients with thrombosis 38 per cent had pulmonary emboli.

DISCUSSION
Incidence of venous thromboembolism
The incidence of deep venous thrombosis (47 per cent) in this study is comparable to the figures quoted by other investigators. In an early autopsy study involving 324 persons over the age of 20 thrombosis occurred in 29 per cent (Rössle, 1937). In subsequent studies of unselected autopsy material the incidence was 34 per cent (McLachlin and Paterson, 1951; Kaij, 1959). In patients who died after a fractured hip the incidence was over 80 per cent (Sevitt and Gallagher, 1959; Sevitt, 1965). The great variation in the incidence of thrombosis seems to be due to the difference in the groups of patients studied.

Thromboembolism

Some authors have reported that the incidence of venous thrombosis is increased with age (Roberts, 1963; Sevitt, 1969). In a consecutive series of 108 patients dying in general medical and surgical wards the incidence of thrombosis increased from 49 per cent in the age group 50–69 to 61 per cent in the age group 70–89 (Roberts, 1963).

In another series, the incidence of thrombosis in various age groups was the same (McLachlin and Paterson, 1951), and in cases of tibial fracture (25-75 years) in which venography was performed, there was no corelation between age and incidence of thrombosis (Hjelmstedt and Bergvall, 1968). In the present series a tendency towards a higher frequency of thrombosis with increasing age was noted but this was not statistically significant.

One explanation about the different results could be that in medical patients there is no difference in the incidence of venous thrombosis in the higher decades. However, an increasing frequency of thrombosis with age, is perhaps more likely to be found in surgical patients. In the present study 95 per cent of all the patients were over the age of 70.

Origin and primary sites of venous thrombi

Early pathoanatomical studies have claimed that most thrombi arise in the iliofemoral veins (Virchow, 1846; Aschoff, 1934). In some subsequent pathoanatomical and clinical reports (Rössle, 1937; Frykholm, 1940; Bauer, 1940; 1944) the opposite concept has been maintained – namely that thrombi as a rule originate in the veins of the calf. According to some authors (Hadfield, 1950; Martin et al., 1956), thrombosis does not occur in the femoral vein unless it is the extension of a thrombus in the deep veins of the lower leg. Bauer (1946) found by venography that in patients with deep venous thrombosis 90 per cent of the thrombi had originated in the lower leg. The concept that practically all postoperative venous thrombi start in the calf has been stressed by recent studies using the ^{125}I-fibrinogen test (Kakkar, 1972; Nicolaides et al., 1972).

It appears that thrombosis in the veins of the calf produces early symptoms in a higher percentage of patients than thrombosis of the iliofemoral veins. Thrombosis in the proximal veins may give rise to more distinct and easily detectable symptoms; their small lumen will be rapidly occluded. It is therefore possible that venographic studies have given rise to a certain selection favouring patients which have the lower leg veins as the primary site of thrombosis.

The finding that thrombi were confined to the iliofemoral region in 29 per cent of legs with thrombosis in the present series suggested that

159

this was their site of origin. The influence of isolated iliofemoral thrombi was higher in some earlier studies (McLachlin and Paterson, 1951; 1956) and lower in others (Sevitt and Gallagher, 1961; Roberts, 1963). It was suggested (Roberts, 1963) that the very high percentage (73 per cent) reported by McLachlin and Paterson in 1951 could be associated, to some degree, with an incomplete dissection of the calf veins.

Authors who have used the ^{125}I-fibrinogen test and venography are against the opinion that a large number of thrombi arise within the proximal veins. They argue that the concept that most thrombi arise in the iliofemoral segment is based on autopsy findings: 'This involves a highly selected group of patients, among which are many who have died some weeks after injury, with prolonged hypotension and widespread venous stasis' (Field *et al.*, 1972). This argument may be valid to some degree but it must be remembered that, 'The major disadvantage of the radioactive fibrinogen test is its inaccuracy in the proximal femoral vein and the region of the pelvis – – ' (Field *et al.*, 1972). Because of this disadvantage of the ^{125}I-fibrinogen test it is likely that investigations performed with it, give a high incidence of thrombosis in the lower leg in relation to the iliofemoral segment where thrombi may escape detection.

Multiple sites of thrombosis
In the present series 24 per cent of the legs with thrombosis had discontinuous thrombi as shown in Figure 10.4. The findings indicate that thrombi may develop independently in the veins of the calf or in the veins of the thigh, and that simultaneous occurrence in both sites is not uncommon. The necropsy findings of Sevitt are in agreement with this opinion: 'The concept of multiple independent sites of thrombosis is supported by necropsy evidence from patients who had been given oral anticoagulant prophylaxis: when prophylaxis was delayed for a few days after injury, so that thrombi may have already begun to form but could not then extend, small thrombi were sometimes found at widely separate foci, – – ' (Sevitt, 1965; 1969).

Extensive, continuous thrombi from the lower leg veins to the femoral or iliac veins may be explained by: (1) retrograde thrombosis from a primary thrombus in a femoral or iliac vein; (2) ascending extension from thrombosed veins in the lower legs; or possibly (3) merging of extending thrombi from independent primary sites in the thigh and the lower leg.

The role of venous valve pockets in thrombogenesis
The importance of the valves in thrombogenesis was emphasised by

many studies (McLachlin and Paterson, 1951; Paterson and McLachlin, 1954; McLachlin *et al.*, 1960; Gibbs, 1957; Hegemann, 1961; Cotton and Clark, 1965; Gedgaudas *et al.*, 1966; Diener *et al.*, 1969; Lund, 1969; Lund *et al.*, 1969; Sevitt, 1969). In the present series a definite localisation of thrombi to valve pockets was found in 5·4 per cent of the thrombosed legs. This may seem to be a relatively small number but many other thrombi arising in valves were possibly not detected due to their subsequent propagation. It seems likely that a thrombus formed in a valve pocket will propagate proximally until it eventually causes venous obstruction. Venous stasis may in turn lead to further propagation both proximally and distally. As the propagated thrombus extends from the level of the valve, its primary site of formation is likely to be obscured. This will also occur by the merging of multiple thrombi propagating from different valve pockets (Figure 10.8).

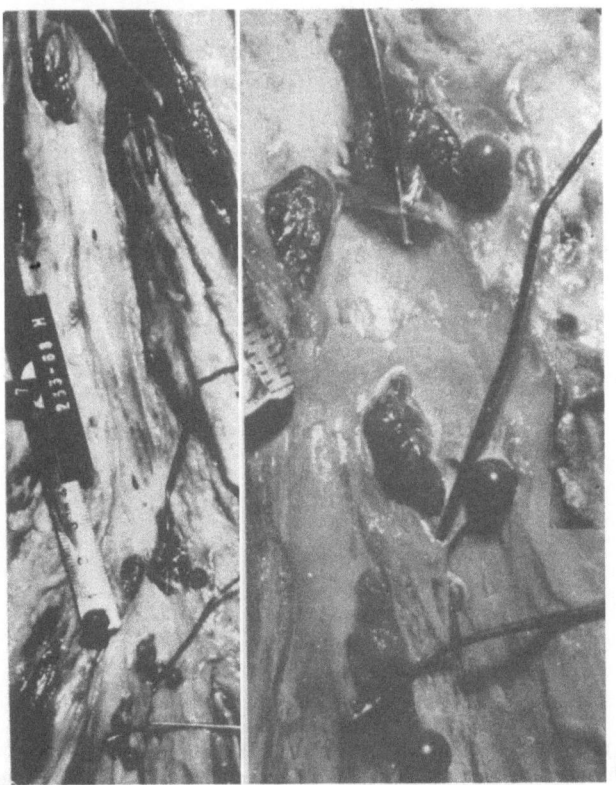

(a)　　　　　　　　　　　　　　　　　　　　　　　　　(b)

Figure 10.8 (a) Multiple thrombi formed in valve pockets. The uppermost lies in the distal part of the femoral vein and the remaining in the popliteal and adjacent regions of lower leg veins. Probes are inserted into valve pockets. (b) Close-up view of lower thrombi

Thrombi were usually attached at, or near, the deepest portion of the valve pockets, where stasis and turbulence were probably most marked. It has been pointed out that retention of contrast medium in valve pockets is seen repeatedly during venography of the lower limbs (McLachlin *et al.*, 1960). India ink injected from above in vertically mounted isolated preparations of cadaveric femoral vein which were perfused through the distal end with a saline solution produced pools of ink at the bottom of the valve pockets with hardly any movement and little diffusion (Cotton and Clark, 1965).

Microscopically the thrombi showed the greatest degree of organisation near the bottom of the valve pocket and they had a more immature structure proximally (Figures 10.9 and 10.10).

The high frequency of thrombi found in multi-valvular veins of the lower extremities and the rarity of primary or isolated thrombi in segments which are avalvular (common iliac and inferior vena cava) or supplied with only a few valves (popliteal and external iliac vein) are further evidence that valve pockets are related to thrombus formation.

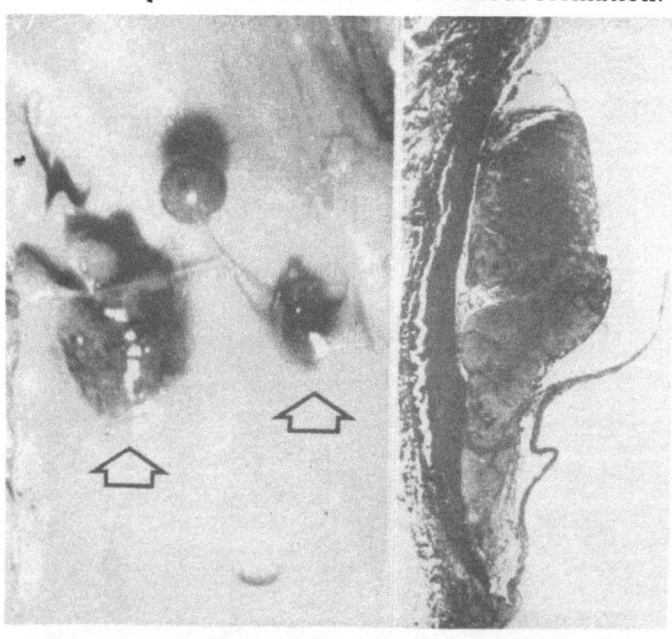

(a)   **(b)**

Figure 10.9 (a) Femoral vein with two small thrombi in valve pockets (arrows). The proximal ends of the thrombi are just protruding out of the pockets. (b) Section of the thrombus in the left valve pocket. The thrombus fills the valve pocket and is partly organised in its deepest portion; it is firmly adherent to the wall of the vein in the organised area. Haematoxylin and eosin. × 7

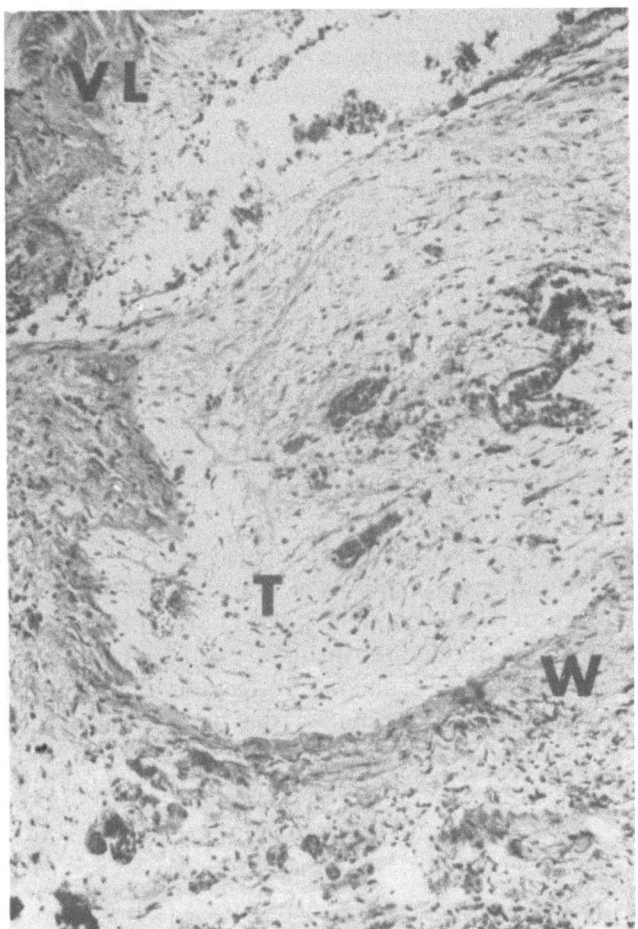

Figure 10.10 Microphotograph showing organisation of thrombus (T) at the deepest portion of a valve pocket. (VL) valve leaflet (W) inner wall of the vein. Haematoxylin and eosin. × 100

Calf muscle veins and anterior tibial veins in thrombogenesis

The muscular veins of the calf constitute another region where thrombi are often formed. When the body is supine they are dependent as dilated saccules with practically no circulation (Browse, 1962; Cotton and Clark, 1965; Nicolaides *et al.*, 1972; Chapter 9). In contrast, isolated thrombi confined to the anterior tibial veins are found very rarely. In the present series none were detected. The absence of thrombi from the anterior tibial veins may be explained by their anatomical arrangement. In the supine position they are placed superiorly to the calf veins and their location in a relatively narrow channel protects them from dilatation and stasis.

Pulmonary embolism

The frequency of venous thromboembolism is high in geriatric patients (Moran, 1947; Towbin, 1954; Kaij, 1959), particularly among geriatric surgical patients (Sevitt and Gallagher, 1961; Sevitt, 1965). Pulmonary embolism is a major – in some series the most common – cause of death in elderly patients (Sevitt and Gallagher, 1961; Smith *et al.*, 1965).

The incidence of 22 per cent of pulmonary embolism in the present study refers to grossly demonstrable thromboemboli. This percentage would be considerably high if 'microemboli' were to be included.

Pulmonary emboli often originate in the lower limbs (Figure 10.7), and the veins of the thigh and pelvis have been pointed out as important sources (Aschoff, 1938; Sevitt and Gallagher, 1961; Mavor and Galloway, 1967; Kakkar *et al.*, 1969).

In the present study, there was no evidence of deep venous thrombosis in 13 cases with pulmonary embolism. However, this does not exclude the lower limbs as a possible source of the embolism. An embolus could have formed from an iliofemoral thrombus which could have embolised in toto without leaving any remnant. At dissection an empty iliofemoral vein would have been found provided the patient did not survive long enough for rethrombosis to occur (Ashoff, 1938; Boyd, 1961; Sevitt and Gallagher, 1961).

References
Arnoldi, C. C. and Bauer, G. (1960). Intraosseous phlebography. *Angiology*, **11**, 44
Arnoldi, C. C. (1961). The function of the venous pump in chronic venous insufficiency. A phlebographic study. *J. Cardiov. Surg.*, **2**, 116
Aschoff, L. (1934). Thrombose und Embolie. *Verhandl. Deutsch. Gesellsch. Kreislaufsforsch*, **7**, 11
Aschoff, L. (1938). Über Thrombose und Embolie. *Wien. Klin. Wchnschr.*, **51**, 1227
Bauer, G. (1940). A venographic study of thromboembolic problem. *Acta Chir. Scand.*, **Suppl. No. 61**
Bauer, G. (1944). Thrombosis following leg injuries. *Acta Chir. Scand.*, **90**, 229
Bauer, G. (1946). Thrombosis. Early diagnosis and abortive treatment with heparin. *Lancet*, **i**, 447
Boyd, W. (1961). *A Textbook of Pathology*, 7th edition, 142 (Philadelphia: Lea and Debiger)
Britton, R. C. (1964). Roentgen anatomy. In: *Vascular Roentgenology*, 658 (New York: A. Schobinger and Macmillan Company)

Thromboembolism

Browse, N. L. (1962). Effect of surgery on resting calf blood flow. *Brit. Med. J.*, **1**, 1714

Coon, W. W. and Coller, F. A. (1959). Clinicopathologic correlation in thromboembolism. *Surg. Gynaecol. Obstet.*, **109**, 259

Cotton, L. T. and Clark, C. (1965). Anatomical localisation of venous thrombosis. *Ann. Roy. Coll. Surg. Engl.*, **36**, 214

Diener, L., Ericsson, J. L. E. and Lund, F. (1969). The role of venous valve pockets in thrombogenesis. In: *Atherogenesis*, 125 (T. Shimamoto and F. Numano, editors) (Excerpta Medica International Congress Series No. 201, Amsterdam)

Diener, L. (1971). Intraosseous phlebography of the lower limb. Postmortem investigation of thrombotic venous disease. *Acta Radiol.*, **Suppl. 304**

Drassner, V. (1946). Intraspongiöse Dauertropfinfusion. *Schweiz. Med. Wchnschr.*, **76**, 36

Field, E. S., Kakkar, V. V. and Nicolaides, A. N. (1972). Deep vein thrombosis after myocardial infarction, prostatectomy and fracture of the femoral neck. In: *Thromboembolism: Diagnosis and Treatment*, 117 (V. V. Kakkar and A. J. Jouhar, editors) (Edinburgh and London: Churchill Livingstone)

Frykholm, R. (1940). The pathogenesis and mechanical prophylaxis of venous thrombosis. *Surg. Gynaecol. Obstet.*, **71**, 307

Gedgaudas, E. and Emerson, E. C. (1966). Indications for phlebography in chronic venous disease and comments on technique. *Vas. Dis.*, **7**, 241

Gibbs, N. M. (1957). Venous thrombosis of the lower limbs with particular reference to bed-rest. *Brit. J. Surg.*, **45**, 209

Greitz, T. (1954). The technique of ascending phlebography of the lower extremity. *Acta Radiol.*, **42**, 421

Hadfield, G. (1950). Thrombosis. *Ann. Roy. Coll. Surg. Engl.*, **6**, 219

Hegemann, G. (1961). Das postthrombotische Syndrom. *Monatskurse Ärztl. Fortb.*, **10**, 610

Hjelmstedt, A. and Bergvall, U. (1968). Incidence of thrombosis in patients with tibial fractures. A phlebographic study. *Acta Chir. Scand.*, **134**, 209

Kaij, K. (1959). Thromboembolifrekvensen i ett obduktionsmaterial. (In Swedish), *Svenska Läk. Tidn.*, **56**, 1437

Kakkar, V. V., Howe, C. T., Flanc, C. and Clarke, M. B. (1969). Natural history of deep vein thrombosis. *Lancet*, **ii**, 230

Kakkar, V. V. (1972). Isotopic detection of deep venous thrombosis. In: *Thromboembolism: Diagnosis and Treatment*, 101 (V. V. Kakkar and A. J. Jouhar, editors) (Edinburgh and London: Churchill Livingstone)

Lindblom, K. (1941). Phlebographische Untersuchung des Unterschenkels bei Kontrastinjektion in eine subkutane Vene. *Acta Radiol.*, **22**, 288

Lund, F. (1969). Postmortal intraoossös flebografi. Ett nytt hjälpmedel vid studier av venös tromboembolism. In: *Trombos och status posttromboticus.* (*In Swedish*), 47 (K. Haeger and B. Robertson, editors) (Lund: Student-literatur)

Lund, F., Diener, L. and Ericsson, J. L. E. (1969). Postmortem intraosseous phlebography as an aid in studies of venous thromboembolism. *Angiology*, **20**, 155

McLachlin, J. and Paterson, J. C. (1951). Some basic observations on venous thrombosis and pulmonary embolism. *Surg. Gynaecol. Obstet.*, **93**, 1

McLachlin, J. and Paterson, J. C. (1956). Observations on venous thrombosis. *A. M. A. Arch. Surg.*, **73**, 606

McLachlin, A. D., McLachlin, J. A., Jory, T. A. and Rawling, E. G. (1960). Venous stasis

Thromboembolism

in the lower extremities. *Ann. Surg.*, 152, 678

Martin, P., Lynn, B. R., Dible, H. J. and Aird, I. (1956). In: *Peripheral Vascular Disorders*, 607 (Edinburgh and London: E. and S. Livingstone Ltd.)

Mavor, G. E. and Galloway, J. M. D. (1967). The iliofemoral venous segment as a source of pulmonary emboli. *Lancet*, i, 871

Moran, T. J. (1947). Thromboembolism. Embolism in nonsurgical patients with prostatic thrombosis. *Amer. J. Clin. Pathol.*, 17, 205

Nicolaides, A. N., Kakkar, V. V., Field, E. S. and Fish, P. (1972). Soleal veins, stasis and prevention of deep vein thrombosis. In: *Thromboembolism: Diagnosis and Treatment*, 69 (V. V. Kakkar and A. J. Jouhar, editors) (Edinburgh and London: Churchill Livingstone)

Paterson, J. C. and McLachlin, J. (1954). Precipitating factors in venous thrombosis. *Surg. Gynaecol. Obstet.*, 98, 96

Roberts, G. H. (1963). Venous thrombosis in hospital patients: A postmortem study. *Scot. Med. J.*, 8, 11

Rogoff, S. M. and De Weese, J. A. (1960). Phlebography of the lower extremity. *J. Amer. Med. Ass.*, 172, 1599

Rössle, R. (1937). Über die Bedeutung und die Entstehung der Wadenvenenthrombosen. *Virchows Arch.*, 300, 180

Sevitt, S. and Gallagher, N. S. (1959). Prevention of venous thrombosis and pulmonary embolism in injured patients. *Lancet* ii, 981

Sevitt, S. and Gallagher, N. G. (1961). Venous thrombosis and pulmonary embolism. A clinico-pathological study in injured and burned patients. *Brit. J. Surg.*, 48, 475

Sevitt, S. (1965). Anticoagulant prophylaxis against venous thrombosis and pulmonary embolism. In: *Pulmonary Embolic Disease*, 265 (A. A. Sasahara and M. Stein, editors) (New York and London: Gruse and Stratton)

Sevitt, S. (1969). Venous thrombosis in injured patients. In: *Thrombosis*, 29 (S. Sherry, K. M. Brinkhous, E. Genton and J. M. Stengle, editors) (Washington D.C.: National Academy of Sciences)

Smith, G. T., Dexter, L. and Dammin, G. J. (1965). Postmortem quantitative studies in pulmonary embolism. In: *Pulmonary Embolic Disease*, 120 (A. S. Sasahara and M. Stein, editors) (New York and London: Gruse and Stratton)

Towbin, A. (1954). Pulmonary embolism. Incidence and significance. *J. Amer. Med. Ass.*, 156, 209

Virchow, R. (1846). Thromboembolism. *Beitr. Exper. Pathol.*, 2, 227

11

Origin and distribution of thrombi in patients presenting with clinical deep venous thrombosis

A. N. Nicolaides and J. D. O'Connell

The purpose of this chapter is to present the results of studies which indicate the site of origin of thrombi and to discuss their significance in relation to pulmonary embolism. Information about the origin of thrombi is of importance in understanding the aetiology of thrombosis (Chapters 2, 7 and 8) and in developing methods of prevention (Chapters 9 and 14). Information about the extension of thrombi and the origin of pulmonary emboli is also essential in the management of patients with deep venous thrombosis (Chapter 19). It has been obtained by anatomico-pathological, isotopic and venographic studies.

ANATOMICO-PATHOLOGICAL STUDIES

Virchow's meticulous anatomico-pathological studies led him to believe that venous thrombi start in the small tributaries and advance towards and into the main venous trunks in the direction of the flow of blood (Virchow, 1860). Yet, by the third decade of the present century, the prevalent theory was that thrombi arose in the large pelvic and femoral veins and extended distally (Aschoff, 1924; Homans, 1934) though four patients with calf thrombosis without occlusion of the femoral veins had been recorded (Homans, 1934). These views persisted into the fifties (McLachlin and Paterson, 1951). The autopsy studies of Sevitt (Sevitt and Gallagher, 1961) led him to recognise six sites of primary lower limb venous thrombosis: the iliac veins, common femoral, deep femoral, popliteal, posterior tibial and soleal veins. Findings also suggesting that thrombi arise at these sites have recently been reported in a series of 400

167

autopsies of geriatric patients (Diener, 1971; Chapter 10), but in the latter series approximately half of the thrombi probably had their origin in the calf.

The observations that gave birth to and sustained the view that thrombi arise in the pelvic and femoral veins were mainly derived from postmortem examinations. In Aschoff's studies dissections were performed only on subjects with clinical thrombosis, pulmonary embolism or both (Aschoff, 1924). It is therefore not surprising that early ·cases of deep venous thrombosis very rarely came under examination. However, other studies in which full dissections of the veins of the pelvis, thigh and calf were performed suggested that the most frequent site of origin was the calf (Rössle, 1937; Newman, 1938; Frykholm, 1940; Hunter *et al.*, 1945; Gibbs, 1957).

In a series of 324 postmortem examinations of medical and surgical patients the incidence of deep venous thrombosis was 25 per cent (Rössle, 1937). In 50 per cent of these there were thrombi in the calf whereas the femoral vein was normal. In 40 per cent thrombi were present in both the calf and femoral vein. Only in 10 per cent of cases was there a thrombus present in the femoral vein without any thrombi in the calf. In another series of 165 postmortem dissections not a single case of thrombosis of the femoral vein was found without simultaneously un-affected calves (Newman, 1938).

In a meticulous dissection of 42 limbs in which not only the pelvic and large limb veins, but also the muscular tributaries were examined, thrombi were present in the veins of the calf in 27 cases (Frykholm, 1940). In one third of these, thrombi were extending into the femoral vein. Only in four cases were thrombi found in the femoral or iliac veins without any thrombi present in the more distal veins. A similar conclusion was reached by others (Hunter *et al.*, 1945). After 400 necropsy dissections of the veins of the lower limb they considered that femoral thrombosis commenced in the veins of the calf because thrombosis in the thigh seldom occurred except in conjunction with thrombosis in the lower leg.

The results of a more recent study of 253 necropsy cases suggested that deep venous thrombosis may occur in two anatomically separate sites – the calf and the thigh. Thrombosis in the thigh veins occurred in approximately 10 per cent of cases with calf vein thrombosis and could have been derived by propagation of thrombus in the calf or by primary thrombosis of the veins of the thigh occurring independently (Gibbs, 1957). In cases where there was thrombosis of the veins of the thigh in continuity with the calf, examples where the thrombus in the superficial femoral vein failed to reach the termination of the latter vein were not seen. It was argued that a primary thrombus laid down adjacent to the termination of the superficial femoral vein with retrograde extension was a more common cause of extensive femoral thrombosis than propagation of the thrombus from the calf. In the same study there was a correlation between the incidence of venous thrombosis and the period of bed rest before death:

'There is a rapid rise in the incidence of venous thrombosis which begins within 3 days of confinement to bed, and reaches a high level in those cases dying after confinement to bed for a period of 2 weeks and is maintained during subsequent weeks. Similarly, the incidence of thigh vein involvement follows an approximate parallel course, with the exception of a high peak occurring in patients dying after 4–5 weeks in bed' (Gibbs, 1957).

It has been suggested that the development of thrombosis in the veins of the calf and thigh is related to different periods of bed rest:

'Comparison of the frequencies of calf and thigh vein thrombi with the periods of bedrest indicates that leg vein thrombi form earlier (Gibbs, 1957; Sevitt and Gallagher, 1961). Thrombosis, in the calf was about twice as frequent as in the thigh among those dying during the first week after injury or burning; thereafter the incidence rose considerably in the calf and thigh and by the end of 1 month and subsequently, thigh vein thrombi (75 per cent of cases) exceeded the frequency of calf vein thrombi' (Hume et al., 1970).

The findings of dissections of the lower limb have also suggested that bilateral thrombosis is twice more common than unilateral (Sevitt and Gallagher, 1961).

STUDIES WITH THE ^{125}I-FIBRINOGEN TEST

Recent studies with the ^{125}I-fibrinogen test have demonstrated that thrombi start in the calf during the first 8–10 days after operation in surgical and after admission to hospital in medical patients (Flanc et al., 1968; Negus et al., 1968; Friend and Kakkar, 1970; Murray et al., 1970; Nicolaides et al., 1971a; Nicolaides, 1972; Ballard et al., 1973; Nicolaides, 1973; Chapter 14). By recording the changes in the radioactivity in the legs it is possible to detect whether a thrombus is lysing or extending. It has been shown that the majority of the thrombi either lyse spontaneously within 72 hours from the operation or remain localised to the calf; only 22 per cent extend into and proximal to the popliteal vein (Kakkar et al., 1969). Clinical pulmonary emboli occur in patients in the latter group

(Kakkar *et al.*, 1969) and only silent small pulmonary emboli occur in the former (Browse *et al.*, 1974).

In another series of 330 general surgical patients studied before and after operation deep venous thrombosis developed in 97 (29·4 per cent) patients. In 89 per cent of the patients with thrombosis the radioactivity was first detected in the calf; in 6·5 per cent in the popliteal fossa and in 4 per cent in the thigh (Nicolaides, 1974).

Unfortunately, the ^{125}I-fibrinogen test cannot detect a thrombus proximal to the inguinal ligament because of the high background radio-activity, and it cannot determine whether a thrombus in the calf is present in the soleal or tibial veins. Information about the iliofemoral segment and the soleal veins may be obtained by venography.

The incidence of bilateral postoperative deep venous thrombosis detected by the ^{125}I-fibrinogen test is much less than unilateral. 542 patients studied at three different hospitals gave an overall incidence of deep venous thrombosis of 28 per cent. Thrombi were bilateral in 9 per cent, right-sided in 9 per cent and left-sided in 10 per cent of patients (Kemble, 1971). Because of the nature of the test and the confinement of the studies to the early postoperative period only early thrombi were detected.

VENOGRAPHIC STUDIES

Bauer was a pioneer in studying the limbs of patients with deep venous thrombosis by serial venography (Bauer, 1940). This was his conclusion:

'Summarising my venographical experiences respecting the starting point of thrombosis, it may be said that the thromboembolic process, if not always, yet in the great majority of cases, manifests itself first in the deep large venous trunks of the lower leg, the posterior and anterior tibial veins as well as the peroneal vein. From these points there occurs a propagation, in the direction of the blood current, to venous trunks of even higher order' (Bauer, 1940).

He was thus repeating what Virchow said over eighty years earlier. However, Bauer was not able to demonstrate the soleal veins and he considered their occasional appearance on the venograms as abnormal. The crucial difficulty in the past has been the lack of a venographic technique which consistently demonstrated the soleal veins and thrombi therein in addition to the rest of the deep veins of the calf, thigh and pelvis (Browse *et al.*, 1967; Browse, 1969). Recently a technique has been developed that would achieve this, and has been used to study 97 patients with clinically suspected deep venous thrombosis (Nicolaides *et al.*, 1970;

Nicolaides *et al.*, 1971b). Of the 97 patients studied 49 had thrombosis. In only one patient there was occlusion of the external iliac veins with normal deep veins distally. With the exception of this single case, whenever there was a thrombus in the more proximal veins there were also thrombi in the soleal veins.

The results of a larger study now in progress (Nicolaides and O'Connell, 1974) provide further information. So far 228 patients presenting with clinical signs suggestive of deep venous thrombosis have been investigated by ascending venography. The diagnosis of thrombosis was made when a constant filling defect was seen on at least two films. Non-visualisation of a vein was not considered diagnostic of thrombosis unless there was a good opacification proximally and distally with the presence of a collateral circulation (De Weese and Rogoff, 1963). Approximately half of the patients were in the medical and the remaining in the surgical wards. Thrombi were detected in 131 (57 per cent) patients (137 limbs). In the remaining there was no evidence of thrombosis. The causes of signs in these patients without thrombosis will be discussed in Chapter 17. The distribution and extent of thrombi in the 137 venograms with thrombosis is summarised in Figure 11.1 and some examples are illustrated in Figures 11.2–11.9.

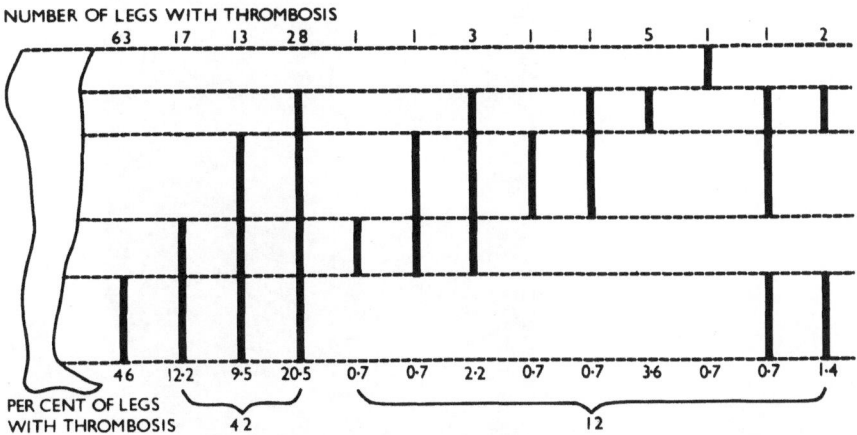

Figuer 11.1 The distribution and extent of thrombi in 137 venograms with thrombosis. The horizontal fields represent calf, popliteal, superficial femoral, common femoral and iliac veins

171

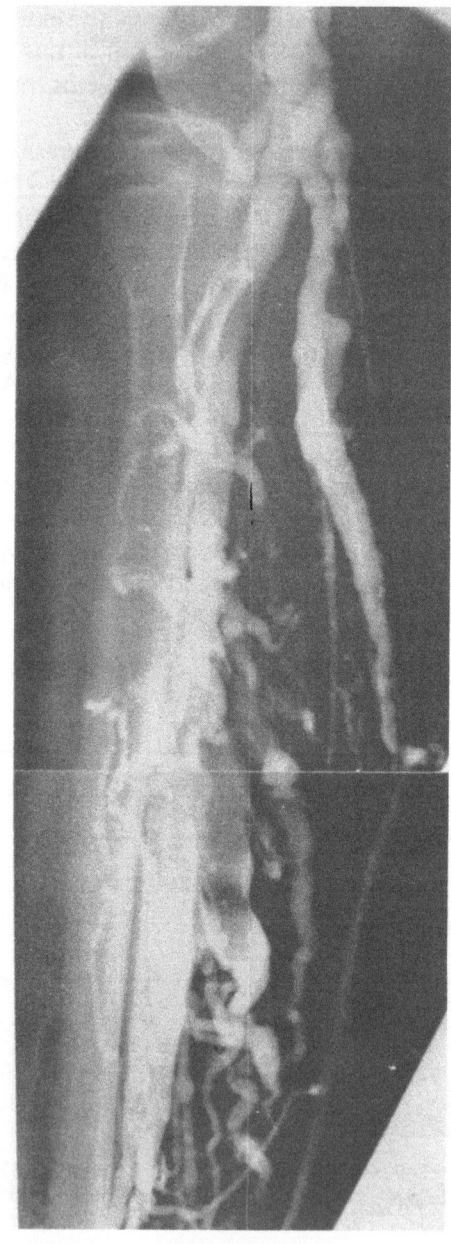

Figure 11.2 Thrombus confined to a soleal vein

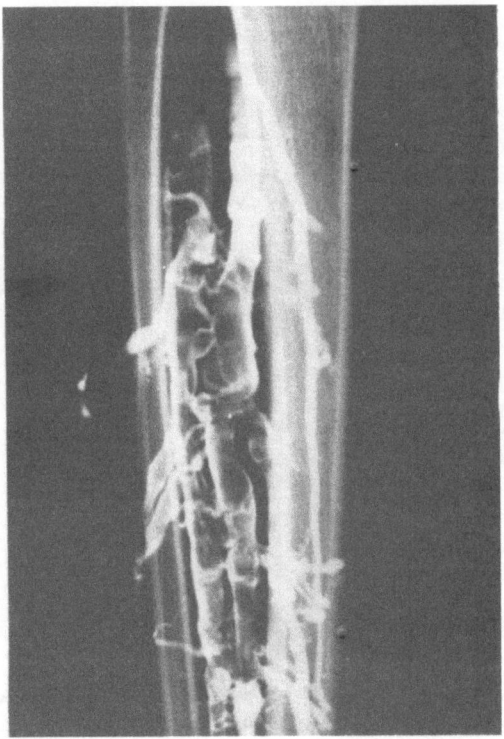

Figure 11.3 Thrombi in soleal and tibial veins

In a retrospective analysis of 430 venograms with thrombosis (Browse and Lea Thomas, 1974) the most common variety of thrombosis was thrombusconfined to the calf (42 per cent) followed by thrombus in the calf continuous withthrombus in the thigh or pelvis (35 per cent). In the remaining venograms (23 per cent) thrombi were arising proximally and independent to the calf. Fifty-eight per cent of the whole group had thrombosis involving the thigh and pelvic veins, but 60 per cent of the thrombi proximal to the knee were continuous with thrombi in the calf. The remaining 40 per cent had arisen independently. In 201 patients in this study (Browse and Lea Thomas, 1974) venography was preformed because of clinical non-lethal pulmonary emboli. This means that venography was performed at a later stage than in the patients of the previous study (Nicolaides and O'Connell, 1974) which was confined to patients with deep venous thrombosis. This difference in the selection of patients may account for the difference in the results. The fact that proximal thrombosis

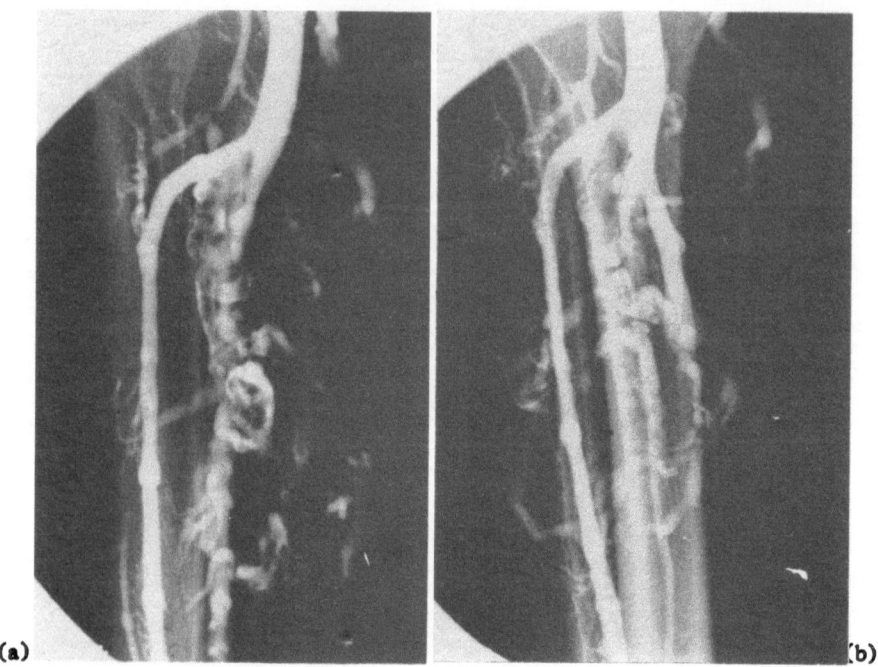

(a)

(b)

Figure 11.4 Thrombi present in soleal, tibial and lower end of popliteal vein. The tail of a thrombus can be seen projecting into the lower end of the popliteal vein in both (a) Anteroposterior and (b) Lateral views

may be more frequent after prolonged confinement to bed is emphasied by a study now in progress (Johnson, 1974) in which venography performed during the 2nd and 3rd weeks after total hip replacement has demonstrated high incidence of thrombosis originating in the pelvic veins.

GENERAL DISCUSSION AND CONCLUSIONS
The fact that in two venographic studies in 42 and 46 per cent of the limbs with thrombosis respectively the thrombi were confined to the calf (Figure 11.1) (Browse and Lea Thomas, 1974; Nicolaides and O'Connell, 1974) means that at least in a proportion of patients thrombi can start there.

It can be argued that the presence of thrombi in the calf whenever there is proximal thrombosis may be due to peripheral extension of thrombi arising in more proximal veins. This, however, does not happen, as shown by studies using the ^{125}I-fibrinogen test in surgical (Flanc *et al.*, 1968; Negus *et al.*, 1968), obstetric (Friend and Kakkar, 1970), gynaecological (Ballard, 1973), and medical (Murray *et al.*, 1970; Nicolaides *et al.*, 1971a)

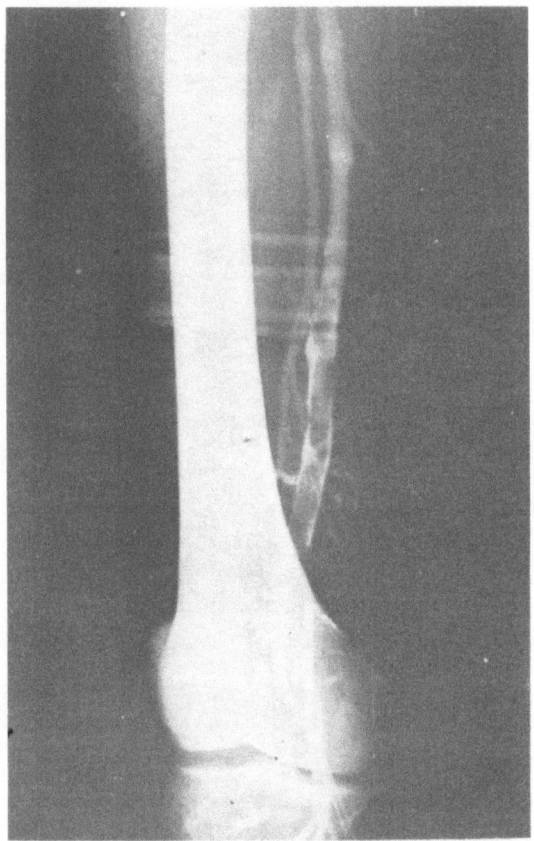

Figure 11.5 Thrombus in the lower third of the superficial femoral in a limb which had thrombi in the soleal, tibial and popliteal veins. The thrombus is not firmly attached to the femoral vein wall so that contrast medium flows round it

patients. These studies have in fact shown that in the early post-operative period and the first week after admission to hospital thrombi start in the calf and extend proximally.

Thrombi started at sites more proximal to the calf in 12 per cent of limbs in one venographic study (Nicolaides and O'Connell, 1974) and 33 per cent in the other (Browse and Lea Thomas, 1974). These limbs constituted one-fifth (Nicolaides and O'Connell, 1974) and two-fifths (Browse and Lea Thomas, 1974) of all the limbs in which the thrombotic process was involving veins proximal to the knee. It has been demonstrated that it is thrombi in the veins proximal to the popliteal that give rise to clinical

175

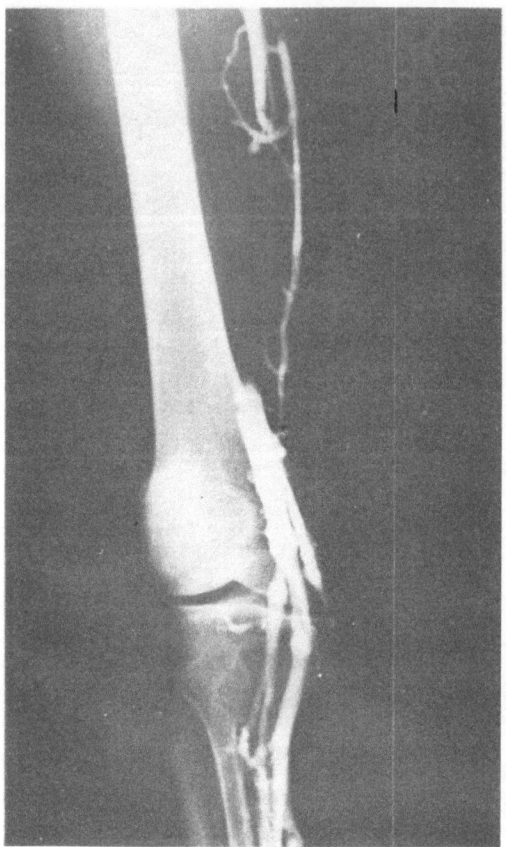

Figure 11.6 Thrombus confined to the superficial femoral vein in a patient who had a hip prosthesis four weeks earlier. On this occasion the patient was re-admitted with clinical pulmonary embolism and a tender calf. There was no calf or pelvic thrombosis on venography

pulmonary embolism (Kakkar *et al.*, 1969) and that thrombi confined to the calf may produce only small silent emboli (Browse *et al.*, 1974).

These findings are not incompatible with the results of the ^{125}I-fibrinogen test in hospital patients and anatomico-pathological studies based on post-mortem examinations. The data from the above venographic studies (Browse and Lea Thomas, 1974; Nicolaides and O'Connell, 1974) support the evidence that thrombi can start practically anywhere in the venous tree of the lower limb. They also support the findings of the ^{125}I-fibrinogen test that the majority of thrombi start in the calf (Chapter 14). The apparently different results obtained by the ^{125}I-fibrinogen test, venography and post-

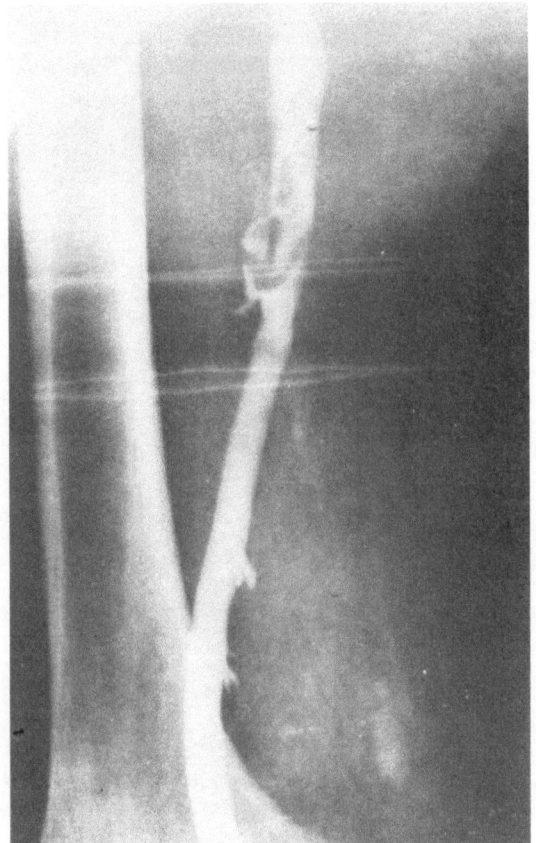

Figure 11.7 Thrombus in the superficial vein in a patient who did not have any other venographic evidence of deep venous thrombosis. The filling defect was constant in three films

mortem examination can be accounted for by the fact that these investigations have been performed in completely different groups of patients at different times in relation to operation and bedrest. In addition postmortem studies are by their nature performed in a selected group of 'high risk' patients. Patients who die are seriously ill, often in shock. The incidence of deep venous thrombosis in patients with hypotension is high (62 per cent) (Nicolaides *et al.*, 1971a) and their poor peripheral perfusion may result in stasis and consequently thrombosis not only in the calf, but also in the proximal veins and their valve pockets (Chapter 9).

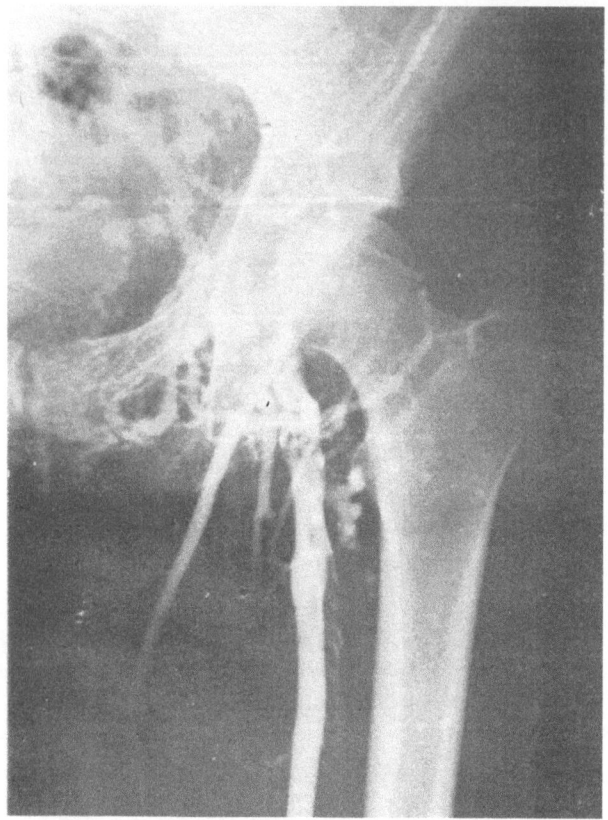

Figure 11.8 Iliofemoral thrombosis in a patient who had spinal fusion three weeks earlier

As far as prevention is concerned one important fact emerges: 67 per cent (Browse and Lea Thomas, 1974) to 78 per cent (Nicolaides and O'Connell, 1974) of the thrombi which are above the knee and constitute a danger of large pulmonary embolism have their origin in the calf. If one can therefore prevent the thrombi that start in the calf one may be eliminating only 67–78 per cent of the thrombi that constitute a risk to life. The evidence that proximal thrombi occur after the first 10 days of confinement to bed (Gibbs, 1957; Sevitt and Gallagher, 1961; Johnson, 1974) suggests that prevention should continue until the patient is fully ambulant or even until discharged from hospital.

Thromboembolism

References

Aschoff, L. (1924). *Lectures in Pathology*, (New York: Hoeber)

Ballard, R. M., Bradley-Watson, P. J., Johnstone, F. D., Kenney, A., McCarthy, T. G., Campbell, S. and Weston, J. (1973). Low doses of subcutaneous heparin in the prevention of deep vein thrombosis after gynaecological surgery. *J. Obstet. Gynaecol.*, **80**, 469

Bauer, G. (1940). A venographic study of thromboembolic problems. *Acta Chir. Scand.*, **suppl. 61**

Browse, N. L., Thomas, M. L. and Solan, M. J. (1967). Management of the source of pulmonary emboli: The value of phlebography. *Brit. Med. J.*, **4**, 596

Browse, N. L. (1969). Deep vein thrombosis: *Diagnosis. Brit. Med. J.*, **4**, 676

Browse, N. L., Clemenson, G. and Croft, D. N. (1974). Fibrinogen – detectable thrombosis in the legs and pulmonary embolism. *Brit. Med. J.*, **1**, 603

Browse, N. L. and Lea Thomas, M. (1974). Source of non-lethal pulmonary emboli. *Lancet*, i, 258

De Weese, J. A. and Rogoff, S. M. (1963). Phlebographic patterns of acute deep venous-thrombosis of the leg. *Surgery*, **53**, 99

Diener, L. (1971). Intraosseous phlebography of the lower limb. *Acta Radiol.*, **suppl. 304**

Flanc, C., Kakkar, V. V. and Clarke, M. B. (1968). The detection of venous thrombosis in the legs using ^{125}I-labelled fibrinogen. *Brit. J. Surg.*, **55**, 742

Friend, J. and Kakkar, V. V. (1970). The diagnosis of deep vein thrombosis in the puerperium. *J. Obstet. Gynaecol. Brit. Comm.*, **77**, 820

Frykholm, R. (1940). The pathogenesis and mechanical prophylaxis of venous thrombosis. *Surg. Gynaecol. Obstet.*, **71**, 307

Gibbs, N. M. (1957). Venous thrombosis of the lower limb with particular reference to bedrest. *Brit. J. Surg.*, **45**, 209

Homans, J. (1934). Thrombosis of deep veins of lower leg causing pulmonary embolism. *New Engl. J. Med.*, **211**, 993

Hunter, W. C., Krygier, J. J., Kennedy, J. C. and Sneeden, V. D. (1945). Etiology and prevention of thrombosis of the deep leg veins. *Surgery*, **17**, 178

Hume, M., Sevitt, S. and Thomas, D. P. (1970). *Venous Thrombosis and Pulmonary Embolism*, (Cambridge, Massachusetts: Harvard University Press)

Johnson, R. (1974). Personal communication

Kakkar, V. V., Howe, C. T., Flanc, C. and Clarke, M. B. (1969). Natural history of deep vein thrombosis. *Lancet*, **ii**, 230

Kemble, J. V. H. (1971). Incidence of deep vein thrombosis. *Brit. J. Hosp. Med.*, **6**, 721

McLachlin, J. and Paterson, J. C. (1951). Some basic observations on venous thrombosis and pulmonary embolism. *Surg. Gynaecol. Obstet.*, **93**, 1

Murray, T. S., Lorimer, A. R., Cox, F. C. and Lawrie, T. D. V. (1970). Leg vein thrombosis following myocardial infarction. *Lancet*, **ii**, 792

Negus, D., Pinto, D. J., Le Quesne, L. P., Brown, N. and Chapman, M. (1968). ^{125}I-Labelled fibrinogen in the diagnosis of deep vein thrombosis and its correlation with phlebography. *Brit. J. Surg.*, **55**, 835

Newman, R. (1938). Ursprungs Zentren und Ewtwickelungsformen der Beinthrombosen. *Virchows Arch. Pathol. Anat.*, **310**, 708

Nicolaides, A. N., Kakkar, V. V., Renney, J. T. G. (1970). The soleal sinuses: origin of deep vein thrombosis. *Brit. J. Surg.*, **57**, 860

Nicolaides, A. N., Kakkar, V. V., Renney, J. T. G., Kidner, P. H., Hutchison, D. C. S. and Clarke, M. B. (1971a). Myocardial infarction and deep vein thrombosis. *Brit. Med. J.*, **1**, 432

Thromboembolism

Nicolaides, A. N., Kakkar, V. V., Field, E. S. and Renney, J. T. G. (1971b). The origin of deep vein thrombosis: a venographic study. *Brit. J. Radiol.*, **44**, 653

Nicolaides, A. N. (1972). *The Prevention of Postoperative Deep Venous Thrombosis* (Jacksonian Prize Essay)

Nicolaides, A. N. (1973). Prevention of deep-vein thrombosis. *Geriatrics*, **28**, 69

Nicolaides, A. N. and O'Connell, J. D. (1974). Unpublished data

Rössle, R. (1937). Uber die Bedentung und entstehung der Wandenvenenthrombosen. *Virchow's Arch. Pathol. Anat.*, **300**, 180

Sevitt, S. and Gallagher, N. G. (1961). Venous thrombosis and pulmonary embolism: A clinico-pathological study in injured and burned patients. *Brit. J. Surg.*, **48**, 475

Virchow, R. (1860). *Cellular Pathology* (London: Churchill)

12

Prospective identification of the pulmonary embolism prone patient employing multi-variable risk factor analysis

Bernard Sigel, W. R. Felix jr., J. R. Justin, G. L. Popky,
Raymond Mark, Jimmie Williams, R. J. Gibson, A. Janet
Parker, Johannes Ipsen and Judith Mausner

Prevention of pulmonary embolism by treatment of *identified* high risk patients is a potentially rewarding endeavour for a number of reasons: First, there are therapies which are probably effective in preventing the occurrence of pulmonary embolism (Chapter 14). Second, because the most effective therapeutic regimens are not free of risks their application is best limited to selected patients in whom pulmonary embolism is likely. Third, the risk for pulmonary embolism probably varies during an individual's lifetime. This implies that vigorous and potentially hazardous prophylactic therapy need not be maintained indefinitely. Fourth, pulmonary embolism is a discrete event which might be prevented by therapy administered for only a brief period of time.

At present we are conducting an epidemiological study whose major objective is the prospective identification of the patient who is prone to pulmonary embolism. The purpose of this chapter is to describe our approach to such a prediction and to illustrate our method by presenting some preliminary results.

In attempting to identify patients at high risk of pulmonary embolism, two types of variables need be considered; dependent and explanatory. The dependent variable is pulmonary embolism, the end-point in our investigation. The explanatory variables consist of conditions, called risk factors, whose presence or absence is associated with the occurrence of pulmonary embolism. In order to predict the outcome, it is necessary to

Supported by funds from the National Institutes of Health (Grant No. HL11774), Part I research funds from the Veterans Administration, and a grant from The John A. Hartford Foundation

record the presence or absence of the explanatory variables when patients do not have evidence of pulmonary embolism, follow the patients for a given period, and determine the occurrence of pulmonary embolism in that peroid. That is, our end point is the rate of occurrence, or incidence of *new* disease in a defined period of time. The task is to develop a set of risk factors which will permit identification of those patients who are likely to develop pulmonary embolism.

The considerations in the selection and application of risk factors, and the relationship of these considerations to the design of our prospective study, will be discussed under the following headings: (1) The natural history of venous thromboembolism; (2) Initial selection of risk factors; (3) Relative risk analysis using single and multiple variables; (4) Multivariate analysis; (5) Usefulness of explanatory variables as predictors; and (6) Measurement of the effectiveness of prediction in a prospective study.

THE NATURAL HISTORY OF VENOUS THROMBOEMBOLISM
Pulmonary embolism is an event which occurs late in a total sequence of events and information about risk factors may be obtained at various stages. For the purposes of this study, thromboembolism has been divided into four stages:

(1) *Susceptibility:* This stage refers to the presence of relatively permanent factors which increase the likelihood of venous thromboembolism in an individual. Examples of these are genetic factors (e.g. ABO blood group), age, sex, race and persisting or permanent disease (e.g. postphlebitic syndrome and diseases of blood coagulation).

(2) *Predisposing Conditions:* This stage refers to factors which are often reversible but which may initiate and enhance the propagation of venous thrombosis. When the effect of these factors is diminished, there is a reduction in the likelihood of pulmonary embolism. Examples of such factors are trauma, inactivity, operation and congestive heart failure.

(3) *Venous Thrombosis:* By definition, this stage precedes the occurrence of pulmonary embolism and may be silent or overt. This stage, too, may be transitory. With resolution of venous thrombosis, the risk of pulmonary embolism also diminishes.

(4) *Pulmonary Embolism:* This stage includes survivors of a previous pulmonary embolism who may be at high risk for the development of subsequent emboli.

With the framework afforded by these stages of disease, it is possible to draw up a list of potential risk factors on the basis of information obtained from history, physical examination, laboratory tests and special examinations. To be useful clinically in prognosticating, the battery of risk factors selected must provide reliable information and be practical to employ.

INITIAL SELECTION OF RISK FACTORS

Multi-variate analysis is necessary for the creation of an effective battery of selected risk factors to estimate an individual's risk for pulmonary embolism. Probably the most important question in initiating an effort to prospectively identify the pulmonary embolism prone patient is: how are the best predictors selected initially? There are many potential risk factors to be considered in the different stages of venous thromboembolism. Essentially, the choice of potential risk factors for our study was pragmatic, the considerations being: to represent adequately all of the epidemiological stages of disease, to minimise the use of factors with obviously great intercorrelation and to heed the limitations of resources available for the study.

In selecting the best potential risk factors, we were guided by references in the literature and by generally accepted clinical tenets. Furthermore, we had completed a prospective epidemiological study of venous disease in patients undergoing elective surgical operations (Sigel *et al.*, 1974). In that study, we determined the relative contribution of over seventy explanatory variables to deep venous thrombosis of the lower extremities.

The decision to include risk factors from the various stages of the disease was based on consideration of the type of subjects expected in our study. These were patients in hospital with suspected or existing potentially serious disease. Because such individuals would be more likely to manifest the later stages of venous thromboembolic disease than the population at large, we selected risk factors for pulmonary embolism from all four stages and not merely the initial ones.

An attempt was made to avoid the use of highly intercorrelated factors. Although the multi-variate analysis used makes allowances for this type of dependency between factors, the presence of such factors tends to weaken its predictive ability and to enlarge the size of the battery of predictors. Some highly intercorrelated factors were evident *a priori*. For other factors, statistical testing was used as an aid for selecting the best potential measure of a particular attribute in the course of disease.

As in almost all studies, we had to consider the limitations of our

183

resources in planning the investigation. We estimated the need to study a population of about 8,000 patients in hospital in order to register an adequate number of new occurrences of pulmonary embolism. This meant that we could not use complicated and expensive tests as potential predictors. These considerations prompted us not to use tests of blood coagulation as risk factors in the stages of susceptibility and predisposition and to use the findings from Doppler ultrasound examination (Sigel *et al.,* 1972) as a risk factor for the stages of venous thrombosis.

RELATIVE RISK ANALYSIS USING SINGLE AND MULTIPLE VARIABLES

The effect of a risk factor can be measured by means of an odds ratio or approximate relative risk (Ipsen and Feigl, 1971; Fleiss, 1973). This is defined as follows:

Let p_1 be the incidence* of the dependent variable in patients in whom a particular explanatory variable is present p_2 be the incidence* of the dependent variable in patients in whom the same explanatory variable is absent.

By definition,

$$q_1 = 1 - p_1$$
$$q_2 = 1 - p_2$$

$$\text{Odds Ratio} = \frac{p_1}{p_2} \ \frac{q_2}{q_1}$$

which, when both p_1 and p_2 are small (i.e. the occurrence of the dependent variable is unlikely whether or not the explanatory factor is present), is a very good approximation to the relative risk. These two terms will be used interchangeably since this approximation is valid in this analysis. For reasons of mathematical accuracy, however, the computed relative risk ratio will follow the odds ratio formula.

The relative risk for any explanatory variable of interest depends on the relative incidence of pulmonary embolism in patients with and without that variable. Relative risk is independent of the actual frequency of pulmonary embolism. Therefore, it is useful for comparing the risk of pulmonary embolism in different populations. Thus, if the relative risk of a factor is 2·5, the presence of the dependent variable is two and one-half times as likely as when that same factor is absent. This is the single variate analysis of relative risk.

In considering multiple explanatory variables which may be associated

*Incidence expressed on a 0·0 to 1·0 scale, 1·0 representing 100 per cent

with pulmonary embolism, it is not sufficient to appraise their effect only through single variate analysis of relative risk. The comparative effect or importance of risk factors is most likely to differ. Consequently, it is necessary to employ a multi-variate analysis which takes this into account by assigning weights to each explanatory variable used in the battery of predictors. However, in doing this, the effect of one explanatory variable may be influenced by another. There are two main inter-relations which must be regarded when the effect of multiple explanatory variables are considered together: intercorrelation and interaction.

Intercorrelation among explanatory variables in a multi-variate analysis is a measure of the degree to which they are all measuring some underlying feature which itself may not be a recognised risk factor but which, nevertheless, is an important predictor of the dependent variable. The simultaneous analysis of risk factors deals with this relationship and this may help in selecting appropriate risk factors. As a result of such an analysis, the importance of certain factors may be significantly reduced or increased from the value suggested in the single variate analysis. In this way, it may be possible to use a smaller number of the best predictors of the dependent variable.

Interaction among explanatory variables results in an effective prediction which is not the additive effect of independent variables as determined in single variate analysis. Interaction may be positive or negative meaning that the combined effect may be greater or less than the simple additive effect.

MULTI-VARIATE ANALYSIS

The purpose of multi-variate analysis is to reduce the multidimensionality of the data to a single scale that best separates the two possible outcomes, occurrence or non-occurrence of pulmonary embolism. In addition to this basic requirement, the weights assigned to each risk factor should be conceptually easy to interpret and should be compatible with our clinical understanding of the disease. To achieve this, it is useful to transform a given patient's score to a percent risk of pulmonary embolism because this is a clinically understandable expression. In our study, we have used percent risk as a means of separating patients into categories termed 'high', 'medium' and 'low' risk for developing pulmonary embolism.

The study was a discriminant-function model, where each risk factor in a battery of factors is given a weight. The weights are selected so that the higher the score, the greater is the risk of pulmonary embolism. Where appropriate, the degree of severity of a present risk factor is also taken into account. We have examined a number of discriminant-function analyses and believe that Berkson's maximum likelihood multi-variate logit function meets our requirements best (Berkson, 1953; Dunn *et al.*, 1970). We now employ this method which is a weighted multiple regression on the logits* or logarithms of the relative risks. The relative risks are logarithmically transformed to simplify calculation by permitting addition rather than multiplication of risk weights in estimating the combined effect of factors. Following calculation, the data are returned to the original antilogarithmic form to permit easier comprehension and comparison. The set of predictors for each individual are assessed in terms of the risk factors in the battery which are present or absent. Each such configuration is weighted by the number of patients similarly involved and the variance of the expected rate of the dependent variable for that configuration.

It is not possible to develop the optimal set of assigned risk weights for a battery of risk factors by direct solution of equations. This is because of the circularity in definition (i.e. the weights for the configurations are not known exactly until the expected rates of pulmonary embolism are known and vice versa). Instead, iterative refinement by means of a series of trial solutions starting from any reasonable initial guess of risk weights is performed until a stable solution of risk estimate is achieved. The end results of this procedure are new risk weights for each of the predictors. These new risk weights have been adjusted for the effects of each of the other risk weights so that their combined effect can be determined by multiplication. In using this model, it is assumed that the odds ratio between each predictor and the dependent variable is constant and independent of the ambient rate of the dependent variable (incidence of pulmonary embolism).

For Berkson's method to be most effective, the following conditions are desirable:

(1) Sample size should be sufficiently large.

(2) No significant interaction should exist between explanatory variables.

(3) Each predictor should express an independent effect (i.e. explanatory variables should not be too highly intercorrelated).

(4) The successive solutions of iterative refinements should converge rapidly and consistently.

---

*A logit is the natural logarithm of the odds: logit $p = \log_e \left(\dfrac{p}{q}\right)$

USEFULNESS OF EXPLANATORY VARIABLES AS PREDICTORS

Potential risk factors for pulmonary embolism may be classified into those which are known and those which are unknown to us at this time. The known potential factors vary in the ease with which they can be obtained. Some can be determined readily; others can be obtained only with some risk or considerable expense to the patient. The question is: can the factors which are both known and readily available be used successfully to predict the occurrence of pulmonary embolism?

To deal with this question, it is appropriate to introduce the concept of a stochastic or error term in the relation between explanatory and dependent variables (Sonquist, 1971). If the variation in Y, the dependent variable (pulmonary embolism), were completely explained by N number of explanatory variables $X_1, X_2, ---, X_N$ used in a particular analysis, the following functional relation would prevail:

$$Y = f(X_1, X_2, ---, X_N)$$

However, if all the variance of Y cannot be explained by the independent variables employed, then it is necessary to introduce a stochastic or error term, e. The functional relationship now becomes:

$$Y = f(X_1, X_2, ---, X_N) + e$$

The objective in selecting potential risk factors is to employ those which maintain e at an acceptable minimum. If e is too large because the predictive risk factors are not known or cannot be used, the analysis becomes of dubious significance.

MEASUREMENT OF EFFECTIVENESS OF PREDICTION IN A PROSPECTIVE STUDY

The ultimate success of prediction is determined by the frequency with which individual subjects are assigned correct risks of developing pulmonary embolism. To illustrate the approach described in this paper, we present some interval results from a prospective study currently in progress. The population studied so far consists of adult patients in three hospitals. The risk of pulmonary embolism in this group is probably slightly higher than would be true of an unselected group of hospitalised patients because it includes patients referred for consultation.

Table 12.1 shows that of 3275 patients entering the study between September 1971 and May 1973, 2928 did not have a diagnosis of pulmonary embolism on admission and were therefore at risk for the development of this complication during a one-month period of observation. During this period, the overall incidence of pulmonary

Tabel 12.1 Course of venous thrombosis study

September 1971 to May 1973		
Total number of patients admitted to study	3,275	
Diagnosis of pulmonary embolism on admission	347	10·6 per cent
Patients at risk of developing initial pulmonary embolism	2,928	
Incidence of pulmonary embolism within one month	134	4·6 per cent

embolism was 4.6 per cent. Pulmonary embolism as defined here includes both suspected and confirmed (positive pulmonary scan and/or positive pulmonary angiogram) cases. When further cases have accumulated, the analysis will be done separately for confirmed and suspected cases.

Table 12.2 Relative risk factors for incidence of pulmonary embolism within one month. Multi-variate analysis of 2,928 patients

Variable	Relative risk	Significance
Inactivity—Any	2·06	***
Inactivity—Total	1·89	*
Congestive heart failure	1·57	**
Lower extremity operations	1·97	**
Previous pulmonary embolism	2·83	**
Ultrasound incompetent valves	1·58	*
Clinical occlusion	1·15	—
Ultrasound occlusion	2·07	**
Trauma—Lower extremity	1·55	*
Maximum relative risk based on above factors	198·94	

Significance levels:
  $* \; p < 0.05$
  $** \; p < 0.01$
  $*** \; p < 0.001$

Table 12.2 shows an array of the best predictors of pulmonary embolism determined to date. These values were derived by the multi-variate discriminant analysis described above based on factors present at the time of initial examination. The individually expressed values of relative risk indicate the comparative importance of a given factor in the battery taking into account dependency between the factors shown. Thus, if an individual patient manifested any significant degree of inactivity, his risk for pulmonary embolism would be 2.06 times greater than if he were normally active. If his inactivity were total (complete bed rest), his risk would be the product of 2.06 (for any inactivity) and 1.89 (for total inactivity) or 3.89 times greater than an individual with normal activity. The model specifies that if all the risk factors shown in Table 12.2 were present in a given patient, the estimated risk of pulmonary embolism would be 198.94 (product of all the relative risks) times greater than for a patient in whom all the factors were absent. However, no patient has been observed who has had all risk factors present. So far, the highest product of relative risks has been 48.

Table 12.3 shows the data for individual patients combined in risk groups. *Risk classification was derived from the initial estimate of per cent risk for each patient.* All patients were listed in descending order of percent risk as estimated from factors present at the time of initial examination. The listing also showed the outcome for each patient in terms of occurrence or non-occurrence of pulmonary embolism within the

Table 12.3 Estimated risk for development of pulmonary embolism*. Based on analysis of 2,928 patients

Risk classification	Number of patients with pulmonary embolism	Number of patients	Incidence of pulmonary embolism in 30 days
High	45 (33·6 per cent)	325 (11·1 per cent)	13·8 per cent
Medium	43 (32·1 per cent)	699 (23·9 per cent)	6·2 per cent
Low	46 (34·3 per cent)	1,904 (65·0 per cent)	2·4 per cent
Total	134 (100 per cent)	2,928 (100 per cent)	4·6 per cent

* Includes confirmed and suspected pulmonary embolism

one-month follow-up period. Starting with the patient with the highest estimated per cent risk, we went down the list and included in the 'high' risk group those patients with the greatest initial risk of pulmonary embolism until we had accounted for approximately one-third of all the pulmonary emboli observed in this study population. This indicated that a third of all the pulmonary emboli occurred in only 11·1 per cent of all the patients in the study. Similarly, we placed patients with the next highest per cent risk into a 'medium' risk group until we had accounted for another third of all the pulmonary emboli. This 'medium' risk group corresponded to 23·9 per cent of all the study patients. By combining the 'high' and 'medium' risk groups, we identified the one-third of the study population which accounted for about two-thirds of all the pulmonary emboli diagnosed during the period of one month. As shown in Table 12.3, the actual incidence of pulmonary embolism was 13·8, 6·2 and 2·4 per cent for the 'high', 'medium' and 'low' risk groups respectively.

As noted above, risk classification was derived from an initial examination of each patient. If serial examinations are done and risk recalculated after each examination, the ability to predict pulmonary embolism is greatly improved.

DISCUSSION

There are many problems associated with the precise prospective identification of patients prone to pulmonary embolism. The description of our approach to prediction has served to illustrate some of the difficulties inherent in the method. As carried out in our study to date, prospective analysis appears to possess moderate accuracy. However, there is still a sizeable error because about a third of pulmonary emboli occurred in patients classified as 'low risk' (Table 12.3). We believe that there are at least three major reasons for such a discrepancy.

First, we may not be using the best risk factors because certain factors were ruled out as impractical for our study. Future research should continue to focus upon identification of the best predictors.

Second, there are problems in defining the dependent variable, pulmonary embolism. The measures of pulmonary embolism used should faithfully reflect the true biological occurrence of this event. Short of operation or autopsy, the diagnosis should be confirmed by either appropriately performed pulmonary isotope scanning or by angiography. This is the intent in our study.

A further problem stems from the fact that confirmatory procedures are performed only when clinical suspicion of pulmonary embolism exists. An increase in the index of suspicion for pulmonary embolism could lead to an increase in requests for confirmatory tests, and thus to an apparent, but not necessarily, true increase in the incidence of pulmonary embolism. These considerations regarding the diagnosis of pulmonary embolism should be taken into account in the design of epidemiological studies.

References

Berkson, J. (1953). A statistically precise and relatively simple method of estimating the bioassay with quantal response, based on the logistic function. *Amer. Stat. Assoc. J.*, **48**, 565

Dunn, J. P., Ipsen, J., Elsom, K. O. and Ohtani, M. (1970). Risk factors in coronary artery disease, hypertension and diabetes. *Amer. J. Med. Sci.*, **259**, 309

Fleiss, J. L. (1973). *Statistical Methods for Rates and Proportions* (John Wiley and Sons)

Ipsen, J. and Feigl, P. (1971). *Bancroft's Introduction to Biostatistics* (New York: Harper and Row)

Sigel, B., Felix, Jr, W. R., Popky, G. L. and Ipsen, J. (1972). Diagnosis of lower limb venous thrombosis by doppler ultrasound technique. *Arch. Surg.*, **104**, 174

Sigel, B., Felix, Jr, W. R. and Ipsen, J. (1974). The epidemiology of lower extremity deep venous thrombosis in surgical patients. *Ann. Surg.* (In press)

Sonquist, J. A. (1971). *Multivariate Model Building: The Validation of a Search Strategy* (University of Michigan, Ann Arbor: Institute for Social Research)

13

Clinical factors and the risk of deep venous thrombosis

A. N. Nicolaides and Doreen Irving

This chapter describes attempts to determine the relationship between clinical factors and the risk of postoperative deep venous thrombosis. Simple methods of prophylaxis which can be used in surgical patients are now available (Chapters 14–16). A method that could determine the risk of deep venous thrombosis in any patient before operation without the need of special haematological tests (Chapters 4–6) would be of great value in selecting the patients who need prophylaxis. In addition by determining the clinical factors predisposing to thrombosis and their relative importance insight to the aetiology of this condition might be obtained.

Evidence has accumulated in the literature that certain clinical factors are associated with a high incidence of deep venous thrombosis. These are: age (Borgstrom, 1950; Coon and Coller, 1959; Sevitt and Gallagher, 1961; Thies, 1961; Hume, 1965; Flanc et al., 1969), immobility and bedrest (Gibbs, 1957; Sevitt and Gallagher, 1961; Roberts, 1963), previous thromboembolism (Barker et al., 1941; Turnbull, 1960), obesity (Snell, 1927; Barker et al., 1941; Coon and Coller, 1959; Sandritter, 1962), congestive cardiac failure (Coon and Coller, 1959; Kucera, 1968), carcinoma (Sproul, 1938; Coon and Coller, 1959; Rosenthal et al., 1963; Byrd et al., 1967), severity of operation (Barker et al., 1940; 1941; Belding, 1965), trauma (Vance, 1934; Bauer, 1944; Aurin and Herrman, 1948; Sevitt and Gallagher, 1961) and possibly blood group A (Jick et al., 1969). The diagnosis of deep venous thrombosis in most of the above studies was based either on clinical signs which we now know to be

193

unreliable (Chapter 17) or on postmortem findings. Recent studies have attempted to confirm the association of clinical factors and deep venous thrombosis using the ^{125}I-fibrinogen test to detect thrombosis in the perioperative period (Kakkar *et al.*, 1970; Nicolaides, 1972; Nicolaides *et al.*, 1973).

SINGLE VARIATE ANALYSIS

In the study of Kakkar and his colleagues (Kakkar *et al.*, 1970) 203 patients undergoing elective surgery were investigated with the ^{125}I-fibrinogen test and an attempt was made to determine the patients who were at a 'great risk' of developing deep venous thrombosis. It was found that the patients who formed the high risk group included those who had a history of previous deep venous thrombosis or pulmonary embolism, varicose veins, malignant disease, an age over 60, obesity and major operation. In this investigation a single variate analysis was performed. Two by two tables were constructed for each of the clinical factors and deep venous thrombosis. The presence of any significant association between a clinical factor and thrombosis was determined by the chi square test. However, this type of analysis had its limitations as it did not take into account any correlations that might exist between the various factors thought to predispose to thrombosis and could not determine their relative importance. For example, there is a high incidence of deep venous thrombosis in patients having major operations and also in patients with malignancy. Practically all patients with malignancy have a major operation and it is impossible to know which one of the two factors may be responsible for the high incidence of thrombosis.

MULTI-VARIATE ANALYSIS

It has been suggested that a multi-variate analysis would overcome the above difficulties and obtain an estimate of the risk as determined by all the clinical factors (Nicolaides *et al.*, 1973). A multi-variate analysis has been performed using the data from a prospective study now in progress (Nicolaides and Irving, 1974). So far 624 patients have been investigated with the ^{125}I-fibrinogen test. None of them had any specific prophylactic measures. A special form has been filled in for every patient on which the following data are recorded: Age, sex, height and weight, type of operation, premedication with omnopon, blood group, history of previous deep venous thrombosis or pulmonary embolism, malignancy, varicose veins and postoperative infection. These factors were selected because of previous reports in the literature. Taking into consideration the sex, height and weight and using the weight-for-height standards (Kensley *et al.*, 1962) the overweight patients (obese) were determined. The operations were classified arbitrarily as minor or major. Operations such as simple mastectomy, herniorrhaphy and haemorrhoidectomy were minor. All abdominal and thoracic operations were classified as major. Prostatectomy, hip operations and vascular on the aortoiliac segment were also classified as major. Infection was considered to be present only if there was bacteriological confirmation of the clinical diagnosis. The patients studied belonged to five main groups shown in Table 13.1.

Table 13.1 Patients studied and incidence of deep venous thrombosis

Group	No DVT	DVT	Total
General surgical	319	111·(26 per cent)	430
Orthopaedic (Hip operations)	47	45 (49 per cent)	92
Urological (Prostatectomy) (Open and TUR)	25	4 (14 per cent)	29
Thoracic	44	10 (19 per cent)	54
Vascular (Aorto-iliac)	15	6 (29 per cent)	21
Total	450	176 (28 per cent)	626

DVT = Deep venous thrombosis

A single variate analysis was first performed. The association between each of the clinical factors and deep venous thrombosis is demonstrated in Table 13.2. This was determined by the chi square test. The following factors were significant: Age, varicose veins, history of previous deep venous thrombosis, infection, history of previous pulmonary embolism, **premedication with omnopon, obesity and severity of operation.**

It has already been mentioned that this type of analysis has its limitations as it does not take into account any intercorrelations or interactions (see Chapter 12) that might exist between the various factors thought to predispose to thrombosis and cannot determine their relative importance. A linear logistic analysis was therefore applied to the data in order to obtain an estimate of the risk as determined by all the clinical factors associated with deep venous thrombosis. This type of multi-variate analysis is suitable for prognostic data, where an individual is classified as 'success' (no deep venous thrombosis) or 'failure' (deep

Table 13.2 The association between clinical factors and deep venous thrombosis

Clinical factor	Number of patients: * With DVT	Without DVT		x^2	p
Sex (Male)	234	83 (26%)		1·05	>0·05
(Female)	215	93 (30%)			
Blood (A)	156	60 (28%)	Compared	0·12	
group (B)	39	17 (30%)	with	0·01	>0·05
(AB)	9	1 (10%)	group	1.00	
(O)	144	61 (30%)	O		
Age (Under 60 years	239	58 (19%)		19·77	<0·0005
(60 years or over	207	116 (36%)			
Obesity (Absent)	349	120 (26%)		6·35	<0·025
(Present)	95	55 (37%)			
Malignancy (Absent)	344	123 (26%)		3·30	>0·05
(Present)	99	52 (34%)			
Varicose (Absent)	414	143 (26%)		19·72	<0·0005
veins (Present)	29	33 (53%)			
History of (Absent)	429	152 (26%)		19·11	<0·0005
previous DVT (Present)	15	23 (61%)			
History of (Absent)	441	168 (28%)		6·76	<0·01
previous PE (Present)	3	7 (70%)			
Severity of (Minor)	112	28 (20%)		5·43	<0·025
operation (Major)	337	148 (31%)			
Jaundice (Absent)	416	164 (28%)		0·00	>0·05
(Present)	19	8 (30%)			
Premedication with Omnopon					
(Not administered)	282	93 (25%)		4·09	<0·05
(Administered)	115	58 (34%)			
Infection in postoperative (Absent)	338	106 (24%)		15·67	<0·0005
period (Present)	63	48 (43%)			

DVT = Deep venous thrombosis

* For some patients information about one or more clinical factor was not available.

venous thrombosis), several variables are observed and the object is to predict the probability of success or failure in terms of the variables.

The linear logistic model used is given by the equation:

$$y = a + b_1x_1 + b_2x_2 + \cdots + b_nx_n \qquad (1)$$

where

$$y = \text{logit } p = \log_e\left(\frac{p}{1-p}\right) = \log_e\left(\frac{p}{q}\right) \qquad (2)$$

and by definition $\frac{p}{1-p}$ is the odds.

196

$x_1, x_2, \ldots, x_n$ denote n explanatory variables (clinical factors) and p is the probability of occurrence of a particular well-defined event (deep venous thrombosis) which depends on the values of the explanatory variables, a is a constant and $b_1, b_2, \ldots, b_n$ are coefficients which represent the natural logarithms of relative risk attributed to the corresponding clinical factors. The constant and the coefficients need to be estimated for any given data.

A standard programme in the library of the Computer Centre of the University of London was used to obtain the estimates of a and $b_1, b_2, \ldots, b_n$ using the method of maximum likelihood (Armitage, 1971). The programme required the values of the clinical factors $x_1, x_2, \ldots, x_n$

Table 13.3 Maximum liklihood estimates of constant and coefficients of the linear logistic model (535 patients*)

Variable	Estimate of coefficient	Estimate of relative risk	t-value	
1. Age increase by 1 year	0·0538	1·055	5·23	
2. Premedication with Omnopon	1·000	2·72	4·00	
3. Varicose veins	1·220	3·39	3·61	
4. Infection	0·894	2·44	3·36	Significant
5. History of previous DVT	1·192	3·30	2·66	
6. Severity of operation	0·758	2·13	2·66	
7. Urological operation	−1·705	0·18	2·60	
8. Thoracic operation	−1·184	0·31	2·43	
9. Orthopaedic operation	0·710	2·04	1·84	
10. History of previous PE	1·515	4·55	1·56	Not significant
11. Malignancy	0·349	1·42	1·31	
12. Obesity	0·276	1·32	1·09	
13. Vascular operation	0·430	1·54	0·73	
14. Jaundice	−0·340	0·71	0·62	

Constant $a = -5\cdot78$

* Only patients for whom complete data were available were included in this analysis.

DVT = Deep venous thrombosis.   PE = Pulmonary embolism.

for each patient and an indication whether deep venous thrombosis occurred or not. With the exception of age which was measured in years the values of all other factors were either zero (factor absent) or one (factor present).

Blood group was not included in the analysis because it was not known for 139 (22 per cent) of the patients and it did not appear to be important in the preliminary analysis shown in Table 13.2.

The results of the linear logistic analysis are shown in Table 13.3. It can be seen that the factors associated with venous thrombosis were: age, premedication with omnopon, varicose veins, infection, history of previous deep venous thrombosis, severity of operation, urological and thoracic operations. The last two were associated in a negative way, i.e. with a low risk. Obesity, malignancy, history of previous pulmonary embolism, jaundice, orthopaedic and vascular operations were not significant. Previous history of pulmonary embolism was not significant probably because of the small number of patients.

In order to improve the predictive ability of the model the analysis was repeated using only the significant factors. The new estimates of the coefficients are listed in Table 13.4. By taking their antilogarithm they have been expressed as relative risk which is more meaningful. The

Table 13.4 Maximum likelihood estimates of constant and coefficients of the linear logistic model using the significant variables (535 patients*)

Variable	Estimate of coefficient	Estimate of relative risk	t-value
1. Age increase by 1 year	0·0617	1·065	6·5
2. Premedication with omnopon	0·966	2·63	3·9
3. Varicose veins	1·257	3·52	3·8
4. History of previous DVT	1·383	3·99	3·3
5. Infection	0·843	2·33	3·2
6. Urological operation	−1·942	0·14	2·9
7. Severity of operation	0·786	2·20	2·8
8. Thoracic operation	−1·152	0·31	2·4

Constant $a = -6·00$

* Only patients for whom complete data were available were included in this analysis

DVT = Deep venous thrombosis.

relationship between relative risk and increase in age could be expressed in graphic form because age was a continuous variable (Figure 13.1). It can be seen that for two patients of the same age the relative risk is 1; for two patients with a difference of 40 years in age the relative risk is 12 i.e. the risk of the older patient developing thrombosis is 12 times greater than the younger.

From the new estimates of the coefficients (Table 13.4) the model became:

$y = -6.00 + (\text{Age} \times 0.0617) + (\text{Varicose veins} \times 1.26)$
$\quad + (\text{Previous history of DVT} \times 1.38) + (\text{Severity of operation} \times 0.79)$
$\quad + (\text{Premedication with omnopon} \times 0.97) + (\text{Infection} \times 0.84)$
$\quad - (\text{Urological operation} \times 1.94) - (\text{Thoracic operation} \times 1.15)$

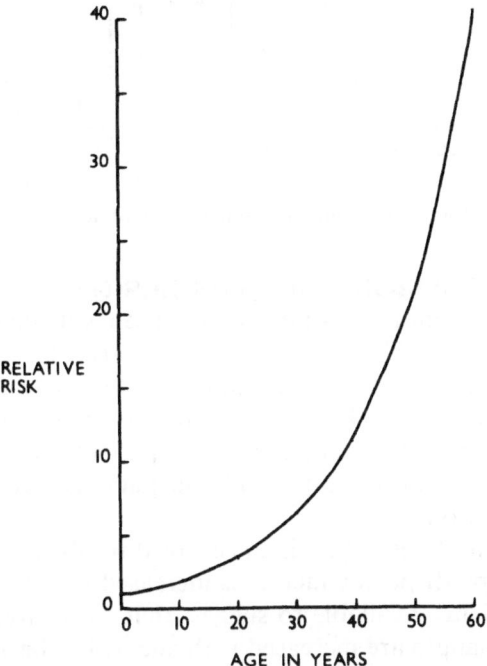

Figure 13.1 The relationship between relative risk and increase in age

Using this equation the logit y was calculated for every patient. The number of patients with or without thrombosis were plotted against the y value (Figure 13.2). The two populations are poorly separated so that y cannot be of diagnostic value unless it is over 2 when the probability of deep venous thrombosis is high or less than -2 when the probability is small. However, for any patient, y can be expressed as the probability or risk of developing thrombosis (Figure 13.2).

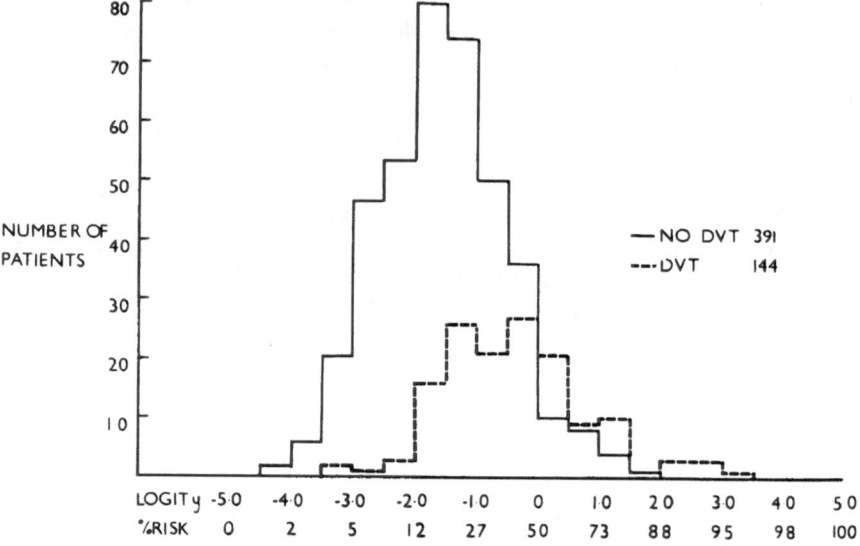

Figure 13.2 Histogram showing the estimated risk of deep venous thrombosis

GENERAL DISCUSSION AND CONCLUSION

The risk of deep venous thrombosis has been calculated for 8 hypothetical patients (Table 13.5) in order to demonstrate how it increases with age and with the presence of other clinical factors. It can be seen that if preventive measures are to be applied in patients with a risk greater than 6 per cent they should be applied to all patients over the age of 40 having a major operation and to all the patients over the age of 60 having any operation.

The association of age with a high risk of thrombosis suggests that the effect of certain predisposing factors is increased in older patients. There is very little evidence available to suggest that stasis, hypercoagulability or endothelial changes are increased with age. It has been suggested that the soleal veins become dilated in older patients (Gibbs, 1957), but the amount of stasis in them is not related to age (Chapter 9). It has been claimed that decreased mobility, occlusive arterial disease and reduction in cardiac output (Hume *et al.*, 1970), increased factor VIII (Cooperberg and Teitelbaum, 1960) and changes in antithrombin III (Von Kaulla and Von Kaulla, 1970) occur with age.

Varicose veins may predispose to stasis and in a number of patients

Table 13.5 The risk of deep venous thrombosis in eight hypothetical patients

Age and other clinical factors present	y	p	Per cent risk
1. Age 20 minor operation	−4·8	0·008	0·8
2. Age 40 minor operation	3·5	0·029	2·9
3. Age 40 major operation	−2·7	0·063	6·3
4. Age 60 minor operation	−2·3	0·91	9·1
5. Age 60 Major operation	−1·5	0·18	18·3
6. Age 60 major operation ─ history of previous deep venous thrombosis	−0·13	0·47	47
7. Age 80 major operation	−0·27	0·43	43
8. Age 80 major operation History of previous DVT, infection, varicose veins	3·21	0·96	96

they may be the result of a subclinical deep venous thrombosis which has damaged the valves of the deep veins. A history of previous thrombosis may reflect a predisposition because of a hypercoagulable state, and the presence of valvular or endothelial damage.

Major operations produce a greater activation of coagulation factors than minor operations (Davidson and Tomlin, 1963; Flute *et al.*, 1972). The fractional and the absolute catabolic rates of fibrinogen are increased in the postoperative period (Atkins and Hawkins, 1969; Lim *et al.*, 1969; Davies *et al.*, 1970; Hickman, 1971). These changes have been interpreted as evidence of the stimulation of coagulation (Flute *et al.*, 1972).

The association of infection and premedication with omnopon, with an increased risk of thrombosis were rather unexpected findings. The significance of the latter is not clear as the criteria for administering it varied amongst the various anaesthetists. The high incidence of thrombosis in patients with postoperative infection is the result of an increase in the number of thrombi occurring after the third postoperative day (Nicolaides *et al.*, 1972). Bacterial endotoxin activates factor IX producing a hypercoagulable state and thrombosis in areas of venous stasis (Thomas and Wessler, 1964). Postoperative infection is often associated with bedrest and relative immobility.

The fact that malignancy, obesity and blood groups were not significant in this series does not mean that they do not predispose to thrombosis in other groups of patients such as medical in whom the tissue trauma is minimal and gynaecological whose average age is low.

The coefficients of the significant risk factors are expressions of relative risk and as such are independent of the incidence of thrombosis. They can be used as weights in order to compare the risk in different groups of patients of randomised controlled studies. Better still, they can be used prospectively to estimate the risk of thrombosis and stratify the patients admitted to a clinical trial before the latter are randomised. This method will ensure a comparable risk in the various groups.

Finally it should be stressed that the linear logistic analysis described has certain disadvantages. It has been performed in one series of patients and the results apply to this particular series only. Even if its validity were tested and confirmed in another prospective similar series it would not be necessarily applicable to a different group of patients in another hospital because of the probable presence of other unknown risk factors.

References

Armitage, P. (1971). *Statistical Methods in Medical Research* (Oxford and Edinburgh: Blackwell Scientific Publications)

Atkins, P. and Hawkins, L. A. (1969). The relationship of fibrinogen to postoperative venous thrombosis of the legs. *Surg. Gynaecol. Obstet.*, **128**, 818

Aurin, F. B. and Herrman, L. G. (1948). Management of venous thrombosis and pulmonary embolism following injury to the extremities. *Amer. J. Surg.*, **116**, 586

Barker, N. W., Nygaard, K. K., Walters, W. and Priestly, J. T. (1940). A statistical study of postoperative venous thrombosis and pulmonary embolism. *Proc. Mayo Clin.*, **15**, 769

Barker, N. W., Nygaard, K. K., Walters, W. and Priestly, J. T. (1941). A statistical study of postoperative venous thrombosis and pulmonary embolism: Predisposing factors. *Proc. Mayo Clin.*, **16**, 117

Bauer, G. (1944). Thrombosis following leg injuries. *Acta Chir. Scand.*, **90**, 229

Belding, H. H. (1965). Use of anticoagulants in prevention of venous thromboembolic disease in postoperative patients. *Arch. Surg.*, **90**, 566

Coon, W. W. and Coller, F. A. (1959). Some epidemiological considerations of thromboembolism. *Surg. Gynaecol. Obstet.*, **109**, 487

Cooperberg, A. A. and Teitelbaum, J. I. (1960). The concentration of antihaemophilic globulin related to age. *Brit. J. Haematol.*, **6**, 281

Davidson, E. and Tomlin, S. (1963). The levels of the plasma coagulation factors after trauma and childbirth. *J. Clin. Pathol.*, **16**, 112

Davies, J. W. L., Liljedahl, S. O. and Reijenstein, P. (1970). Fibrinogen metabolism following injury and its surgical treatment. *Injury*, **1**, 178

Flanc, C., Kakkar, V. V. and Clarke, M. B. (1969). Postoperative deep vein thrombosis. Effect of intensive prophylaxis. *Lancet*, **1**, 477

Flute, P. T., Kakkar, V. V., Renney, J. T. G. and Nicolaides, A. N. (1972). The blood and venous thromboembolism. In: *Thromboembolism*, (V. V. Kakkar and A. J. Jouhar, editors) (Churchill Livingstone)

Thromboembolism

Gibbs, N. M. (1957). Venous thrombosis of the lower limbs with particular reference to bedrest. *Brit. J. Surg.*, **45**, 209

Hickman, J. A. (1971). A study of the metabolism of fibrinogen after surgical operations. *Clin. Sci.*, **41**, 141

Hume, M. (1965). The relation of 'hypercoagulability' to thrombosis. *Monogr. in Surg. Sciences*, **2**, 133

Hume, M., Sevitt, S. and Thomas, D. P. (1970). *Venous Thrombosis and Pulmonary Embolism* (Cambridge, Massachusetts: Harvard University Press)

Jick, H., Sloane, D., Westerholm, B., Inman, W. H. W., Vessey, M. P., Shapiro, S., Lewis, G. P. and Worcester, J. (1969). Venous thromboembolic disease and ABO blood type. *Lancet*, **1**, 539

Kakkar, V. V., Howe, C. T., Nicolaides, A. N. Renney, J. T. G. and Clarke, M. B. (1970). Deep vein thrombosis of the leg – is there a 'high risk' group. *Amer. J. Surg.*, **120**, 527

Kemsley, W. F. F., Billewicz, W. Z. and Thomson, A. N. (1962). A new weight-for-height standard. *Brit. J. Prev. Soc. Med.*, **16**, 189

Kucera, M. (1968). Some problems of venous thromboembolism in patients with heart disease. *Rev. Czech. Med.*, **14**, 1

Lim, R. C. Jr, Appelgren, L., Bergentz, S. E. and Leander, L. (1969). The turnover of fibrinogen in aortic surgery. An experimental study in dogs. *Acta Chir. Scand.*, **135**, 363

Nicolaides, A. N. (1972). The prevention of postoperative deep venous thrombosis. *Jacksonian Prize Essay*

Nicolaides, A. N., Kakkar, V. V., Field, E. S. and Spindler, J. (1972). Antibiotics, postoperative infection, and deep vein thrombosis. *Brit. J. Surg.*, **60**, 312

Nicolaides, A. N. Irving, D., Pretzell, M., Dupont, P., Lewis, J., Desai, S., Douglas, J. N., Kakkar, V. V. and Field, E. S. (1973). The risk of deep-vein thrombosis in surgical patients. *Brit. J. Surg.*, **60**, 312

Nicolaides, A. N. and Irving, D. (1974). Unpublished data

Roberts, G. H. (1963). Venous thrombosis in hospital patients. A postmortem study. *Scot. Med. J.*, **8**, 11

Rosenthal, M. C., Niemetz, J. and Wish, N. (1963). Hemorrhage and thrombosis associated with neoplastic disorders. *J. Chronic Dis.*, **16**, 667

Sandritter, W. (1962). Die pathologische anatomic der thrombose und lungembolic. *Sonderdruck Benzinghnerke – Mitteil*, **41**, 37

Sevitt, S. and Gallagher, N. G. (1961). Venous thrombosis and pulmonary embolism. A clinico-pathological study in injured and burned patients. *Brit. J. Surg.*, **48**, 475

Snell, A. M. (1927). The relation of obesity to fatal postoperative pulmonary embolism. *Arch. Surg.*, **15**, 237

Sproul, E. E. (1938). Carcinoma and venous thrombosis. The frequency of association of carcinoma of the body or tail of the pancreas with multiple venous thrombosis. *Amer. J. Cancer*, **24**, 566

Thies, H. A. (1961). 13 years of postoperative thrombosis-prophylaxis with coumarin derivatives. In: *Proc. Dijkzigt Conf. on Prevention of Thromboembolism in Surgery*, 18 (Amsterdam: Excerpta Medica)

Thomas, D. and Wessler, S. (1964). Stasis thrombi induced by bacterial endotoxin. *Circ. Res.*, **14**, 486

Turnbull, A. C. (1960). Prophylaxis by anticoagulants after gynaecological operations. In: *Thrombosis and Anticoagulant Therapy*, 61 (W. Walker, editor) (London: Livingstone)

Thromboembolism

Vance, B. M. (1934). Thrombosis of veins of lower extremity and pulmonary embolism as a complication to trauma. *Amer. J. Surg.*, **26,** 19

Von Kaulla, E. and Von Kaulla, K. M. (1970). Oral contraceptives and low antithrombin activity. *Lancet,* **i,** 36

14

A rational approach to prevention

A. N. Nicolaides and Ian Gordon-Smith

The magnitude of the problem of deep venous thrombosis of the legs and its consequences has become apparent in the last few years (Chapter 1). The development of the ^{125}I-fibrinogen test (Hobbs and Davies, 1960; Atkins and Hawkins, 1965; Flanc et al., 1968; Negus et al., 1968; Kakkar et al., 1970a), which is an objective and sensitive method for diagnosing and studying thrombosis, has demonstrated that the incidence of the disease is high not only in surgical (Atkins and Hawkins, 1965; Flanc et al., 1968; Negus et al., 1968; Kakkar et al., 1970b; Friend, 1971; Field et al., 1972; Nicolaides et al., 1972c), but also in medical patients (Murray et al., 1970; Maurer et al., 1971; Nicolaides et al., 1971b).

If the mortality due to pulmonary embolism and the morbidity due to the destruction of venous valves by deep venous thrombosis were to be significantly reduced, effective methods of prevention should be developed and applied to the patients at risk (Chapter 13). Recent progress in understanding the pathogenesis of deep venous thrombosis has gone some way towards devising preventive measures. Before, however, any attempts are made at prophylaxis, the following questions should be answered: when, where and why thrombi start, what is their fate and which patients are particularly at risk? Answers to these questions are essential preliminary steps in any rational attempt to prevent deep venous thrombosis.

PATHOGENESIS
[125]I -fibrinogen test
This is the most sensitive test to detect the presence of a developing

Table 14.1 Incidence of deep venous thrombosis in patients studied with the [125] I-fibrinogen test

Type of patients	Incidence (per cent)	Reference
General surgical	35	Flanc et al., 1968
	35	Negus et al., 1968
	30·5	Kakkan et al., 1970a
	41	Williams, 1971
	42	Gordon-Smith et al., 1972
	23	Nicolaides et al., 1972b
	14·5	Gallus et al., 1973b
Patients undergoing a thoracotomy	26	Nicolaides et al., 1972b
Gynaecological	17	Friend, 1971
	15	Bonnar et al., 1972
	29	Ballard et al., 1973
Patients with fractured neck of femur	47	Field et al., 1971
	54	Kakkar et al., 1972
	56	Gallus et al., 1973a
Patients undergoing elective hip operations	42	Gallus et al., 1973a
	37	Nicolaides et al., 1974b
Patients undergoing prostatectomy	30	Nicolaides et al., 1972c
	38	Mayo et al., 1972
Patients with myocardial infarction	34	Murray et al., 1970
	38	Nicolaides et al., 1971a
	29	Handley et al., 1972
	17·2	Warlow et al., 1973
	22·5	Gallus et al., 1973b
Medical patients in shock	68	Nicolaides et al., 1971a

thrombus and can accurately determine its progress, whether extending or lysing. The test is based on the work of Hobbs and Davies who first demonstrated experimentally that [131] I-fibrinogen injected into the circulation was incorporated into a developing thrombus as [131] I-fibrin which could be detected by an external scintillation counter (Hobbs and Davies, 1960). Atkins and Hawkins substituted the isotope ^{125}I for [131]I (Atkins and Hawkins, 1965). Because ^{125}I emits a softer gamma radiation, lighter and more mobile apparatus could be used. The accuracy of this test has been confirmed by venography (Flanc *et al.*, 1968; Negus *et al.*, 1968; Field *et al.*, 1972), and by using a ratemeter (Kakkar *et al.*, 1970b) it has become a simple test suitable for the routine screening of a large number of patients. This test has demonstrated that clinical signs are unreliable and that the true incidence of deep venous thrombosis in several groups of patients is much higher than previously thought (Table 14.1). It has also played a vital part in answering the following questions:

When do thrombi occur? By screening a large number of surgical patients with the [125] I-fibrinogen test it was demonstrated that 45 per cent of the thrombi occurred on the day of operation, 43 per cent during the first four postoperative days and the remaining 12 per cent during the subsequent five days (Nicolaides, 1972). The time thrombosis was first detected in patients and in individual limbs is shown in Figures 14.1 and 14.2. Bilateral thrombosis tended to occur in the early postoperative period (Figure 14.1). With the exception of two patients whenever thrombi occurred in both limbs, they occurred within 24 hours of each other. Most studies with the [125] I-fibrinogen test have been limited to the first seven to ten postoperative days. Information about the frequency of thrombosis during the subsequent postoperative period is not available. However, a recent venographic study in patients having elective hip operations has suggested that 50 per cent of the patients have thrombi in the leg veins during the second and third postoperative weeks (Johnson, 1974) and that many of the thrombi are in the femoral and more proximal veins. It can therefore be concluded that preventive measures must be applied during the operation as well as in the postoperative period. They should probably be continued until the patient is discharged from hospital.

Where do thrombi start? The site in the legs where the increased radioactivity first occurs in patients studied with the [125] I-fibrinogen test is the site where a thrombus starts. Of 330 general surgical patients studied before and after operation deep venous thrombosis developed in 98 (29·7 per cent) patients (Nicolaides, 1972). In 89 per cent of the patients with thrombosis the radioactivity was first detected in the calf. In 6·5 per

Thromboembolism

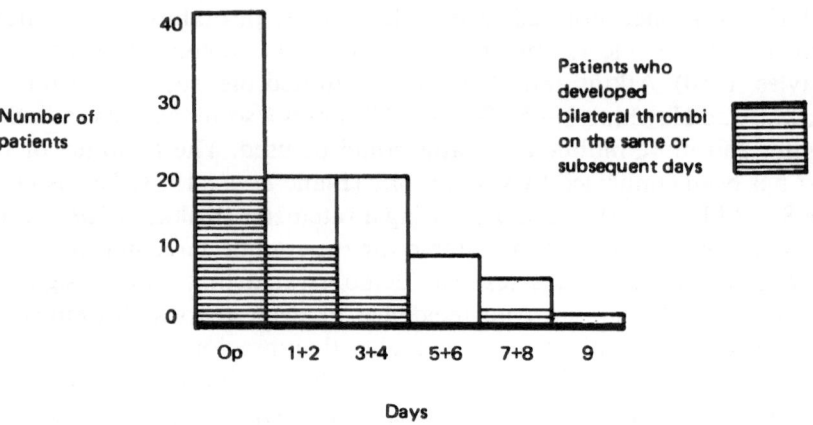

Figure 14.1 The time thrombosis was detected

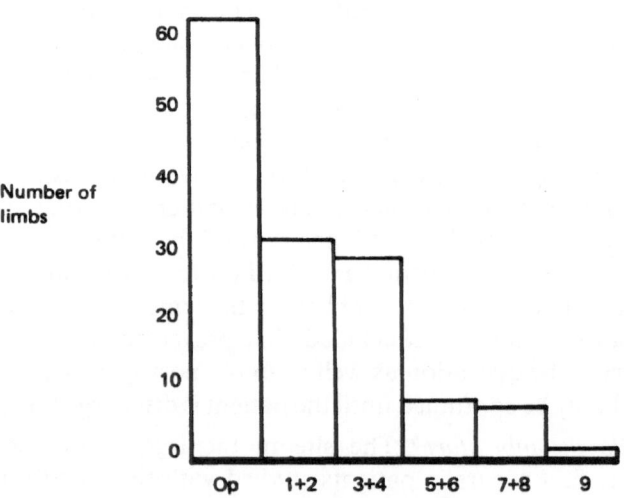

Figure 14.2 The time thrombi started

cent it was first detected in the popliteal fossa and in 4 per cent in the thigh. Thrombosis was bilateral in 35 and unilateral in 63 patients. There were 72 right and 59 left legs with thrombosis.

Unfortunately, the [125] I-fibrinogen test cannot detect a thrombus proximal to the inguinal ligament because of the high background radioactivity and it cannot determine whether a thrombus in the calf is present in a soleal or a tibial vein. Information on the exact site of origin of thrombi is of importance for several reasons. Any attempt at prophylaxis would have to take into account where the thrombus commences, whether it is related to stasis and, if so, how stasis can be prevented. Using a venographic technique that could demonstrate the soleal veins consistently in the presence or absence of thrombosis evidence has been produced that the majority of calf thrombi which start in the calf, start in the soleal veins (Nicolaides *et al.*, 1971a; Nicolaides, 1972; Chapter 11).

Anatomico-pathological studies (Chapter 10) have demonstrated that thrombi can start practically anywhere in the deep veins of the lower limb. However, a venographic study of the distribution and extent of thrombi in 137 limbs of patients in hospital (Chapter 11) has suggested that in 46 per cent of limbs thrombosis was confined to the calf; in 42 per cent thrombi had probably started in the calf but had extended proximally; in only 12 per cent was there evidence that thrombi had started in veins proximal to the calf. If one can therefore prevent thrombi that start in the calf one would be eliminating 88 per cent of all thrombi and 78 per cent of the proximal which constitute a risk to life (see below : What is the fate of thrombi?). Proximal thrombi must also be prevented and methods that prevent the hypercoagulable state are probably more likely to succeed in this than methods which prevent venous stasis in the lower leg.

What is the fate of thrombi? The early natural history of post operative thrombosis has been studied using the [125] I-fibrinogen test (Kakkar *et al.*, 1969). The majority of thrombi (78 per cent) either lyse spontaneously or remain localised to the calf, while only 22 per cent extend into and proximal to the popliteal vein. Large clinical pulmonary emboli occur in patients in the latter group (Kakkar *et al.*, 1969) and only small silent emboli in patients with thrombi confined to the calf (Browse *et al.*, 1974a). Thus for the first time it has become possible to select the patients whose life is at risk.

Why do thrombi start? There is good clinical evidence that in surgical patients the maximum risk of deep venous thrombosis is at the time of operation or soon afterwards when the majority of thrombi start (Figure

14.1). This means that factors responsible for intravascular coagulation produce their maximum effect at this particular time. *In vitro* experiments have shown that, immediately after operation, clotting factors are found circulating in the blood in an activated form. The hypercoagulable state produced by these activated clotting factors and the significance of Factor X, its plasma inhibitor, phospholipid, heparin, venous stasis and platelets whose interplay may result in the production of thrombin and deposition of fibrin have been discussed in Chapter 2. The production of thrombi depends mainly on the action of activated clotting factors in an area of stasis. Thrombosis is not produced by stasis alone or by activated factors alone, but by the combination of the two (Wessler and Yin, 1968; Chapter 2). Stasis in the soleal veins is considerable when the patient is supine with the leg horizontal and immobile (Chapter 9) and may explain why the majority of thrombi start in the soleal and not in the tibial veins.

Recent studies of the venous endothelium using scanning electron microscopy have demonstrated that stasis produces white cell migration and damage to the endothelium particularly if there is associated tissue trauma, even at a distant site (Chapter 8).

If the incidence of deep venous thrombosis is to be reduced by preventing the hypercoagulable state induced by operation, then it must be done when this state is at its maximum, during and immediately after operation. If the incidence of venous thrombosis is to be reduced by preventing stasis, then prophylactic measures must be directed towards the prevention of stasis in the soleal veins, particularly during operation. The efficacy of different methods of preventing stasis in the soleal veins has been discussed in Chapter 9.

It has been suggested that trauma, surgery and other clinical states which predispose to thrombosis produce an initial transient activation of fibrinolysis followed by a period of inhibition lasting up to 10 days (Innes and Sevitt, 1964; Flute, 1965; Pinson *et al.*, 1965; Leandoer, 1968; Chakrabarti *et al.*, 1968). When the dilute blood clot lysis time (Fearnley *et al.*, 1957) was measured in 92 general surgical patients studied with the [125] I-fibrinogen test there was no difference in fibrinolytic activity between those who did and those who did not develop thrombosis in the post-operative period (Flute *et al.*, 1972). Measurements of the fibrinolytic activity in studies such as the above, made using the euglobulin lysis time (von Kaulla, 1963) and the dilute blood clot lysis time (Fearnley *et al.*, 1957), are influenced by the concentration of fibrinogen which forms the substrate (Blix, 1961; Gallimore and Shaw, 1969; Hickman,

1971) and is markedly increased in the postoperative period (Egeburg, 1962; Flute et al., 1972). Recently, a technique has been deveoped for the measurement of blood fibrinolytic activity employing [125] I-fibrinogen in vivo (Hickman and Gordon-Smith, 1972) which is independent of the fibrinogen concentration (Hickman et al., 1973). Using this technique the changes in the blood fibrinolytic activity were studied in 50 patients undergoing major operations (Gordon-Smith et al., 1974). A phase of enhanced fibrinolytic activity occurred at the time of operation, but no evidence of sustained fibrinolytic shut down was demonstrated. However, patients who developed thrombosis had a significantly lower fibrinolytic activity on the first postoperative day than patients without thrombosis. There was no difference in the fibrinolytic activity in the two groups during the subsequent six postoperative days. This has confirmed the similar previous findings of another study (Mansfield, 1972) based on measurements of the dilute blood clot lysis time and euglobulin lysis time.

In a recent study (Nicolaides et al., 1972a) the fibrinolytic activity of the endothelium of the femoral, popliteal and soleal veins obtained soon after death has been compared using a histochemical technique. The results suggest that the fibrinolytic activity in the soleal veins may be low when compared with the femoral and popliteal. It has already been stated that stasis in the soleal veins is considered to be an important factor predisposing to deep venous thrombosis. The relatively low fibrinolytic activity found in these veins and any low activity that may occur in the postoperative period may play a part in determining whether a small early thrombus will propagate or lyse; diminished fibrinolytic activity is unlikely to be responsible for the initiation of thrombosis. A recent trial (Fossard et al., 1973) has demonstrated that a preoperative course of oral phenformin and ethylestrenol which stimulated the fibrinolytic activity in the blood was ineffective in preventing deep venous thrombosis.

Urokinase with its specific inhibitor forms an integral part of the fibrinolytic mechanism (Bernik and Kwaan, 1971). This specific inhibitor was found to be high in platelets (Kwaan and Sawanwela, 1971) and in the plasma in late pregnancy (Brakman and Astrup, 1963), in patients with carcinoma (Soong and Miller, 1970; Kwaan, 1973) and sickle cell disease (Kwaan, 1973). This finding may be an important aetiological factor in the pathogenesis of venous thrombosis in patients with these conditions. It may also explain why passive compression of legs with pneumatic cuffs did not increase the fibrinolytic activity in the blood of patients with malignant disease (Allenby et al., 1974) and did not prevent thrombosis, while it did in patients without malignancy.

Thromboembolism

The number of platelets and their stickiness is increased after operation and in certain medical conditions. Platelet aggregation and adhesion can be produced by small amounts of thrombin and polymerising fibrinogen (Chapters 2, 7 and 8). When the platelet count and adhesiveness were studied in surgical patients screened with the ^{125}I-fibrinogen test, no correlation was found with deep venous thrombosis (Flute *et al.*, 1972). It seems that the increase in platelet count and adhesiveness which occurs after operation is a normal response to trauma. It reaches its maximum approximately one week after operation, but by then most of the thrombi have already formed (Figure 14.1). The available evidence (Chapters 2, 7 and 8) suggests that though platelet aggregation is important for the evolution of venous thrombi it is a secondary phenomenon following the activation of clotting factors. It is therefore not surprising that antiplatelet drugs have a limited success in preventing venous thrombosis (see below).

Bacterial endotoxin activates Factor XI which produces a hyper-coagulable state and thrombosis in areas of venous stasis. (Thomas and Wessler, 1964; Chapter 2). This can be prevented experimentally by as little as 10 units of heparin per kilogram, injected intravenously, a dose insufficient to prolong the clotting time. In a recent series of 400 surgical patients screened with the ^{125}I fibrinogen test, the incidence of deep venous thrombosis was 20 per cent in patients without evidence of infection and 55 per cent in patients who had postoperative infection (Nicolaides *et al.*, 1972e). The increased incidence in the latter group was due to a large number of thrombi occurring between the third and eighth postoperative days.

The evidence available suggests that in surgical patients the hyper-coagulable state produced by tissue trauma and venous stasis are the most important factors responsible for the initiation of thrombosis, while other factors mentioned above may play a secondary part in the formation of thrombi (Chapter 2). However, some factors such as low levels of antithrombin III in women on the pill (Fagerhol *et al.*, 1970), high levels of urokinase inhibitor in patients with carcinoma (Soong and Miller, 1970; Kwaan, 1973) and low fibrinolytic activity in patients with recurrent idiopathic venous thrombosis (Nilsson, 1968) may be of importance in medical or low risk surgical patients.

Which patients are at risk? The aim of prophylaxis in surgical patients is to prevent the deep venous thrombosis which occurs in a proportion of patients (Table 14.1) and its sequelae. Though methods of prophylaxis may soon become simple and safe, it is highly desirable to be able to select the high risk patients and avoid treating everybody. The clinical factors associated with a high incidence of pulmonary embolism and deep venous thrombosis have already been discussed in Chapters 12 and 13, where it has been demonstrated how the risk of pulmonary embolism and deep venous thrombosis for a patient can be estimated using clinical information.

METHODS OF PROPHYLAXIS
It follows from the above that the incidence of deep venous thrombosis is likely to be reduced by methods which prevent either venous stasis or the hypercoagulable state. There have been many attempts to prevent thrombosis in the past, but in most trials the diagnosis of thrombosis was based on clinical signs which we now know to be unreliable (Chapters 11 and 17). The review which follows is limited mainly to recent clinical trials in which the diagnosis of thrombosis was made using objective methods such as the [125] I-fibrinogen test and venography.

Methods of preventing venous stasis
Specific attempts to reduce the incidence of deep venous thrombosis by preventing venous stasis have produced variable results. Passive compression of the legs using elastic stockings and leg elevation, each used on its own, have been ineffective in preventing thrombosis in surgical patients scanned with the [125] I-fibrinogen test (Rosengarten et al., 1980): Rosengarten and Laird, 1971; Browse et al., 1974b). When leg elevation was used in combination with elastic stockings and frequent supervised active leg exercises, it was found to reduce the incidence of thrombosis by approximately 50 per cent in patients over the age of 60 undergoing major operations (Flanc et al., 1969). Better results were obtained in a subsequent study using the same regimen (Tsapogas et al., 1971), but the work involved in supervising the patients undergoing intensive prophylaxis would strain the resources of the department of physical medicine and school of nursing of any hospital.

Active intermittent compression of the calf by enclosing the leg in a pneumatic bag during and after operation has prevented deep venous thrombosis in several controlled clinical trials (Sabri et al., 1971b; Hills et al., 1972; Roberts et al., 1972; Allenby et al., 1973). However, it was not always effective in patients with malignant disease. The main disadvantage of this method is the logistic problem of applying the pneumatic bags, not only at operation but also during the postoperative period.

213

Passive dorsiflexion of the foot during operation by motor driven pedals has reduced the incidence of deep venous thrombosis by 77 per cent during the first three postoperative days (Roberts *et al.*, 1971; Sabri *et al.*, 1971a). There is not any evidence, however, that it has an effect during the subsequent postoperative period.

Electrical stimulation of the calf muscles during operation produced a 61 per cent reduction in the incidence of deep venous thrombosis in an exemplary trial using the [125] I-fibrinogen test (Browse and Negus, 1970). However, this has not been confirmed by others (De Jode *et al.*, 1970; Moloney *et al.*, 1972). The difference in the results may be due to the different stimuli used.

Cinephlebographic studies have shown that the soleus muscle and its veins act as a peripheral pump, filling during relaxation and emptying during contraction (stroke volume) (Almen and Nylander, 1962). By recording the changes in the blood velocity in the femoral vein it was possible to determine the most effective electrical calf stimulus which produces the maximum stroke volume which can be maintained during the operation (Nicolaides *et al.*, 1972d). It has become clear that the most important rate of stimulation which prevents stasis in the soleal veins by alternately emptying them and allowing them to refill is once every four seconds. Stimuli more frequent than this produce a progressive fall in the stroke volume because the short interval between them does not allow complete filling of the soleal veins. When this stimulus was used in a controlled clinical trial in patients scanned with the [125] I-fibrinogen test during the first nine postoperative days, it produced a 92 per cent reduction in the incidence of deep venous thrombosis (Nicolaides *et al.*, 1972d).

Physical methods of prophylaxis present certain difficulties. They cannot be used during orthopaedic operations, in patients in the lithotomy position, and in patients undergoing lateral thoracotomy. They are impractical or extremely inconvenient for the surgeon. It may well be that methods which prevent blood hypercoagulability may prove more practical in these patients.

METHODS ALTERING THE COMPOSITION OF BLOOD
Dextran

Experimental work with Dextran has demonstrated that it prevents thrombi in injured vessels (Bryant *et al.*, 1963; Just-Viera and Veager, 1964; Sawyer *et al.*, 1965), but for non traumatic experimental thrombosis the evidence has been conflicting (Borgstrom *et al.*, 1959; Gurewich and Thomas, 1965; Gruber and Bergentz, 1966). It is thought that Dextran-70 acts by coating the venous endothelium and the formed elements of the blood, and by interfering with the platelet adhesiveness and aggregation (Bygdeman, 1968; Dhall et al., 1968; Bygdeman, 1969; Atik et al., 1970).

In the first controlled clinical trial reported (Koekenberg, 1961) all cases of thrombosis and 11 other cases of embolism were diagnosed among the 105 controls, and only 4 cases of thrombosis among the 94 patients receiving Dextran-70. Subsequent trials by other workers confirmed the beneficial effect of Dextran-70 not only in general surgical patients (Jansen, 1968; Sawyer, 1968; Stadil, 1968; London and Cross-fill, 1969) but also in patients with a fractured neck of femur (Ahlberg et al., 1968; Johnson et al., 1968). The diagnosis of venous thrombosis in these trials was based mainly on clinical signs although sometimes venography was employed (Johnson et al., 1968).

With the advent of the [125] I-fibrinogen test further trials were performed using this test to diagnose thrombosis. Matheson, Lambie and their co-workers compared the effect of warfarin begun on the second postoperative day with Dextran-70 administered during operation and on subsequent days in a series of 80 gynaecological patients (Matheson, 1969; Lambie et al., 1970). The incidence of thrombosis in the warfarin group was 12/40 and in the Dextran-70 group 4/70. However, subsequent workers using the [125] I-fibrinogen test and Dextran-70 obtained conflicting results (Renney et al., 1970; Bonnar et al., 1972).

As the number of patients in each of the trials published was too small to permit statistical analysis on the incidence of fatal pulmonary embolism, Bygdeman and his colleagues combined the results of all the controlled studies available at the time (Bygdeman et al., 1970). There were 18 patients with fatal pulmonary embolism out of 1381 in the control groups and only four out of 1321 patients in the treated groups ($\chi^2 = 7 \cdot 18$; $p < 0 \cdot 01$). The results of the clinical trials with Dextran-70 taken as a whole suggest that the incidence of deep venous thrombosis and pulmonary embolism is diminished, but it is by no means abolished. The absence of bleeding complications and the lack of laboratory control are advantages, while the intravenous route and the danger of overloading the circulation are serious disadvantages.

Recently a regimen of 1000 ml of Dextran-40 daily for 10 days starting just before operation has been used in a controlled clinical trial of patients having elective hip operations (Evarts and Feil, 1971). Venograms were performed routinely before operation and at 10 to 12 days after operation. The incidence of deep venous thrombosis was 55·6 per cent in the control group (36 patients) as compared with 6·4 per cent in the test group (31 patients). The high doses of Dextran-40 used had the dangers of causing haemodilution and congestive cardiac failure.

Antiplatelet agents other than Dextran
Dipyridamole inhibits ADP-induced platelet aggregation in man and prevents thrombosis in rabbit vessels subjected to trauma (Emmons *et al.*, 1965). However, a double blind trial has failed to demonstrate any protective effect against postoperative venous thrombosis (Browse and Hall, 1969).

Hydroxychloroquine also inhibits ADP-induced platelet aggregation in man (Carter *et al.*, 1971) and red cell 'sludging' (Madow, 1960). In a controlled clinical trial involving 565 patients undergoing major operations the incidence of pulmonary embolism was 6 per cent in the controls and 1 per cent in the test group (Carter *et al.*, 1971). There was a highly significant difference in the incidence of deep venous thrombosis as determined by clinical signs and venography. These promising results may be due to the combined antiplatelet and antisludging effect of hydroxychoroquine.

Aspirin inhibits ADP and collagen induced platelet aggregation (Wiess and Aledort, 1967; Zucker and Paterson, 1968). The efficacy of aspirin and dipyridamole in preventing thrombosis has been compared (Saltsman *et al.*, 1971). Aspirin was the most promising, but was not found to prevent deep venous thrombosis in other studies (O'Brien *et al.*, 1971; Sherry, 1971; Report of the Steering Committee of a Trial Sponsored by the Medical Research Council, 1972).

Anticoagulants
Heparin was found to be valuable in preventing thromboembolism (Wetterdall, 1941; Bauer, 1946) soon after it was isolated. However, the difficulties of its administration and control and the risk of bleeding prevented its widespread use in surgical but not in medical patients.

Later, when oral anticoagulants became available, they were found to be more acceptable. The first controlled trial by Sevitt and Gallagher in patients with fractured hips showed a marked reduction in clinical thrombosis and pulmonary embolism in the treated patients (Sevitt and Gallagher, 1959). It soon became apparent that the main disadvantage of oral anticoagulants was that the dose had to be controlled by a properly organised hospital laboratory, and this was essential if the incidence of bleeding and haematoma formation was to be kept to the minimum. A small haematoma at the hip would not be a grave complication, but at the site of an intestinal anastomosis might prove fatal. In addition reversal of an oral anticoagulant takes some time and this is undesirable in surgical patients.

The most promising form of prophylaxis reported is the use of low doses of subcutaneous heparin (Chapters 15 and 16). The basis for this method of prophylaxis stems from the identification of a potent, naturally occurring inhibitor to activated Factor X in Human plasma (Yin and Wessler, 1970; Chapter 2) and the observation that the activity of this inhibitor is enhanced by heparin (Chapter 2). Activated Factor X occupies a key position in the intrinsic and extrinsic coagulation mechanisms. If heparin is administered before the tissue trauma activates Factor X, then low doses of heparin are quite adequate in preventing thrombosis. Such doses would be quite safe as they would have no effect on the clotting time. Other possible actions of small dose subcutaneous heparin include reduced postoperative platelet adhesiveness and increased lipoprotein lipase activity. (Chapter 15). Its efficacy in the various clinical trials recently performed, its relative safety and possible dangers are discussed in Chapters 15 and 16. There is little doubt that small dose subcutaneous heparin is effective in preventing deep venous thrombosis in general surgical, thoracic and gynaecological patients.

In six of the randomised trials of small dose subcutaneous heparin recently reported (Chapter 16) data are available about the incidence of thrombi extending into the popliteal and more proximal veins (Table 14.2). There were 22 proximal thrombi in 512 patients in the control groups and 3 in the test groups ($\chi^2 = 12\cdot4$; $p< 0\cdot0005$). It is interesting to note that the three proximal thrombi in the heparin-treated group had occurred in orthopaedic patients: one after elective and two after emergency hip operations. It has already been stated that if thrombosis is limited to the calf the risk of large clinically detectable pulmonary emboli is for all practical purposes negligible, but if the popliteal and more proximal veins are involved the risk of pulmonary embolism is rapidly increased to 50 per cent (Kakkar *et al.*, 1969). It has been demonstrated (Chapter 11) that the proximal extensions of the thrombi which start in the calf constitute approximately two-thirds of all the thrombi involving the proximal veins from which pulmonary emboli arise. It can therefore be argued that the reduction in the incidence of the proximal extensions by small dose subcutaneous heparin will also result in the reduction of the incidence of pulmonary embolism. This argument is indirect, but it is supported by the results reported by Sharnoff (Sharnoff and deBlazio, 1970; Chapter 15). Direct evidence

Table 14.2 The incidence of proximal thrombi in randomised trials of small dose subcutaneous heparin in surgical patients

Randomised trials with available data about proximal thrombi	Number of patients in trials	Number of patients with thrombi extending into the popliteal and more proximal veins	
		Control group	Heparin group
Williams, 1971	56	1	0
Nicolaides et al., 1972b	244	9	0
Gordon-Smith 1972	100	3	0
Gallus et al., 1973b	419	6	3*
Ballard et al., 1973	110	0	0
Nicolaides et al., 1974b	60	3	0
Total	989	22 (4.1 per cent)	3 (0·6 per cent)

x^2 (with Yates correction) $= 12·4$; $p < 0·0005$

*Thrombi occurred in one patient after elective hip surgery and in two patients after emergency hip surgery

about the efficacy of small dose subcutaneous heparin on the incidence of pulmonary embolism cannot be obtained from trials in which the [125] I-fibrinogen is used, however large they may be, because whenever proximal thrombosis is detected conventional anticoagulation therapy is administered. It would be unethical to do otherwise.

Direct evidence has recently been produced by studying small dose heparin prophylaxis against fatal pulmonary embolism in a controlled prospective trial now in progress in patients over the age of 50 having major operations (Sagar, 1974). In this study all patients who die come to necropsy. A dose of 5000 units of heparin is given subcutaneously two hours before operation and then twelve-hourly for five days. Fatal pulmonary embolism did not occur in any of the 156 patients in the test group, whereas 6 (4·2 per cent) patients of the 144 in the control group died of pulmonary embolism. This difference was significant. There was no increase in perioperative bleeding or in the formation of wound haematomas in the treated group.

A number of questions remain unanswered and some of them point the direction further research should follow: heparin has been isolated from the vessel wall (Gore and Larkey, 1960). Its unique property to

218

potentiate the naturally occurring inhibitor to activated Factor X suggests that it forms a critical barrier against activated coagulation factors at the vessel wall interface. It may prove useful to investigate the resistance of the vascular endothelium to thrombosis in relation to the heparin bound to it (Damus *et al.*, 1973). The sensitive method of measuring heparin blood levels based on the action of heparin on the inhibitor to activated Factor X (Yin *et al.*, 1973) has been simplified (Denson and Bonnar, 1973). It is therefore possible to study the blood levels produced by the various regimens of heparin used empirically until now. Information is required on the blood levels of heparin in patients who develop thrombosis while on a prophylactic regimen; on the maximum blood levels of heparin produced when 5000 units of subcutaneous heparin are administered eight-hourly; and on the effect of the patient's age, weight and tissue trauma on these blood levels. Answering questions such as these would be a rational approach to the development of a safe and effective regimen of subcutaneous heparin, not only in general surgical, but also in orthopaedic and medical patients.

Most of the advances in prophylaxis achieved in recent years have been made mainly by studies in surgical patients. The problem of thromboembolism is also great in medical patients, for example, 13 per cent of cardiac patients who die, die from pulmonary embolism (Coon and Coller, 1959) and probably more die in the geriatric wards (Gilchrist and Tulloch, 1956). It has been suggested that studies in these patients might be even more rewarding (Nicolaides *et al.*, 1974a).

References .

Ahlberg, A., Nylander, G., Robertson, B., Cronberg, S. and Nilson, I. M. (1968). Dextran in prophylaxis of thrombosis in fractures of the hip. *Acta Chir. Scand., Suppl.* **387,** 83

Allenby, F., Calnan, J. S. and Pflug, J. J. (1973). The use of pneumatic compression in the swollen leg. *J. Physiol. (London),* **231,** 65

Allenby, F., Boardman, L., Pflug, J. J. and Calnan, J. S. (1973). Effects of external pneumatic compression on fibrinolysis in man. *Lancet,* **ii,** 1412

Almen, T. and Nylander, G. (1962). Serial phleborgraphy of the normal lower leg during muscular contraction and relaxation. *Acta Radiol.,* **57,** 264

Atik, M., Harkess, J. W. and Wichman, H. (1970). Prevention of fatal pulmonary embolism. *Surg. Gynaecol. Obstet.,* **130,** 403

Atkins, P. and Hawkins, L. A. (1965). Detection of venous thrombosis in the legs. *Lancet,* **2,** 1216

Ballard, R. M., Bradley-Watson, P. J., Johnstone, F. D., Kenney, A., McCarthy, T. G., Campbell, S. and Weston, J. (1973). Low doses of subcutaneous heparin in the prevention of deep vein thrombosis after gynaecological surgery. *J. Obstet. Gynaecol.,* **80,** 469

Bauer, G. (1946). Thrombosis: Early diagnosis and abortive treatment with heparin. *Lancet,* **i,** 447

Thromboembolism

Bermik, M. B. and Kwaan, H. C. (1971). Inhibitors of fibrinolysis in human tissues in culture. *Amer. J. Physiol.*, **221**, 916

Blix, S. (1961). The fibrinolysis of plasma clots under various conditions. *Acta Med. Scand.*, **169**, 495

Bonnar, J. and Walsh, J. (1972). Prevention of thrombosis after pelvic surgery by British dextran 70. *Lancet*, **i**, 614

Borgstrom, S. Gelin, L. E. and Zederfeldt, B. (1959). Formation of vein thrombi following tissue injury. *Acta Chir. Scand.*, **Suppl. 247**

Brakman, P. and Astrup, T. (1963). Selective inhibition in human pregnancy blood of urokinase induced fibrinolysis. *Scand. J. Clin. and Lab. Invest.*, **15**, 603

Browse, N. L. and Hall, J. H. (1969). Effect of dipyridamole on the incidence of clinically detectable deep vein thrombosis. *Lancet*, **ii**, 718

Browse, N. L. and Negus, D. (1970). Prevention of postoperative leg vein thrombosis by electrical muscle stimulation. An evaluation with ^{125}I-labelled fibrinogen. *Brit. Med. J.*, **3**, 615

Browse, N. L., Clemenson, G. and Croft, D. N. (1974a). Fibrinogen-detectable thrombosis in the legs and pulmonary embolism. *Brit. Med. J.*, **1**, 603

Browse, N. L., Jackson, B. T., Mayo, M. E. and Negus, D. (1974b). The value of mechanical methods of preventing postoperative calf vein thrombosis. *Brit. J. Surg.*, **61**, 219

Bryant, M. F., Bloom, W. L. and Brewer, S. S. (1963). Experimental study of the anti-thrombotic properties of dextrans of low molecular weight. *Amer. Surg.*, **29**, 256

Bygdeman, S. (1968). Experimental studies on the antithrombotic effect of dextran. *Acta Chir. Scand.*, **Suppl. 387**, 44

Bygdeman, S. (1969). Prevention and therapy of thromboembolic complications with dextran. In: *Progress in Surgery*, vol. VII p. 14 (Basel: Karger)

Bygdeman, S., Svenjo, E. and Tollerz, C. (1970). Prevention of venous thrombosis. *Lancet*, **ii**, 419

Carter, A. E., Eban, R. and Perrett, R. D. (1971). Prevention of postoperative deep venous thrombosis and pulmonary embolism. *Brit. Med. J.*, **1**, 312

Chakrabarti, R., Hocking, E. D., Fearnley, G. R., Mann, R. D., Attwell, T. N. and Jackson, D. (1968). Fibrinolytic activity in coronary heart disease. *Lancet*, **i**, 987

Coon, W. W. and Coller, F. A. (1959). Some epidemiological consideration of thromboembolism. *Surg. Gynaecol. Obstet.*, **109**, 487

Damus, P. S., Hicks, M. and Rosenberg, R. R. (1973). Anticoagulant action of heparin. *Nature (London)*, **246**, 355

De Jode, L. R., Khuzshid, M. and Walter, W. W. (1970). Postoperative leg vein thrombosis. *Brit. Med. J.*, **4**, 56

Denson, K. W. E. and Bonnar, J. (1973). The measurement of heparin. A method based on the potentiation of antifactor Xa. *Thromb. Diath. Haemorrh. (Stuttg.)* **30**, 171

Dhall, D. P., Bennett, P. N. and Matheson, N. A. (1968). Effect of dextran on platelet behaviour after abdominal operations. *Acta Chir. Scand.*, **Suppl. 387**, 75

Egeburg, O. (1962). Changes in the coagulation system following major surgical operations. *Acta Med. Scand.*, **171**, 679

Emmons, P. R., Harrison, M. J. G., Honour, A. J. and Mitchell, J. R. A. (1965). Effect of dipyridamole on human platelet behaviour. *Lancet*, **ii**, 603

Evarts, C. M. and Feil, E. J. (1971). Prevention of thromboembolic disease after elective surgery of the hip. *J. Bone Joint Surg. (A.M.)*, **53**, 1271

Thromboembolism

Fagerhol, M. K., Abilgaard, V., Bergsje, P. and Jacobsen, J. H. (1970). Oral contraceptives and low antithronmbin III concentration. *Lancet*, **i**, 1175

Fearnley, G. R., Balmforth, G. and Fearnley, E. (1957). Evidence of a diurnal rhythm; with a simple method of measuring natural fibrinolysis. *Clin. Sci.*, **16**, 645

Field, E. S., Nicolaides, A. N., Kakkar, V. V. and Crellin, R. Q. (1972). Deep-vein thrombosis in patients with fractures of the femoral neck. *Brit. J. Surg.*, **59**, 377

Flanc, C., Kakkar, V. V. and Clarke, M. B. (1968). The detection of venous thrombosis of the legs using 125I-labelled fibrinogen. *Brit. J. Surg.*, **55**, 742

Flanc, C., Kakkar, V. V. and Clarke, M. B. (1969). Postoperative deep-vein thrombosis: Effect of intensive prophylaxis. *Lancet*, **i**, 477

Flute, P. T. (1965). Fibrinolysis in relation to thrombosis. *Ann. Roy. Coll. Surg. Engl.*, **36**, 225

Flute, P. T., Kakkar, V. V., Renney, J. T. G. and Nicolaides, A. N. (1972). The blood and venous thromboembolism. In: *Thromboembolism* (V. V. Kakkar and A. J. Jouhar, editors) (Churchill Livingstone)

Fossard, D. P., Corrigan, T. P., Field, E. S., Friend, J., Kakkar, V. V. and Flute, P. T. (1973). The effect of stimulating fibrinolytic activity on the incidence of postoperative deep vein thrombosis. *IVth Int. Cong. Thromb. Haemost.* (Abstracts), **248**, 283

Friend, J. (1971). Personal communication

Gallimore, M. J. and Shaw, J. T. B. (1969). The influence of various plasma components on the lysis of dilute human blood clots. *Thromb. Diath. Haemorrh.*, **22**, 223

Gallus, A. S., Hirsh, J., Turpre, A. G. G. and Tuttle, R. (1973a). Prevention of venous thrombosis with small doses of subcutaneous heparin. *IVth Int. Cong. Thromb. Haemost.* (Abstracts), 276

Gallus, A. S., Hirsh, J., Tuttle, R. J., Trebilcock, R., O'Brien, S. E., Carroll, J. J., Minden, J. H. and Hudecki, S. M. (1973b). Small subcutaneous doses of heparin in prevention of venous thrombosis. *New Eng. J. Med.*, **288**, 545

Gilchrist, A. R. and Tulloch, J. A. (1956). An evaluation of anticoagulant therapy in acute myocardial infection. *Scot. Med. J.*, **1**, 1

Gordon-Smith, I. C. (1972). Personal communication

Gordon-Smith, I. C., Grundy, D. J., Le Quesne, L. P., Newcombe, J. F. and Bramble, F. J. (1972). Controlled trial of two regimens of subcutaneous heparin in prevention of post-operative deep vein thrombosis. *Lancet*, **i**, 1133

Gordon-Smith, I. C., Hickman, J. A. and Le Quesne, L. P. (1974). Postoperative fibrinolytic activity and deep vein thrombosis. *Brit. J. Surg.*, **61**, 213

Gore, I. and Larkey, B. J. (1960). Functional activity of aortic mucopolysaccharides. *J. Lab. Clin. Med.*, **56**, 839

Gruber, V. F. and Bergentz, S. E. (1966). The anti-thrombotic effect of dextran. *J. Surg. Res.*, **6**, 379

Gurewich, V. and Thomas, D. P. (1965). Pathogenesis of venous thrombosis in relation to its prevention by dextran and heparin. *J. Lab. Clin. Med.*, **66**, 604

Handley, A. J., Emerson, P. A., Fleming, P. R. (1972). Heparin in the prevention of deep vein thrombosis after myocardial infarction. *Brit. Med. J.*, **2**, 436

Hickman, J. A. (1971). A study of the metabolism of fibrinogen after surgical operations. *Clin. Sci.*, **41**, 141

Hickman, J. A. and Gordon-Smith, I. C. (1972). Timed fibrin digestion: a simplified technique for the measurement of the fibrinolytic activity of the blood. *J. Clin. Pathol.*, **25**, 191

221

Thromboembolism

Hickman, J. A., Gordon-Smith, I. C., Whitfield, P. and Godfrey, S. (1973). The relationship of the dilute whole blood lysis time to the fibrinolytic activity of blood: effect of change in plasma fibrinogen. *J. Clin. Pathol.*, **26**, 189

Hills, N. H., Pflug, J. J., Jeyasingh, K., Boardman, L. and Calnan, J. S. (1972). Prevention of deep vein thrombosis by intermittent pneumatic compression of calf. *Brit. Med. J.*, **1**, 131

Hobbs, J. T. and Davies, J. W. L. (1960). Detection of venous thrombosis with 131I-labelled fibrinogen in the rabbit. *Lancet*, **ii**, 134

Innes, E. and Sevitt, S. (1964). Coagulation and fibrinolysis in injured patients. *J. Clin. Pathol.*, **17**, 1

Jansen, H. (1968). Dextran as a prophylactic against thromboembolism in general surgery. *Acta Chir. Scand.*, **Suppl. 387**, 86

Johnson, S. R., Bygdeman, S. and Eliason, R. (1968). Effect of dextran on post-operative thrombosis. *Acta Chir. Scand.*, **Suppl. 387**, 80

Johnson, R. (1974). Personal communication

Just-Viera, J. O. and Yeager, G. H. (1964). Prevention from thrombosis in large veins. *Surg. Gynaecol. Obstet.*, **118**, 354

Kakkar, V. V., Howe, C. T., Flanc, C. and Clarke, M. B. (1969). Natural history of deep vein thrombosis. *Lancet*, **ii**, 230

Kakkar, V. V., Howe, C. T., Nicolaides, A. N., Renney, J. T. G. and Clarke, M. B. (1970a). Deep vein thrombosis of the leg—Is there a "high risk" group. *Amer. J. Surg.*, **120**, 527

Kakkar, V. V., Nicolaides, A. N., Renney, J. T. G., Friend, J. and Clarke, M. B. (1970b). 125I-labelled fibrinogen test adapted for routine screening for deep-vein thrombosis. *Lancet*, **i**, 540

Kakkar, V. V., Corrigan, T., Spindler, J., Fossard, D. P., Flute, P. T., Crellin, R. Q., Wessler, S. and Yin, E. T. (1972). Efficacy of low doses of heparin in prevention of deep-vein thrombosis after major surgery. *Lancet*, **2**, 101

Koekenberg, L. J. L. (1961). Experimental use of Macrodex as a prophylaxis against postoperative thromboembolism. In: *Proc. Dijkzigt Conf. on Prevention of Thromboembolism in Surgery*, 123 (Amsterdam: Excerpta Medica)

Kwaan, H. C. and Suwanwela, N. (1971). Inhibitors of fibrinolysis in platelets in polycythaemia vera and thrombocytosis. *Brit. J. Haematol.*, 21, **3**, 313

Kwaan, H. C. (1973). Inhibitors of fibrinolysis. *Thromb. Res.*, **2**, 31

Lambie, J. M., Barber, D. C., Dhall, D. P. and Matheson, M. A. (1970). Dextran 80 in prophylaxis of postoperative venous thrombosis. A controlled trial. *Brit. Med. J.*, **2**, 144

Leandoer, L. (1968). Fibrinogen in blood and lymph after massive haemorrhage in dogs. *Acta Chir. Scand.*, **134**, 511

London, D. and Crossfill, M. L. (1969). The effect of dextran-70 on post-operative deep vein thrombosis. *Brit. J. Clin. Prac.*, **23**, 158

Madow, B. P. M. (1960). Use of antimalarial drugs as "disludging" agents in vascular disease processes. J. Amer. Med. Ass., **172**, 1630

Mansfield, A. O. (1972). Alteration in fibrinolysis associated with surgery and venous thrombosis. *Brit. J. Surg.*, **59**, 754

Matheson, N. A. (1969). In: *Round Table Conference on Deep Vein Thrombosis* (Brit. Orthop. Ass.)

Thromboembolism

Maurer, B. J., Wray, R. and Shillingford, J. P. (1971). Frequency of venous thrombosis after myocardial infarction. *Lancet*, **ii**, 1385

Mayo, M. E., Halil, T. and Browse, N. L. (1972). The incidence of deep vein thrombosis after prostatectomy. *Brit. J. Urol.*, **43**, 738

Moloney, G. E., Morrell, M. T. and Fell, R. H. (1972). Postoperative leg vein thrombosis. *Brit. Med. J.*, **4**, 244

Murray, T. S., Lorimer, A. R., Cox, F. C. and Lawrie, T. D. V. (1970). Leg vein thrombosis following myocardial infarction. *Lancet*, **ii**, 792

Negus, D., Pinto, D. J., LeQuesne, L. P., Brown, N. and Chapman, M. (1968). ^{125}I-labelled fibrinogen in the diagnosis of deep-vein thrombosis and its correlation with phlebography. *Brit. J. Surg.*, **55**, 835

Nicolaides, A. N., Kakkar, V. V., Field, E. S. and Renney, J. T. G. (1971a). The origin of deep-vein thrombosis: a venographic study. *Brit. J. Radiol.*, **44**, 653

Nicolaides, A. N., Kakkar, V. V., Renney, J. T. G., Kidner, P. H., Hutchison, D. C. S., Clarke, M. B. (1971b). Myocardial infarction and deep-vein thrombosis. *Brit. Med. J.*, **1**, 432

Nicolaides, A. N. (1972). The prevention of postoperative deep venous thrombosis. *Jacksonian Prize Essay*

Nicolaides, A. N., Clark, C. T., Thomas, R. D. and Lewis, J. D. (1972a). Soleal veins and local fibrinolytic activity. *Brit. J. Surg.*, **59**, 914

Nicolaides, A. N., Dupont, P. A., Desai, S., Lewis, J. D., Douglas, J. N., Dodsworth, H., Fourides, G., Luck, R. J. and Jamieson, C. W. (1972b). Small doses of subcutaneous sodium heparin in preventing deep venous thrombosis in major surgery. *Lancet*, **2**, 890

Nicolaides, A. N., Field, E. S., Kakkar, V. V., Yates-Bell, A. J., Taylor, S. and Clarke, M. B. (1972c). Prostatectomy and deep-vein thrombosis. *Brit. J. Surg.*, **59**, 487

Nicolaides, A. N., Kakkar, V. V., Field, E. S. and Fish, P. (1972d). Optimal electrical stimulus for prevention of deep-vein thrombosis. *Brit. Med. J.*, **3**, 756

Nicolaides, A. N., Kakkar, V. V., Field, E. S. and Spindler, J. (1972e). Antibiotics, postoperative infection and deep-vein thrombosis. *Brit. J. Surg.*, **59**, 302

Nicolaides, A. N. (1973). Prevention of deep vein thrombosis. *Geriatrics*, **28**, 69

Nicolaides, A. N., Dupont, P. A., Desai, S., Lewis, J. D., Dodsworth, H., Fourides, G., Luck, R. J., Jamieson, C. W. (1974a). Annotation—Small doses of subcutaneous heparin in preventing postoperative deep venous thrombosis. *Amer. Heart J.*, **87**, 261

Nicolaides, A. N., Dupont, P. A., Parsons, D., Appleberg, M., Horan, F. T., Esah, K. M. and Walker, C. J. (1974b). Small dose subcutaneous sodium heparin in preventing deep venous thrombosis after elective hip surgery. *Brit. J. Surg.*, **61**, 320

Nilsson, I. M. (1968). Changes in the coagulation and fibrinolytic systems predisposing to thrombosis. *Acta Chir. Scand.*, **Suppl. 387**, 15

O'Brien, J. R., Tulevski, V. and Etherington, M. (1971). Two *in vivo* studies comparing high and low aspirin dosage. *Lancet*, **i**, 399

Pinson, J., Boyan, C. P. and Cliffton, E. E. (1965). Fibrinolytic activity in patients during operation. *J. Amer. Med. Assoc.*, **191**, 1026

Renney, J. T., Kakkar, V. V. and Nicolaides, A. N. (1970). The prevention of postoperative deep-vein thrombosis, comparing dexran-70 and intensive physiotherapy. *Brit. J. Surg.*, **57**, 388

Report of the Steering Committee of a Trial sponsored by the Medical Research Council. (1972). Effect of Aspirin on postoperative venous thrombosis. *Lancet*, **ii**, 442

Roberts, V. C., Sabri, S., Pietroni, M. C., Gurewich, V., Cotton, L. T. (1971).

Thromboembolism

Passive flexion and femoral vein flow: a study using a motorised foot mover. *Brit. Med. J.*, **3,** 78

Roberts, V. C., Sabri, S., Beeley, A. H. and Cotton, L. T. (1972). The effect of intermittently applied external pressure on the haemodynamics of the lower limb in man. *Brit. J. Surg.*, **59,** 223

Rosengarten, D. S., Laird, J., Jeyasingh, K. and Martin, P. C. (1970). The failure of compression stockings (Tubigrip) to prevent deep venous thrombosis after operation. *Brit. J. Surg.*, **57,** 296

Rosengarten, D. S. and Laird, J. (1971). The effect of leg elevation on the incidence of deep-vein thrombosis after operation. *Brit. J. Surg.*, **58,** 182

Sabri, S., Roberts, V. C. and Cotton, L. T. (1971a). Prevention of early postoperative deep vein thrombosis by passive exercise of leg during surgery. *Brit. Med. J.* **3,** 82

Sabri, S., Roberts, V. C. and Cotton, L. T. (1971b). Prevention of early postoperative deep vein thrombosis by intermittent compression of the leg during surgery. *Brit. Med. J.*, **4,** 394

Sagar, S. (1974). Heparin prophylaxis against fatal postoperative pulmonary embolism. *Brit. Med. J.*, **2,** 153

Saltzman, E. W., Harris, W. H. and de Sanctis, R. W. (1971). Reduction in venous thromboembolism by agents affecting platelet function. *New Eng. J. Med.*, **248,** 1287

Sawyer, R. B., Moncrief, J. A. and Canajaro, P. C. (1965). Dexran therapy in thrombophlebitis. *J. Amer. Med. Ass.*, **191,** 740

Sawyer, R. B. (1968). Clinical experiences with dextran treatment. *Acta Chir. Scand.,* **Suppl. 387,** 58

Sevitt, S., and Gallagher, N. G. (1959). Prevention of venous thrombosis and pulmonary embolism in injured patients: A trial of anticoagulant prophylaxis with phenindione in middle-aged and elderly patients with fractured necks of femur. *Lancet,* **ii,** 981

Sharnoff, J. G. and de Blasio, G. (1970). Prevention of fatal postoperative thromboembolism by heparin prophylaxis. *Lancet,* **ii,** 1006

Sherry, S. (1971). Thrombosis prevention. *New Eng. J. Med.*, **284,** 1324

Soong, B. C. F. and Miller, S. P. (1970). Coagulation disorders in cancer. III. Fibrinolysis and inhibitors. *Cancer*, **25,** 867

Stadil, F. (1968). Macrodex prophylaxis in postoperative thrombosis. A preliminary communication. *Acta Chir. Scand.*, **Suppl. 387,** 88

Tsapogas, M. J., Goussous, H., Peabody, R. A., Karmody, A. M. and Eckert, C. (1971). Postoperative venous thrombosis and the effectiveness of prophylactic measures. *Arch. Surg.*, **103,** 561

Von Kaulla, K. N. (1963). *Chemistry of Thrombolysis: Human Fibrinolytic Enzymes,* 79 (Springfield, Ill.: Thomas)

Warlow, C., Beattie, A. G., Terry, G., Ogston, D., Kenmure, A. C. F. and Douglas, A. S. (1973). A double-blind trial of low doses of subcutaneous heparin in the prevention of deep-vein thrombosis after myocardial infarction. *Lancet,* **ii,** 934

Wessler, S. and Yin, E. T. (1968). On the mechanism of thrombosis. *Progr. Haematol.*, **6,** 201

Weiss, H. J. and Aledort, L. M. (1967). Impaired platelet-connective-tissue reaction in man after aspirin ingestion. *Lancet,* **ii,** 495

Wetterdall, P. (1941). Use of heparin as a prophylactic following gynaecological operations. *Acta Med. Scand.*, **107,** 123

Thromboembolism

Williams, H. T. (1971). Prevention of postoperative deep-vein thrombosis with perioperative subcutaneous heparin. *Lancet*,**ii**, 950

Yin, E. T. and Wessler, S. (1970). Heparin-accelerated inhibition of activated factor X by its natural plasma inhibitor. *Biochem. Biophys. Acta*, **201**, 387

Yin, E. T., Wessler, S. and Butler, J. V. (1973). Plasma heparin: A unique, practical, submicrogram-sensitive assay. *J. Lab. Clin. Med.*, **81**, 298

Zucker, M. B. and Paterson, J. (1968). Inhibition of adenosine diphosphate-induced secondary aggregation and other platelet functions by acetylsalicylic acid ingestion. *Proc. Soc. Exp. Biol. Med.*, **127**, 547

15

Small dose subcutaneous heparin. A safe regimen

J. G. Sharnoff

There is now evidence that deep venous thrombosis and fatal pulmonary embolism are preventable with small doses of subcutaneous heparin, especially in patients having an operation (Chapters 14 and 16). The increased incidence of thromboembolism in recent years (Chapter 1; Sharnoff, 1973) has made the need for prophylaxis most urgent. This chapter will describe what prompted the author to develop a regimen of small doses of subcutaneous heparin and the results obtained when this regimen was administered to surgical patients.

In 1957, it was observed that three patients who died from thrombotic thrombocytopaenic purpura had what was then presumed to be megakaryocytes trapped in their pulmonary precapillaries and capillaries (Sharnoff, 1957). These large cells were first observed in the pulmonary capillaries by Aschoff who described them as an "effete" phenomenon having escaped from the bone marrow and of no significance (Aschoff, 1893). Subsequent studies (Sharnoff and Kim, 1958a; 1958b; Sharnoff and Scardino, 1960) confirmed that they were truly megakaryocytes and could be seen in all stages of fragmentation in the pulmonary capillary vessels of man and other mammals. They are trapped in the capillaries because of their size. Eventually, they are forced through by the repeated pulsations of the right heart to emerge in the peripheral blood as platelets and often as casts of the capillaries (Sharnoff, 1959). The megakaryocytes were frequently found in samples of blood from the pulmonary arteries during chest surgery (Scheinin and Koivuniemi, 1963).

A marked increase in the number of entrapped megakaryocytes in sections of the lungs of patients dying of some form of thrombotic disease has been noted (Sharnoff, 1959). It has been postulated that the marked increase in capillary entrapped megakaryocytes could act as a priming effect and when followed by a sudden increase in pulmonary artery pressure and heart rate in stressful situations these cells could be forced more rapidly through and fragment into platelets, entering the peripheral blood causing thrombocytosis which in turn would cause a hyper-coagulable state and eventually thrombosis. This hypothesis was tested in rabbits by sampling the blood of the right and left ventricles. It was found that the normally active rabbits showed no difference in the platelet count in samples from both ventricles, but the rabbits which were completely immobilised by hibernating in severe cold, when stressed revealed a marked increase in the number of platelets in the blood from their left ventricle. The increased number of platelets in samples from the left ventricles was sometimes two to three times the number in samples from the right ventricle (Sharnoff and Scardino, 1960). A subsequent study of changes in the platelet count and Lee–White coagulation times performed before, during and daily after major operations was under-taken in 41 patients (Sharnoff, 1966). There were three fatalities, all associated with a significant increase in the number of platelets and shorter than normal coagulation times during surgery. The remaining 38 patients had a less marked thrombocytosis and coagulation times only to the lower limits of normal. Two of the three fatal cases came to autopsy. One died on the second postoperative day as a result of a massive pulmonary embolism. The other died on the twelfth postoperative day as a result of coronary artery thrombosis and acute myocardial infarction which occured on the day of operation. Both were female over the age of 60 and had bowel resections for carcinoma. The third fatal case was a 53-year-old man who had a partial gastrectomy for a benign ulcer. He died suddenly from a clinically massive pulmonary embolism when he first got out of bed.

It was soon realised that it was not possible to determine in advance which patients will develop a thrombocytosis and decreased coagulation time as a result of the stress of surgery. The small difference in coagulation times observed in the patients who died with thrombosis compared to the remaining 38 patients suggested that only small quantities of anticoagulant would be necessary to maintain normo-coagulation (Sharnoff et al., 1962). Sodium heparin, a natural substance, not affecting wound healing, having a limited and predictable action and in contrast to oral anticoagulants (Cucinell et al., 1965; Aggeler *et al.*, 1967) not affected by other medication, was chosen as the anticoagulant most suitable for a trial (Sharnoff *et al.*, 1962) in patients undergoing major operations. The study included one test and two control groups. There were 140 patients in the test, 92 in the first control and 1396 in the second control group. The patients in the test and first control groups were all over the age of 60 and deemed at "high risk" because of age, cardiac disease, previous history of thrombosis and varicose veins. The second control group consisted of "low risk" patients because of a lower mean age and absence of other risk factors. The patients in the test group received 10 000 units of heparin sub-cutaneously, approximately 10 hours before operation. After operation 2500 to 5000 units of heparin were administered every 6 hours, depending on their weight, until discharge. The first control group received the same regimen except the preoperative dose which was omitted. Heparin was not administered to the second control group. There were nine deaths in the test group with neither clinical nor postmortem evidence of pulmonary embolism. In the first and second control groups there was a postmortem incidence of fatal pulmonary embolism of 62·5 and 68·1 percent respectively (Sharnoff *et al.*, 1962).

Control of heparin dosage to maintain normocoagulation was considered essential. Initially, this was accomplished with the Lee–White method. Later the Dale and Laidlaw coagulometer (Sharnoff, 1963) was the only method of control used. It was found to be reliable, reproducible, simple to perform requiring only a small drop of blood and was more accurate than the Lee–White method. The Dale and Laidlow method has a normal coagulation time of 1·5 to 2·5 minutes; most frequently it gave times below 2 minutes. The test was performed before heparin administration, immediately after operation and then daily just before the 6-hourly administration of heparin with the dose adjusted if necessary as indicated by the times obtained. Following the administration of 10 000 units of heparin a prolongation of coagulation time to slightly beyond normal levels for two to three hours and maintainance of normal coagulation times for approximately twelve hours occurred.

Prophylaxis with the regimen of subcutaneous heparin described has been continued (Sharnoff and DeBlazio, 1970) and a total of 1750 patients have been treated successfully with only two exceptions. The patients treated had predominantly elective operations such as chole-cystectomy, gastrectomy, exploratory laparotomy, bowel resection, hysterectomy, herniorrhaphy, mastectomy, thoracotomy, hip operations including pinning of the hip and knee replacement. Haemorrhage was seldom a problem except in rare instances when errors were made in heparin administration or when heparin was administered too close to surgery. The two exceptions had evidence of pulmonary embolism confirmed by autopsy. In both patients the circumstances were identical. A male of 87 years and a female of 96 years with fractures of the femur were immoblised for eight days and no heparin was given until the day before operation. This suggested that heparin administration in patients with fractures should start upon admission to the hospital and continue until they are fully ambulant or discharged.

Pulmonary embolism is also common in medical patients especially when cardiac disease is present (Coon and Coller, 1959; Kucera, 1966; 1968; Chapter 14). Its incidence in patients with myocardial infarction who die can be as high as 25 percent (Sharnoff, 1974). Fatal pulmonary emboli in these patients are often interpreted clinically as a second coronary thrombosis. Patients with malignancy, limb paralysis and superficial phlebitis are also at risk and are in need of prophylaxis. Small doses of subcutaneous heparin in medical patients may prove as effective in preventing thromboembolism as in surgical patients.

References

Aggeler, P. M., O'Reilly, R. A., Leong, L. and Kowitz, P. E. (1967). Potentiation of anticoagulant effect of warfarin by phenylbutazone. *New Eng. J. Med.,* **276,** 496

Aschoff, L. (1893). Ueber capillare embolic riesenkernhaltigen zellen. *Arch. Path. Anat.,* **134,** 11

Coon, W. W. and Coller, F. A. (1959). Some epidemiological considerations of thromboembolism. *Surg. Gynec. Obstet.,* **109,** 487

Cucinell, S. A., Conney, A. H., Sansur, M. and Burns, J. J. (1965). Drug interactions in man. 1. Lowering effect of phenobarbital on plasma levels of bishydroxycoumarin (Dicoumarol) and diphenylhydantoin (Dilantin). *Clin. Pharmacol. Therap.,* **6,** 420

Kucera, M. (1966). Incidence and importance of venous thromboembolic disease in cardiacs. *Vnitrni Lekarstvi,* **12,** 209

Kucera, M. (1968). Some problems of venous thromboembolism in patients with heart disease. *Rev. Czech. Med.,* **14,** 1

Scheinin, T. M. and Koivuniemi, A. P. (1963). Megakaryocytes in the pulmonary circulation. *Blood,* **22,** 82

Sharnoff, J. G. (1957) Thrombotic thrombocytopenic purpura. *Amer. J. Med.,* **23,** 270

Sharnoff, J. G. (1959). Increased pulmonary megakaryocytes—probable role in postoperative thromboembolism. *J. Amer. Med. Ass.,* **169,** 688

Sharnoff, J. G. (1963). An evaluation of the Dale and Laidlow coagulometer in the heparin control of thromboembolism. *Proc. N.Y. State Assoc. Pub. Health Lab.,* **43,** 10

Sharnoff, J. G. (1966). Results in the prophylaxis of postoperative thromboembolism. *Surg. Gynec. Obstet.,* **123,** 303

Thromboembolism

Sharnoff, J. G. (1973). Prevention of thromboembolism. *Bull. N.Y. Acad. Med.*, **49**, 655

Sharnoff, J. G. (1974). Unpublished data.

Sharnoff, J. G. and DeBlazio, G. (1970). Prevention of fatal postoperative thromboembolism by heparin prophylaxis. *Lancet*, **2**, 1006

Sharnoff, J. G., Kass, H. H. and Mistica, B. A. (1962). A plan of heparinization of the surgical patient to prevent postoperative thromboembolism. *Surg. Gynec. Obstet.*, **115**, 75

Sharnoff, J. G. and Kim, E. S. (1958a). Evaluation of pulmonary megakaryocytes. *Arch. Path.*, **66**, 176

Sharnoff, J. G. and Kim, E. S. (1958b). Pulmonary megakaryocyte studies in rabbits. *Arch. Path.*, **66**, 340

Sharnoff, J. G. and Scardino, V. (1960. Platelet count differences in blood of the rabbit right and left heart ventricles. *Nature*, **187**, 334

16

Small dose subcutaneous heparin in preventing deep venous thrombosis

Alex Gallus and Jack Hirsh

Treatment with small doses of subcutaneous heparin before and after operation is a promising approach to the prevention of venous thromboembolism (Chapter 14). It is the purpose of this chapter to describe the various regimens evaluated, their effects on *in vitro* coagulation tests and on bleeding, to compare their results and draw some conclusions about their usefulness in various clinical situations.

Anticoagulants, in their conventional therapeutic doses, have repeatedly been shown to prevent venous thromboembolism in surgical and medical patients. (Sevitt and Gallagher, 1959; Saltzman *et al.*, 1966; Harris *et al.*, 1967; Skinner and Saltzman, 1967; Report of the Working Party on Anticoagulant Therapy in Coronary Thrombosis to the Medical Research Council, 1969; Handley *et al.*, 1972). Sevitt and Gallagher showed that perioperative oral anticoagulant treatment with phenindione in doses sufficient to prolong the prothrombin time after operation to between 2 and 3 times normal levels, markedly reduced both the clinical and post-mortem incidence of deep venous thrombosis and pulmonary embolism in elderly patients operated on for fracture of the femoral neck (Sevitt and Gallagher, 1959). In addition there was a reduced mortality in the treated patients during their stay in hospital. Similar results with oral anticoagulants have been reported by a number of other investigators in patients who had surgery after fracture of the hip (Slazman *et al.*, 1966) and in patients who had elective general surgical (Skinner and Saltzman, 1967) and orthopaedic operations (Harris *et al.*, 1967). However, prophylaxis with full doses of oral anticoagulants carries an increased

This work was supported in part by Ontario Provincial Government Health research grants, PR33OC and 143, and by Ontario Heart Foundation grant T, 15–5; 72.

risk of bleeding and although this has been reported to be acceptable (Sevitt and Gallagher, 1959; Skinner and Saltzman, 1967), the fear of bleeding has prevented its wide use in the perioperative period.

Treatment with small doses of subcutaneous heparin was suggested as an alternative approach to prophylaxis by Sharnoff and DeBlasio (Sharnoff, 1969; Sharnoff and DeBlasio, 1970). They gave heparin subcutaneously before and after operation in doses aimed at preventing the accelerated blood coagulation which they had observed without prolonging the whole blood clotting time above normal levels.

Their studies suggested that their regimen of 10 000 units of heparin 10 hours before operation followed by 2500 or 5000 every six hours after surgery prevented postoperative thromboembolism without causing perioperative bleeding (Chapter 15).

A number of modifications of this regimen have now been evaluated in controlled randomised studies using the ^{125}I-fibrinogen test to detect

Table 16.1 Incidence of deep venous thrombosis detected by ^{125}I-fibrinogen test in patients having elective abdominal and thoracic operations reported in clinical trials of small dose heparin

Author	Heparin regimen	Leg vein thrombosis	
		Control group	Treated group
Williams, 1971	10 000 U 9–10 hours preop. 2500–5000 U 6-hourly postop. × 7 days	12/29 (41%)	4/27 (15%)
Kakkar et al., 1972	5000 U 2 hours preop. 5000 U 12-hourly postop. × 7 days	17/39 (42%)	3/39 (8%)
Nicolaides et al., 1972	5000 U 2 hours preop. 5000 U 12-hourly postop. × 7 days	29/122 (24%)	1/122 (0·8%)
Ballard et al., 1973	5000 U 2 hours preop. 5000 U 12-hourly postop. × 7 days	16/55 (29%)	2/55 (3·6%)
Gordon-Smith et al., 1972	5000 U 1 hour preop. 5000 U 12-hourly postop. × 1 day	21/50 (42%)	7/52 (15·5%)
Gordon-Smith et al., 1972	5000 U 1 hour preop. 5000 U 12-hourly postop. × 5 days	21/50 (42%)	4/48 (8·3%)
Gallus et al., 1973a	5000 U 2 hours preop. 5000 U 8-hourly postop. × 7 days	25/171 (14·5%)	2/167 (1·2%)

deep venous thrombosis in patients after elective major abdominal and thoracic operations (Williams, 1971: Gordon-Smith *et al.*, 1972; Kakkar *et al.*, 1972; Nicolaides *et al.*, 1972; Ballard *et al.*, 1973; Gallus *et al.*, 1973b). All of these studies have shown a marked reduction in the incidence of venous thrombosis in treated patients (Table 16.1).

Williams, used a regimen very similar to that of Sharnoff's. This consisted of 10 000 units of sodium heparin given subcutaneously 9–10 hours before operation followed by 2500 or 5000 units of heparin six-hourly for seven days, the dose depending on the patient's weight. He found a reduction of leg vein thrombosis from 41 per cent in the untreated to 15 per cent in the treated patients (Williams, 1971). Two subsequent studies (Kakkar *et al.*, 1972; Nicolaides *et al.*, 1972) using a regimen of 5000 units of calcium or sodium heparin respectively given subcutaneously two hours before operation then twelve-hourly, demonstrated a reduction of leg vein thrombosis from 42 per cent in the untreated to eight per cent in the treated patients in the first study (Kakkar *et al.*, 1972) and from 24 per cent to one per cent in the second study (Nicolaides *et al.*, 1972). Ballard and his colleagues using calcium heparin given in a similar schedule, were also able to show a reduction of leg vein thrombosis from 29 per cent in the untreated to 3·6 per cent in the treated patients after gynaecological operations (Ballard *et al.*, 1973).

Gordon-Smith and his colleagues have evaluated the effect of the duration of heparin prophylaxis on the incidence of thrombosis and found that there was less protection when heparin treatment was discontinued after the first postoperative day than when it was continued for five days (Gordon-Smith *et al.*, 1972).

Finally, we have evaluated the use of more frequent injections of subcutaneous heparin. Our regimen consisted of 5000 units of sodium heparin given two hours before operation followed by 5000 units eight-hourly starting six to eight hours after the operation and continuing for a minimum of one week. (Gallus *et al.*, 1973b; Gallus *et al.*, 1973a). We found a reduction of leg vein thrombosis from 15 per cent in the untreated to one per cent in the treated patients after major elective abdominal and thoracic operations (Gallus *et al.*, 1973b; Gallus *et al.*, 1973a), and from 42 per cent to nine per cent after elective hip replacement (Gallus *et al.*, 1973a). In a more recent controlled trial, the same regimen used in patients having elective hip replacement reduced the incidence of deep venous thrombosis from 40 per cent in the control group to four per cent in the test group (Nicolaides *et al.*, 1974).

The results of prophylaxis with low dose heparin have been disappointing in patients with fractured hips (Table 16.2). Kakkar and his colleagues using twelve-hourly injections of 5000 units of heparin, found a 40 per cent incidence of thrombosis in treated and a 54 per cent incidence in a similar previous group of untreated patients (Kakkar et al., 1972). We found a 23 per cent incidence of thrombosis in patients treated with eight-hourly injections of heparin after hip fracture compared with a 56 per cent incidence in untreated (Gallus et al., 1973a).

Table 16.2 Incidence of deep venous thrombosis detected by the ^{125}I-fibrinogen test in patients having an operation for hip fracture reported in clinical trials of small dose heparin

Author	Heparin regimen	Leg vein thrombosis	
		Control group	Treated group
Kakkar et al., 1972	5000 U 12-hourly	27/50 (54%)	20/50 (40%)
Gallus et al., 1973a	5000 U 8-hourly	18/32 (56%)	6/26 (23%)

The results of teatment with low dose heparin after myocardial infarction have been conflicting (Table 16.3). In one study, twelve-hourly injections of heparin had no effect on the incidence of leg vein thrombosis detected with the I-fibrinogen test (Handley, 1972). The same regimen in another study reduced the incidence from 17.2 per cent in the control group of 3.2 per cent in the heparin group (Warlow et al., 1973). We found a reduction of thrombosis detected with the ^{125}I-fibrinogen test during the patient's stay in hospital from 22.5 per cent in untreated patients to 2.6 per cent in patients treated with eight-hourly injections of heparin (Gallus et al., 1973b). The difference between the results may be due to the different regimens used.

Table 16.3 Incidence of deep venous thrombosis detected by the ^{125}I-fibrinogen test in patients with myocardial infarction reported in controlled clinical trials of small dose heparin

Author	Heparin regimen	Leg vein thrombosis	
		Control group	Treated group
Handley, 1972	5000 U 12-hourly	7/24 (29%)	6/26 (23%)
Warlow et al., 1973	5000 U 12-hourly	11/64 (17·2%)	2/63 (3·2%)
Gallus et al., 1973b	5000 U 8-hourly	9/40 (22·5%)	1/38 (2·6%)

The majority of thrombi detected in all of these studies were calf thrombi which carry a low morbidity (Kakkar et al., 1969; Chapter 14). Nicolaides and his colleagues, have reported a reduced incidence of thrombi detected by the ^{125}I-fibrinogen test in the femoral and popliteal vein in patients given twelve-hourly heparin after major elective operations (Nicolaides et al., 1972; Chapter 14) and we have had similar results with heparin given eight-hourly (Gallus et al., 1973a). Thrombi in the femoral and popliteal vein appear to carry a high risk of clinical pulmonary embolism (Kakkar et al., 1969) and their reduction by low dose subcutaneous heparin suggests that this prophylaxis should reduce the incidence of pulmonary embolism (Chapter 14). A multicentre study now in progress is designed to answer the question whether low doses of heparin (5000 units of subcutaneous heparin given eight-hourly) will prevent pulmonary embolism detected clinically and at postmortem, and in particular whether it will prevent massive fatal pulmonary embolism (Kakkar, 1974). It has already been demonstrated that the number and size of postoperative pulmonary embolism detected by perfusion scans is reduced by the twelve-hourly regimen (5000 units two to five hours before operation and then every twelve hours for five days) (Lahnborg et al., 1974). Preliminary results of another trial in which all patients who die come to postmortem have also suggested that the incidence of fatal pulmonary embolism is reduced by the same regimen (Sagar, 1974; Chapter 14).

A number of explanations have been proposed for the effectiveness of low dose heparin prophylaxis. It was initially suggested by Sharnoff that small doses of heparin prevented thromboembolism by preventing the postoperative shortening of the whole blood clotting time measured with a Dale and Laidlaw coagulometer rather than by producing a measurable anticoagulant effect (Sharnoff et al., 1962; Sharnoff, 1966; Chapter 15). Subsequent reports confirmed that subcutaneous injections of 5000 units of heparin do not prolong the whole blood clotting time (Williams, 1971) and suggested that they do not affect the thrombin clotting time either (Kakkar et al., 1971). However, the use of a thrombin clotting time assay made more sensitive to the presence of heparin by performing it without recalcification (Bonnar et al., 1972), and of an assay based on the inhibition of Factor Xa (Kakkar et al., 1972) showed that measurable concentrations of heparin may persist for up to eight hours after subcutaneous injection of 5000 units of heparin in normal volunteers (Kakkar et al., 1972) and patients with placental insufficiency (Bonnar et al., 1972), but for a shorter time after elective operations (Kakkar et al., 1972). We have reported a statistically significant increase of the partial thromboplastin time for five hours after a subcutaneous injection of 5000 units of sodium heparin (Gallus et al., 1973b). Thus, the mean partial thromboplastin

237

time increased from 43 sec before treatment to between 50 and 53 sec for the following five hours. In the great majority of patients this increase was slight or moderate but in a few the partial thromboplastin time was prolonged to levels which we would normally associate with therapeutic doses of heparin given for established venous thromboembolism (Basu et al., 1972; Gallus et al., 1973b).

Other effects of small doses of heparin have also been described. These include reduced postoperative platelet adhesiveness (Negus et al., 1971), impaired postoperative platelet aggregation (O Brien et al., 1972) and increased lipoprotein-lipase activity (Negus et al., 1971).

It seems most likely that small dose prophylactic heparin exerts its effect by potentiating antithrombin III a naturally occurring inhibitor of activated Factor X (Yin et al., 1971). In this context it is of interest that untreated patients with a high-normal partial thromboplastin time before and after elective operations are at a low risk of postoperative thrombosis detected with the ^{125}I-fibrinogen test compared with similar patients with a shorter pre- and postoperative partial thromboplastin time (Gallus et al., 1973). Thus, even a slight to moderate prolongation of the partial thromboplastin time to levels which would not be considered adequate for the treatment of established venous thromboembolism may be sufficient to protect against venous thrombosis.

Sharnoff reported that low dose heparin prophylaxis was safe and did not carry any increased risk of bleeding (Sharnoff and DeBlasio, 1970). This has been substantially confirmed by subsequent investigators (Williams, 1971; Gordon-Smith et al., 1972; Kakkar et al., 1972; Nicolaides et al., 1972; Ballard et al., 1973) though there have been sporadic reports of excessive bleeding when small dose heparin prophylaxis was used in patients having hip operations (Arden et al., 1972; Charnley, 1972; Levay, 1972), admittedly in conjunction with Dextran in one instance (Charnley, 1972).

We have compared blood loss in patients treated with 5000 units of heparin eight-hourly commencing two hours before major operations with blood loss in untreated patients (Gallus et al., 1973b). The parameters recorded were the surgeon's impression of perioperative blood loss, the haematocrit fall during the first postoperative week and transfusion requirements during and after operation (Table 16.4).

The surgeons' reports of operative blood loss suggested that there was no noticeable increase of perioperative bleeding. Similarly there was no increase in the percentage of patients requiring transfusion, either after elective abdominal and thoracic operations or after elective or emergency

238

Table 16.4 Bleeding during small dose heparin prophylaxis (5000 U 8-hourly) (Gallus *et al.*, 1973b; Gallus and Hirsh, 1973). **Differences between the treated and untreated patients were assessed by chi square or unpaired t-test.**

Surgical procedure	Bleeding parameter	Control patients (Mean and range)	Treated patients (Mean and range)	p value
Elective abdominothoracic operation	Patients transfused	17/80 (21%)	17/68 (25%)	>0.05
	Amount transfused (litres)	1·1 (0·5–2·0)	1·6 (0·5–3·5)	<0.05
	Postop. haematocrit fall (%)	5·1 (0–14)	6·5 (0–20)	<0.05
Elective hip operation	Patients transfused	16/16 (100%)	8/10 (80%)	>0.05
	Amount transfused (litres)	1·5 (0·5–3·0)	1·6 (0·6–2·5)	>0.05
	Postop. haematocrit fall (%)	8·6 (2–14)	10·8 (2–20)	>0.05
Operation for hip fracture	Patients transfused	17/32 (53%)	16/26 (62%)	>0.05
	Amount transfused (litres)	1·2 (0·5–3·5)	1·5 (0·5–2·5)	>0.05
	Postop. haematocrit fall (%)	8·3 (0–18)	8·3 (0–18)	>0.05

hip operations. However, there was a moderate and significant increase of blood requirements in those patients who needed transfusion from a mean of 1100 ml in the untreated group, to 1600 ml in the treated group after elective abdominal and thoracic operations. Blood transfusion requirements in transfused patients were similar in the two groups after elective or emergency hip operations, but there was a slightly greater, but significant, fall of the mean postoperative haematocrit (5·1 per cent in untreated and 6·5 per cent in treated patients) after elective abdominal and thoracic operations. However, the increased fall of postoperative haematocrit (8·6 per cent in untreated and 10·8 per cent in treated patients) after elective hip operations was not statistically significant and the haematocrit fall was similar in treated and untreated patients after operations for hip fracture (Gallus and Hirsh, 1973). Finally, there was an increase in the number of wound haematomas from three per cent in untreated to 19 per cent in treated patients after hip fracture, though again this was not statistically significant (Gallus and Hirsh, 1973).

It appears that treatment with eight-hourly heparin is associated with a slightly increased postoperative blood loss which is not clinically significant in the majority of patients. We have also observed that unexpected postoperative wound bleeding has generally been associated with excessive prolongation of the partial thromboplastin time after heparin injection (Gallus and Hirsh, 1973). Thus, while one of the attractive features of prophylaxis with small doses of heparin has been the hope that it will not need to be monitored with *in vitro* clotting tests, it may be necessary to check for excessive anticoagulant action if occasional episodes of un-expected bleeding are to be avoided.

Because of the relatively poor results of small dose heparin prophylaxis in patients undergiong operations after hip fracture operations, we attempted to combine the eight-hourly regimen with the use of perioperative Dextran infusion in a small number of patients (Gallus and Hirsh, 1973). This combination led to excessive bleeding and we now feel that treatment with concurrent small doses of heparin and Dextran is dangerous.

GENERAL RECOMMENDATIONS

Small doses of subcutaneous heparin are very effective in preventing deep venous thrombosis after elective general operations. Although the usefulness of this regimen for preventing minor and major pulmonary embolism after surgery has not been fully assessed, preliminary results suggest that it will be effective.

Good results have been reported with all the regimens used, but we feel that the injection of heparin two hours before operation is more likely to be protective during the operation than the injection 9–10 hours earlier and a sustained heparin effect is more likely to be produced by the eight-hourly than the twelve-hourly regimen. This feeling is supported by the rapid clearance of heparin in some patients after operation (Kakkar *et al.*, 1972) and by our observation that there is a measurable effect on the partial thromboplastin time for only five hours after a postoperative injection of 5000 units of heparin (Gallus *et al.*, 1973b). However, equally good results have been reported with twelve-hourly injections (Nicolaides *et al.*, 1972) and the optimal regimen will only be determined by formal comparison of the available dosage schedules with the concurrent estima-tion of heparin blood levels.

Treatment with small doses of heparin before and after elective hip operations is still under evaluation though preliminary results are promis-ing (Gallus *et al.*, 1973a; Nicolaides *et al.*, 1974). The results of small dose heparin prophylaxis in patients after hip fracture are unsatisfactory and the best available prophylactic regimen in those patients is still oral anticoagulant treatment (Sevitt and Gallagher, 1959; Salzman *et al.*, 1966). The results of small dose heparin prophylaxis in medical patients are promising, but further trials are necessary, particularly in high risk seriously ill patients.

Thromboembolism

References

Arden, G. P., Powell, H. D. W. and Fell, R. H. (1972). Subcutaneous heparin treatment. *Brit. Med. J.*, **4**, 486

Ballard, R. M., Bradley-Watson, P. J., Johnstone, F. D., Kenney, A., McCarthy, T. G., Campbell, S. S. and Weston, J. (1973). Low doses of subcutaneous heparin in the prevention of deep vein thrombosis after gynaecological surgery. *J. Obtest. Gynaecol., Brit. Comm.*, **80**, 469

Basu, D., Gallus, A., Hirsh, J. and Cade, J. (1972). A prospective study of the value of monitoring heparin treatment with activated partial thromboplastin time. *New Eng. J. Med.* **287**, 324

Bonnar, J., Denson, K. E. W. and Biggs, R. (1972). Subcutaneous heparin and prevention of thrombosis. *Lancet*, **ii**, 539

Charnley, J. (1972). Prophylaxis of postoperative thromboembolism. *Lancet*, **ii**, 134

Gallus, A. S. and Hirsh, J. (1973). Unpublished observation

Gallus, A. S., Hirsh, J. and Gent, M. (1973). Relevance of pre and postoperative blood tests to postoperative leg vein thrombosis. *Lancet*, **ii**, 805

Gallus, A. S., Hirsh, J., Turpie, A. G. G. and Tuttle, R. (1973a). Prevention of venous thrombosis with small doses of subcutaneous heparin. *Proc. IVth Int. Congr. Thrombosis and Haemostasis, Vienna, Austria*, 276

Gallus, A. S., Hirsh, J., Tuttle, R. J., Trebilcock, R., O'Brien, S. E., Carrol, J. J., Minden, J. H. and Hudecki, S. M. (1973b). Small subcutaneous doses of heparin in prevention of venous thrombosis. *New Eng. J. Med.*, **288**, 545

Gordon-Smith, I. C., Grundy, D. J., LeQuesne, L. P., Newcombe, J. F. and Bramble, F. J. (1972). Controlled trial of two regimens of subcutaneous heparin in prevention of postoperative deep-vein thrombosis. *Lancet*, **i**, 1133

Handley, A. J. (1972). Low-dose heparin after myocardial infarction. *Lancet*, **ii**, 623

Handley, A. J., Emerson, P. A. and Fleming, P. R. (1972). Heparin in the prevention of deep vein thrombosis after myocardial infarction. *Brit. Med. J.*, **2**, 436

Harris, W. H., Salzman, E. W. and DeSanctis, R. W. (1967). The prevention of thromboembolic disease by prophylactic anticoagulation. A controlled study in elective hip surgery. *J. Bone, Joint Surg.*, **49A**, 81

Kakkar, V. V., Howe, C. T., Flanc, C. and Clarke, M. B. (1969). Natural history of postoperative deep-vein thrombosis. *Lancet*, **ii**, 230

Kakkar, V. V., Field, E. S., Nicolaides, A. N., Flute, P. T., Wessler, S. and Yin, E. T. (1971). Low-doses of heparin in prevention of deep-vein thrombosis. *Lancet*, **ii**, 669

Kakkar, V. V., Corrigan, T., Spindler, J., Fossard, D. P., Flute, P. T., Crellin, R. Q., Wessler, S. and Yin, E. T. (1972). Efficacy of low doses of heparin in prevention of deep-vein thrombosis after major surgery. A double-blind randomised trial. *Lancet*, **ii**, 101

Kakkar, V. V. (1974). Personal communication

Lahnborg, G., Bergström, K., Friman, L. and Lagerglen, H. (1974). Effect of low-dose heparin on incidence of postoperative pulmonary embolism detected by photoscanning. *Lancet*, **i**, 329

LeVay, D. (1972). Low-dose heparin, *Lancet*, **ii**, 229

Negus, D., Pinto, D. J. and Slack, W. W. (1971). Effect of small doses of heparin on platelet adhesiveness and lipoprotein-lipase activity before and after surgery. *Lancet*, **i**, 1202

Nicolaides, A. N., Dupont, P. A., Desai, S., Lewis, J. D., Douglas, J. N., Dodsworth, H.,

Thromboembolism

Fourides, G., Luck, R. J. and Jamieson, C. W. (1972). Small doses of subcutaneous sodium heparin in preventing deep venous thrombosis after major surgery. *Lancet*, ii, 890

Nicolaides, A., Dupont, P., Parsons, D., Appleberg, M., Horan, F. T., Esah, K. M. and Walker, C. J. (1974). Small dose subcutaneous sodium heparin in preventing deep venous thrombosis after elective hip surgery. *Brit. J. Surg.*, 61, 320

O'Brien, J. R., Etherington, M., Jamieson, S. and Klaber, M. R. (1972). Platelet function in venous thrombosis and low-dosage heparin. *Lancet*, i, 1302

Report on the Working Party on Anticoagulant Therapy in Coronary Thrombosis to the Medical Research Council. (1969). Assessment of short-term anticoagulant administration after cardiac infarction. *Brit. Med. J.*, 1, 335

Saltzman, E. W., Harris, W. H. and DeSanctis, R. W. (1966). Anticoagulation for prevention of thromboembolism following fractures of the hip. *New Eng. J. Med.*, 275, 122

Sevitt, S. and Gallagher, N. G. (1959). Prevention of venous thrombosis and pulmonary embolism in injured patients. *Lancet*, ii, 981

Sharnoff, J. G., Kass, H. H. and Mistica, B. B. (1962). A plan of heparinisation of the surgical patient to prevent postoperative thromboembolism. *Surg. Gynaecol. Obstet.*, 115, 75

Sharnoff, J. G. (1966). Results in the prophylaxis of postoperative thromboembolism. *Surg. Gynaecol. Obstet.*, 123, 303

Sharnoff, J. G. (1969). Prevention of sudden cardiopulmonary arrest in the perioperative period with prophylactic heparin. *Lancet*, ii, 292

Sharnoff, J. G. and DeBlasio, G. (1970). Prevention of fatal postoperative thromboembolism by heparin prophylaxis. *Lancet*, ii, 1006

Skinner, D. B. and Saltzman, E. W. (1967). Anticoagulant prophylaxis in surgical patients. *Surg. Gynaecol. Obstet.*, 125, 741

Warlow, C., Beattie, A. G., Terry, G., Ogston, D., Kenmure, A. C. F. and Douglas, A. S. (1973). A double-blind trial of low doses of subcutaneous heparin in the prevention of deep-vein thrombosis after myocardial infarction. *Lancet*, ii, 934

Williams, H. T. (1971). Prevention of postoperative deep-vein thrombosis with perioperative subcutaneous heparin. *Lancet*, ii, 950

Yin, E. T., Wessler, S. and Stoll, P. J. (1971). Identity of plasma-activated factor X inhibitor with antithrombin III and heparin cofactor. *J. Biol. Chem.*, 246, 3712

17

The value of clinical signs in the diagnosis of deep venous thrombosis

A. N. Nicolaides, Jeanette Meadway and Doreen Irving

The ^{125}I-fibrinogen test and venography have demonstrated that the clinical diagnosis of deep venous thrombosis is unreliable. Approximately half of the postoperative patients who develop thrombosis detected by the [125] I-fibrinogen test do not have any signs (Flanc et al., 1968; Negus et al., 1968) and half of the patients with clinically suspected thrombosis have normal deep veins on venography (Fishman, 1962; Philips, 1963; Haeger, 1965; 1969; Haeger and Nylander, 1967; Nicolaides et al., 1971; Nicolaides, 1972; Chapter 11). One conclusion has been that a venogram should be performed in every case of clinically suspected thrombosis in order to establish the presence or absence of thrombi (Murray and Kakkar, 1972; Nicolaides, 1972). Others have argued that such practice would strain the resources of a busy radiological department. This chapter describes an attempt to assess the importance of symptoms, signs and other clinical factors and to use the ones which are significant to estimate the probability of thrombosis for any patient with clinical signs.

Swelling is considered to be the most valuable symptom and sign as demonstrated by postmortem and venographic studies (McLachlin et al., 1962; DeWeese and Rogoff, 1963). Local tenderness has been described as one of the earliest signs (Veal and Hussey, 1945; Moser, 1946). It was present in 93 per cent of patients with iliofemoral, 91 per cent of patients with femoral and 81 per cent with calf thrombosis in one study (DeWeese and Rogoff, 1963). Homans' sign (Homans, 1944) is unreliable. It was positive only in half of the patients with venographic evidence of deep venous thrombosis (DeWeese and Rogoff, 1963). None of these signs are diagnostic because they can be produced by conditions other than

243

deep venous thrombosis. Dependency with immobility (e.g. paralysed limb) or cardiac failure may cause oedema; contusion, muscular strain, cellulitis, cramps may cause calf tenderness and a positive Homans' sign (Moser, 1946; Dumphy and Botsford, 1964). There is no doubt that the diagnosis of massive thrombosis when the limb is very swollen and tense is not difficult, but there are many examples of extensive deep venous thrombosis involving the femoral vein without any signs. Provided the superficial system of veins and lymphatics is normal, oedema may not occur until the thrombus extends up to and occludes the saphenofemoral junction (Nicolaides, 1974).

In the venographic study reported in Chapter 11, 97 (43 per cent) of the 228 patients presenting with positive clinical signs had normal deep veins. Of the 97 patients who had clinical, but not venographic evidence of thrombosis there were 34 (35 per cent) in whom the signs could be attributed to causes other than deep venous thrombosis. They were congestive cardiac failure, superficial thrombophlebitis, venous insufficiently, muscle strain, cellulitis, haematoma of the calf and cramp.

In a prospective study of 242 patients, ascending venography (Chapter 11) was performed in 281 limbs. Two-hundred and twenty-nine patients presented with clinical deep venous thrombosis and 13 with symptoms and signs suggestive of pulmonary embolism (chest pain, haemoptysis breath-signs elicted and the presence of any predisposing clinical factors were recorded on a special form before venography (Table 17). The results have been analysed by first using a single variate analysis followed by a multivariate analysis.

SINGLE VARIATE ANALYSIS
The association between each of the clinical factors and deep venous thrombosis is shown in Table 17.1 Of the symptoms studied, leg swelling and proximal extension of symptoms were associated with a high incidence of deep venous thrombosis. Of the recorded signs, extension of signs proximal to the calf, deep induration in the calf muscles, oedema distal to the knee, positive Homans sign, high tenderness and thigh oedema were also associated with a high incidence of deep venous thrombosis. Of the predisposing factors, the presence of superficial thrombophlebitis and the finding of a cause other than deep venous thrombosis responsible for the signs were associated with a low incidence. Surgical patients, malignancy and the presence of a period of hypotension (systolic less than 100 mmHg) during the 5 days prior to the onset of symptoms were associated with a high incidence of thrombosis.

Thromboembolism

Table 17.1 The association between clinical factors and deep venous thrombosis

Clinical factor		Number of patients		x^2	p
(a) *Symptoms*		*Without D.V.T.*	*With D.V.T.*		
Leg pain	Absent	22	31(58%)	0·94	> 0·05
	Present	94	93(50%)		
Leg swelling	Absent	72	49(41%)	10·34	< 0·005
	Present	46	75(62%)		
Extent of symptoms	Confined to Calf	98	85(46%)	11·94	< 0·001
	Proximal Extension	7	28(80%)		

(b) *Signs*		*Number of limbs*			
Extent of signs	Confined to Calf	110	92(46%)	14·51	<0·0005
	Proximal Extension	8	32(80%)		
Calf tenderness	Absent	46	29(39%)	1·42	>0·05
	Present	108	98(48%)		
Deep induration	Absent	138	77(36%)	30·94	<0·0005
	Present	16	50(76%)		
Oedema distal to knee	Absent	98	50(34%)	15·48	<0·0005
	Present	56	77(58%)		
Homans sign	Absent	103	62(38%)	8·64	<0·005
	Present	51	65(56%)		
Thigh tenderness	Absent	146	109(43%)	5·66	<0·025
	Present	8	18(69%)		
Thigh oedema	Absent	147	97(40%)	20·52	<0·0005
	Present	7	30(81%)		

(c) *Predisposing factors*					
Malignancy	Absent	116	114(50%)	3·94	<0·05
	Present	2	10(83%)		
Cardiac failure	Absent	109	112(51%)	0·11	>0·05
	Present	9	12(57%)		
Limb paralysis	Absent	116	118(50%)	1·02	>0·05
	Present	2	6(75%)		
Superficial phlebitis	Absent	106	121(53%)	4·98	<0·05
	Present	12	3(20%)		
Hypotension	Absent	118	118(50%)	4·02	<0·05
	Present	0	6(100%)		
Obvious other cause of signs	Absent	71	121(63%)	49·37	<0·0005
	Present	47	3(6%)		
Group of patients	Medical	83	59(42%)	12·34	<0·0005
	Surgical	33	63(66%)		
Chest infection	Absent	112	110(50%)	2·31	>0·05
	Present	6	14(70%)		

MULTIVARIATE ANALYSIS

A multivariate analysis was performed on the 229 patients presenting with clinical deep venous thrombosis using 15 variables which consisted of the clinical signs and predisposing factors recorded (Table 17.1). The analysis was based on the linear logistic model $y = a \ b_1 x_1 + b_2 x_2 + \dots + b_n x_n$ described in Chapters 12 and 13. Estimates were obtained of a and b_1, b_2, ... b_{15} (Table 17.2) using the method of maximum likelihood (Armitage, 1971). By taking their antilogarithm they have been expressed as relative risk which is more meaningful. A reliable estimate of relative risk and a t-value were not obtainable for hypertension, because all 6 patients with transient hypotension had thrombosis on venography.

Table 17.2 Maximum likelihood estimates of constant and coefficient of the linear logistic model (229 patients)

Variable	Estimate of coefficient	Estimate of relative risk	t-Value	
1. Hypotension	7·815	—*	—*	
2. Obvious cause other than DVT	−3·164	0·04	4·49	
3. Deep induration	1·635	5·13	3·61	
4. Patient's group (surgical)	1·301	3·67	3·28	Significant
5. Extension of signs proximal to calf	2·747	15·60	2·38	
6. Thigh tenderness	−2·232	0·10	1·90	
7. Chest infection	0·997	2·71	1·69	
8. Superficial phlebitis·	−1·261	0·28	1·65	
9. Malignancy	1·454	4·28	1·51	
10. Limb paralysis	1·059	2·88	1·26	Not significant
11. Homans sign	0·455	1·58	1·08	
12. Cardiac failure	0·444	1·56	0·87	
13. Thigh oedema	0·540	1·72	0·66	
14. Oedema distal to knee	0·065	1·07	0·17	
15. Calf tenderness	−0·066	0·94	0·12	

Constant $a = -4·027$

*Reliable estimate not obtainable because all six patients with hypotension had DVT
DVT = Deep venous thrombosis.

In order to simplify the model the analysis was repeated using only the significant factors (Table 17.2). The new estimates of the coefficients are listed in Table 17.3. From the new estimates the model became:

$y = -2 \cdot 5 -$ (Obvious cause other than **DVT** $\times 3 \cdot 1$)

$+$ (Deep induration $\times 1 \cdot 7$) $+$ (Proximal extension of signs $\times 1 \cdot 7$)

$+$ (Surgical group $\times 1 \cdot 0$)

$+$ (Hypotension $\times \cdot 7 \cdot 5$)

Table 17.3 Maximum likelihood estimates of constant and coefficient of the linear logistic model using the significant variables (229 patients)

Variable	Estimate of coefficient	Estimate of relative risk	t-Value
1. Hypotension	7·495	—*	—*
2. Obvious cause other than DVT	−3·128	0·04	4·78
3. Deep induration	1·747	5·74	4·66
4. Extension of signs proximal to calf	1·658	5·25	3·51
5. Patient's group (surgical)	1·024	2·78	3·20

Constant $a = -2 \cdot 483$

*Reliable estimate not obtainable because all six patients with hypotension had DVT
DVT = Deep venous thrombosis.

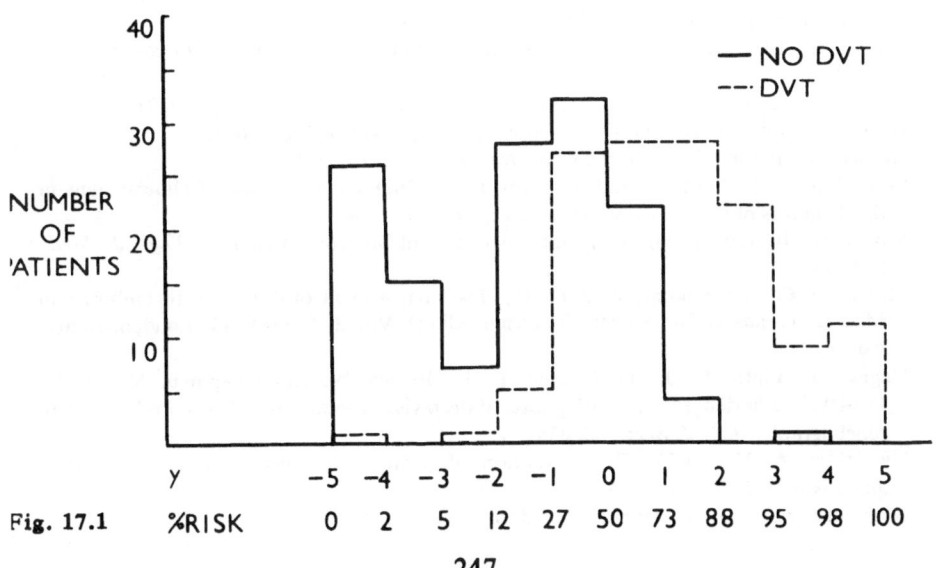

Fig. 17.1

247

Thromboembolism

Using this equation the logit y was calculated for every patient by substituting the clinical factors with 0 or 1 depending on whether they were absent or present. Y was expressed as a percentage risk (Figure 17.1). There was considerable overlap between the two groups: the patients with thrombosis and those without. However, when y was less than -2 the probability of thrombosis was very small. This was so in 20 per cent of the patients. When y was greater than 2 the probability of thrombosis was very high. This was so in 16 per cent of patients.

This study indicates a method of assessing the probability of deep venous thrombosis for patients in whom deep venous thrombosis is clinically suspected. Where this probability is found to be very low, venography may be avoided and it may be relatively safe to use objective diagnostic test such as the ^{125}I-fibrinogen test and doppler ultrasound examination, and clinical observation in these patients (Chapter 19).

References

Armitage, P. (1971). Statistical methods in medical research. Blackwell scientific publications, Oxford and Edinburgh

DeWeese, J. A. and Rogoff, S. M. (1963). Phlebographic patterns of acute deep venous thrombosis of the leg, *Surgery*, **53**, 99

Dunphy, J. E. and Botsford, T. W. (1964). Physical examination of the surgical patient, 3d ed. Philadelphia, Saunders

Fishman, L. G. (1962). Erroneous diagnosis of thrombophlebitis of the lower extremities. *Khirwigiya*, **38**, 58

Flanc, C., Kakkar, V. V. and Clarke, M. B. (1968). The detection of venous thrombosis of the legs using [125] I-labelled fibrinogen. *Brit. J. Surg.*, **55**, 742

Haeger, K. (1965). Den Kliniska thrombodiagnostikens ö Tillracklighet, *Lukartidningen*, **62**, 1067

Haeger, K. (1969). Problems of acute deep venous thrombosis. *Angiology*, **20**, 219

Haeger, K. and Nylander, G. (1967). Acute phlebography. *Triangle*, **8**, 18

Homans, J. (1944). Disease of the veins. *New Engl. J. Med.*, **231**, 51

McLachlin, J., Richards, T. and Paterson, J. C. (1962). An evaluation of clinical signs in the diagnosis of venous thrombosis. *Arch. Surg.*, **85**, 738

Moses, W. R. (1946). The early diagnosis of phlebothrombosis. *New Engl. J. Med.*, **234**, 288

Murray, J. G. and Kakkar, V. V. (1971). The management of deep vein thrombosis: in **Modern Trends in Surgery** (W. T. Irvine, editor), Vol. 3, Chapter 11, London, Butterworths.

Negus, D., Pinto, D. J., Le Quesne, L. P., Brown; N. and Chapman, M. (1968). ^{125}I-labelled fibrinogen in the diagnosis of deep vein thrombosis and its correlation with phlebography. *Brit. J. Surg.*, **55**, 835

Nicolaides, A. N. (1972). The prevention of postoperative deen venous thrombosis. *Jacksonian Prize Essay*

Nicolaides, A. N. (1974). Unpublished data

Thromboembolism

Nicolaides, A. N., Kakkar, V. V., Field, E. S. and Renney, J. T. G. (1971). The origin of deep vein thrombosis: A venographic study. *Brit. J. Radiol.*, **44**, 653

Nicolaides, A. N., Meadway, J., Irving, D. and Dupont, P. A. (1974). Clinical factors in the diagnosis of deep venous thrombosis. *Brit. J. Surg.*, (In Press)

Phillips, R. S. (1963). Prognosis in deep venous thrombosis. *A.M.A. Archives of Surgery*, **87**, 732

18

The place of thrombolytic and defibrinating agents in the treatment of venous thromboembolism

H. C. Kwaan and G. N. Grumet

The development of fibrinolytic agents for clinical use during the past decade is a major advance in the treatment of thromboembolism. This has been achieved through a better understanding of the mechanics of thrombus formation, propagation and resolution. In order to obtain an up to date perspective on the clinical use of the various available therapeutic agents some consideration must be given to the three major factors influencing the natural history of thrombosis postulated by Virchow (Virchow, 1871). Firstly, alterations in the content of blood can producea 'hypercoagueable' state that increases the tendency of thrombosis (Capters 2-7). Such alterations (Table 18.1) have been documented in a wide variety of clinical conditions (Table 18.2). Secondly, much importance is now given to haemodynamic factors. At low blood velocity, such as occurs at near stagnant venous flow, the thrombus that may be formed is rich in fibrin and red cells. In contrast, at higher flow rates, particularly at sites with turbulance such as occurs around prosthetic valves and narrowed atherosclerotic arteries, thrombi tend to be rich in platelets (Chapters 7 and 8). Thirdly, the thrombogenic effect of diseased vessel wall is being recognised (Chapter 8). Normal endothelial lining offers resistance to thrombus formation or adhesions through its ionic charge and its content of fibrinolytic activity. The protective function will be lost whenever the intima is damaged. Although there is still much that needs to be known about the nature of the initial nidus of thrombus formation, consideration of these factors will provide a rational approach to the prevention and treatment of a given form of thrombosis. The recognition of the importance of platelets and the

251

Table 18.1 Laboratory findings observed in the hypercoagulable state

Increased fibrinogen
Increased cryofibrinogen
Increased clotting factors (VII, VIII, IX, X)
Increased inhibitors of fibrinolysis
Increased platelet adhesiveness and aggregation
Increased viscosity
Increased platelets

Table 18.2 Clinical conditions associated with a hypercoagulable state

Pregnancy and puerperium
Oral contraceptives, oestrogens
Chronic infection
Surgery and trauma
Prolonged bed rest
Cancer
Congestive heart failure
Ulcerative colitis
Hyperviscosity
Polycythaemia

discovery of drugs that can interfere with platelet aggregation and adhesiveness may have opened the way to the prevention and treatment of platelet-rich thrombi. Because fibrin is present in all forms of thrombi, though to a varying degree, an important therapeutic attack is directed at fibrin formation and dissolution. In this chapter, two approaches will be discussed: fibrinolytic and defibrination therapies.

FIBRINOLYTIC AGENTS

The physiological function and regulation of fibrinolytic activity in blood has been extensively reviewed (Sherry *et al.*, 1959; Fletcher and Sherry, 1966; Pharmacology Society Symposium, 1966; Sherry, 1966; Kwaan, 1972), and will not be discussed at length. In brief, fibrinolysis *in vivo* is brought about by the conversion of an enzyme precursor, plasminogen, into a proteolytic enzyme, plasmin, by specific plasminogen activators. There is evidence that plasminogen activator derived from the vascular endothelium contributes significantly to the fibrinolytic activity of circulating blood (Kwaan and McFadzean, 1957; Todd, 1959; Warren, 1964; Kwaan, 1969). Attenpts have been made to stimulate the release of the vascular plasminogen activator to produce an enhanced plasma fibrinolytic activity for therapeutic purposes. Such stimulating agents include nicotinic acid (Wiener *et al.*, 1958) and its analogues, sulphonylureas, phenformin, testosterone and other anabolic steroids (Fearnely, 1964). Such drugs may increase transiently the level of blood fibrinolytic activity to a moderate degree. No long-term thrombolytic effect has been observed, though several reports of improvement in cutaneous vasculitis have appeared in recent literature (Dodman *et al.*, 1973). Other fibrinolytic agents are listed in Table 18.3. Of these only two plasminogen activators, urokinase and streptokinase, have undergone extensive experimental and clinical studies.

Table 18.3 Fibrinolytic agents

Plasmin
    Streptokinase-activated
    Trypsin-activated
Plasminogen activator
    Urokinase
        Tissue culture urokinase
    Streptokinase
    Streptokinase–plasmin complex

Mode of action

Urokinase has been available for therapeutic purposes since it was first isolated in relative purity from human urine. The native enzyme in urine was found to consist of a polypeptide chain of molecular weight 54 000 (Lesuk *et al.*, 1965). The purified active product (White *et al.*, 1966) having a specific activity of 35 000 CTA* units/mg protein is a smaller fragment with a molecular weight of 36 000. It is rather stable in the lyophilised form. It tends to adsorb to glass surfaces and to foam during the preparation for injection. Human albumin is therefore added in the clinical preparations for stabilisation.

*CTA = Committee on Thrombolytic Agents, National Heart and Lung Institute

Streptokinase is derived from filtrates of cultures of the beta-haemolytic streptococcus. Earlier preparations containing pyrogenic components are no longer used. Few reactions are seen with recently more purified material.

Both streptokinase and urokinase act enzymatically as potent activators of plasminogen. The reaction between streptokinase and plasmin has been studied in great detail (Robbins and Summaria, 1971). It must be noted that plasminogen activators have no lytic action on fibrin themselves. Their pharmacological effect on fibrinolysis depends on the availability of plasminogen either from the fibrin clot itself or, *in vivo*, from the circulating plasma. During therapy with plasminogen activators an excessive dosage may deplete the circulating plasminogen so that new clots formed subsequently will be lacking in plasminogen and thus be refractory to further actions by plasminogen activators. An equimolecular complex of streptokinase and plasmin can be formed. This complex acts as a plasminogen activator but does not have any fibrinolytic action of its own. Thus, it is possible to have a mixture in which all the plasminogen is converted to plasmin while an excess of streptokinase combines with the plasmin to form streptokinase–plasmin complex. The resulting enzymes will be those that are potent as plasminogen activators but have no therapeutic fibrinolytic effect.

In vivo activity
The susceptibility of various forms of thrombi to lysis by fibrinolytic agents depends on several factors. The thrombi that are predominantly fibrin and have rich plasminogen content are most suitable for lysis. Inhibitors of fibrinolysis may be present and may impede this process. It has been shown that platelets contain both inhibitors to plasmin and to urokinase (Kwaan and Suwanwela, 1971). Thus, one would expect platelet thrombi to be relatively resistant to thrombolysis.

Mode of administration
Either urokinase or streptokinase is usually given systemically, although attempts have been made to infuse either agent locally. In the case of urokinase, a loading dose of 2100 CTA units/lb of body weight is given intravenously, followed by the continuous intravenous infusion of amounts of 2100 CTA units/lb body weight/h. This dosage may be adjusted in order to maintain a euglobulin lysis time of 15–20 min. The individual variations to the pharmacological effect of urokinase, namely drug resistance, are not commonly encountered. If this level of induced

plasma fibrinolytic activity is maintained for 8–12 h, most thrombi in the body that are amenable to lysis should be optimally affected. In the case of streptokinase, a different problem in dosage may arise from previous immunisation to beta-haemolytic streptococcus. A high antistreptokinase antibody level may be encountered in patients having recent streptococcal infections and in those who have recently received streptokinase treatment. In these patients the initial dose is titrated *in vitro* by the determination of the amount of streptokinase required to lyse, in 10 min, 1·0 ml of a patient's citrated plasma, after clotting by calcium chloride. This titrated dose multiplied by the total plasma volume would be the amount of loading dose and should overcome the circulating antistreptokinase activity. In the absence of such antibody, the initial loading dose of 250 000 units should be adequate for a 70 kg adult. Because streptokinase is antigenic, the possibility of an anaphylactoid reaction must be kept in mind. As a precaution, most investigators advocate that the loading dose should be given over 30 min by slow intravenous infusion and that 100 mg of hydrocortisone be given intravenously prior to streptokinase therapy. The loading dose is followed by a continuous intravenous infusion at the rate of 100 000 units/h.

Laboratory monitoring
In the earlier clinical studies, a wide variety of tests were performed to assess the pharmacological action of these agents. The findings are summarised in Table 18.4. For simplified clinical monitoring the euglobulin lysis time provides adequate information on the pharmacological

Table 18.4 Comparative merits of streptokinase and urokinase

	Urokinase	Streptokinase
Fibrinogen	A slight fall if given over eight hours	Early fall
Plasminogen	A marked fall to less than one-half if given over eight hours	Marked early fall
Euglobulin lysis time	Satisfactorily maintained at 15–30 min	Not suitable. See text
Thrombin time	Prolongation	Prolongation
Prothrombin time	Prolongation	Prolongation
Platelet count	No change	Not affected

effect of urokinase. In the case of streptokinase, however, because of the formation of streptokinase–plasmin complex as discussed above, one would like to measure the activity of plasmin and not that of plasminogen. Thus, the euglobulin lysis time is not suitable. Since plasmin causes proteolysis of fibrinogen, the levels of fibrinogen degradation products in the plasma would reflect the ultimate pharmacological action; a simplified laboratory test commonly used is the thrombin time. This should be prolonged to 2–3 times the control value.

Because the level of circulating plasminogen may be depleted after a course of thrombolytic therapy, particularly with streptokinase, re-formation of thrombi with low plasminogen content may occur. Theoretically these are refractory to further action of plasminogen activators. Therefore, an effort should be made to provide adequate heparin therapy following thrombolytic therapy. The time heparin therapy should be started would depend on the patient's thrombin time. At the end of thrombolytic therapy, sufficient fibrinogen degradation products may be present in the circulation to prove too risky for additional heparin administration. One should wait until the thrombin time is less than twice the control value before heparin is given.

Complications

The major complication of urokinase therapy is bleeding. Most of the bleeding is minor, consisting of oozing from sites of venipuncture. There may be greater blood loss from recent wounds, particularly after orthopaedic surgery. Bleeding may also occur in the gastrointestinal tract. In the early clinical trials, unexplained falls in haematocrit values were observed. This was at the time believed to be haemolysis occurring when urokinase was given in conjunction with radiopaque contrast media for angiographic studies. The complication has not been seen subsequently. Urokinase, being homologous in origin, is not antigenic to man, but the use of streptokinase has the additional risk of anaphylactoid reactions. Furthermore, reactions related to impurities that vary with different batches of the drug may be encountered, such as fever, vasomotor collapse and urticaria.

Relative merits of urokinase and streptokinase

Because both preparations are available for clinical use, their relative merits should be considered. It is believed that urokinase has a higher affinity for plasminogen in the thrombus than in the circulation. Hence, it will preferentially cause plasmin release locally in the thrombus rather than in the circulation. This concept is supported by observations of plasminogen depletion and plasmin excess (as indicated by fall in circulating fibrinogen and by excess fibrinogen degradation products) in circulation, if given for under 8 h. Also, being non-antigenic, urokinase dosage is not subjected to alterations by pre-existing antibodies in blood. Repeated courses of the same agent could be given if indicated. A limiting factor for the use of this much more attractive thrombolytic agent is the high cost of preparation and the difficulty of obtaining a sufficient source of the material. The following may illustrate the difficulties involved in the manufacturing: To obtain materials for six hours of therapy for a 70 kg man, approximately three million CTA units are required. The average urokinase activity in urine is about 6 CTA units/ml. Assuming that a 40 per cent recovery is achieved, 2·4 CTA units/ml would be obtained. Then: $\dfrac{3 \times 10^6}{2\cdot4 \times 10^3} = 1250$ l of urine would be needed for this six hour dose. If 1·25 l is the mean urine output for an individual, then 1000 man-urine days would be required.

Recently, successful attempts have been made to obtain a plasminogen activator with characteristics antigenically and physically similar to urinary urokinase from a culture of human foetal kidneys. The cost of this material can be reduced to one twentieth of that required for the extraction from urine.

Clinical experience

The most extensive clinical study with urokinase to date is the Urokinase Pulmonary Embolism Trial sponsored by the National Heart and Lung Institute (Hyers, 1971; The Urokinase Pulmonary Embolism Trial, 1973).

Patients were randomised into two 12 h infusion groups. One group received urokinase and the second group heparin. Urokinase was given intravenously in a loading dose of 2000 CTA units/lb body weight followed by 2000 CTA units/lb for 12 h by intravenous infusion. In the second group, 75 CTA units/lb of heparin was used as a loading dose followed by 10 units/lb/h. At the end of the 12 h infusion period, heparin was started in both groups for five days and this in turn was followed by heparin or warfarin for 14 days. Pulmonary angiography and lung scanning at 2, 3, 5, 7, and 14 days were performed. Seventy-eight patients were randomised to the heparin group, and 82 patients to the urokinase group. Urokinase with subsequent heparin proved to be more effective when measured by complete resolution of lung scan abnormality: 6·2 per cent of the urokinase treated patients compared with only 2·5 per cent of the heparin treated patients. However, by the seventh day the results were identical. This similarity continued to be evident at 3, 6, and 12 months postperfusion. Haemodynamic data including right atrial mean pressure, right ventricular end-diastolic pressure, right ventricular systolic pressure, pulmonary artery mean pressure and total pulmonary resistance showed greater improvement at 24 h in the urokinase treated patients. The improvement in partial pressure of oxygen (P_{O_2}) showed a strong trend in favour of the urokinase treated group but was not statistically significant. Clinical changes were not as striking as objective data. In the group with massive embolism, the dyspnoea and the accentuated pulmonary closure sound disappeared more quickly in the urokinase treated patients.

Morbidity consisted of bleeding with 45 per cent incidence in the urokinase treated group and 27 per cent in the heparin treated group. Early bleeding, that is in the first 24 h, was seen in the urokinase group while the heparin group was less predictable. Analysis of the type of bleeding was as follows: In the heparin treated group 11 of the 21 cases had severe and 10 of the 21 cases had moderate bleeding. In the urokinase group, 22 of the 37 patients had severe and 15 of the 37 patients had moderate bleeding. In summary, most of the bleeding in the urokinase treated patients was localised to the cut-down site, and was nearly three times as frequent as in the heparin treated patients. The incidence of gastrointestinal bleeding was equal in the two groups. It was always severe in the urokinase group, but was severe in only half of the instances of bleeding in the heparin group. Retroperitoneal haemorrhage was five times more common in the heparin treated group. Severe retroperitoneal haemorrhage was three times more common in the heparin treated group than in the urokinase treated patients. Recurrent embolism in the two-week post infusion period occurred in 7·2 per cent in the urokinase treated patients and in 22 per cent of the heparin treated patients. Seven per cent of the urokinase patients died, whereas 9 per cent of the heparin treated patients died during the two week period of treatment.

These results tend to illustrate the fact that it is the patient with massive embolism who is most likely to benefit from urokinase therapy especially if systemic hypotension is present. Thus in the patient in whom surgical embolectomy might be indicated, 'medical embolectomy' may tend to improve the surgical mortality rate. The use of urokinase may prove to be a significant therapeutic advance since the surgical mortality for embolectomy is in the range of 52 to 68 per cent (Cross and Mowlem, 1967; Chapter 20).

ANCROD AND REPTILASE

As previously mentioned, fibrin formation and dissolution can be influenced by preventing fibrin deposition through defibrination as well as by thrombolysis. Two derivatives from snake venom have been shown to have a potential clinical application for this purpose. They are Ancrod, derived from the venom of *Agkistrodon rhodostoma* and Reptilase, from that of *Bothrops atrox*. Details on the biochemical and pharmacological characteristics have been described elsewhere (Esnouf and Tunnah, 1967; Reid and Chan, 1968; Sharp *et al.*, 1968; Blomback *et al.*, 1971; Kwaan, 1973; 1974).

Their main action is that of converting fibrinogen to fibrin. In contrast to the proteolytic action of thrombin, which results in splitting the arginyl-glycyl bonds linking the fibrinopeptides A and B to the rest of the fibrin monomer (Chapter 3), Ancrod and Reptilase release only the fibrinopeptide A from the a chain, while the β and γ chains remain unchanged. A different conformational change then takes place. The thrombin-induced fibrin monomer polymerises end-to-end as well as side-to-side but the Ancrod- or Reptilase-induced monomer polymerises only end-to-end. The resulting fibrin polymer produced by thrombin may be expressed as $[(a\beta\gamma)_2]_n$ while that produced by Ancrod or by Reptilase would be $[(a\beta(B)\gamma)_2]_n$. Under electron microscopy, these two types of polymers are morphologically different. The thrombin-induced type $[(a\beta\gamma)_2]_n$ fibrin appears as thick interconnected fibers, while the Ancrod- or Reptilase-induced type $[(a\beta(B)\gamma)_2]_n$ appears as very thin filaments.

As the result of structural differences between Ancrod- or Reptilase-induced fibrin and thrombin-induced fibrin, the first is more susceptible to plasmin proteolysis (Kwaan and Barlow, 1971a; 1971b). Increased lysis occurs with the Ancrod- and Reptilase-induced fibrin when compared with thrombin-induced fibrin on exposure to the same amount of urokinase. This characteristic of Ancrod-induced fibrin was confirmed by others (Mattock and Esnouf, 1971; Pizzo *et al.*, 1971). Ancrod may have additional proteolytic action on the a chain at cleavage sites different from those of plasmin. These findings are of considerable practical significance because they would explain the benign nature of the *in vivo* defibrination by Ancrod and Reptilase (Kwaan and Barlow, 1971a).

Effects on other clotting factors are surprisingly few. Reptilase, but not

Ancrod, activates Factor XIII and possibly Factors II and X (Eagle, 1937)
Neither compound causes direct lysis of fibrin nor increases the plasma
fibrinolytic activity after intravenous administration. However, recent
findings suggest that both compounds may enhance the activation of
plasminogen by various plasminogen activators such as urokinase and
streptokinase (Kwaan and Grumet, 1973). In man, after an intravenous
dose of 2 units/kg body weight of Ancrod or 0·175 units/kg body
weight of Reptilase, the plasma fibrinogen level decreases rapidly within
one-half to one hour to unmeasurable levels, remaining low for periods of
12 h and then slowly returning to normal levels around 24 h. Since defibrination is produced by transformation of the entire body content of
fibrinogen to fibrin, the rapid intravenous administration of a large dose
may produce sudden death associated with widespread formation of
thrombi (Silberman et al., 1971). If this dose is not excessive and is given
slowly over 15–30 min, safe defibrination can be achieved without
production of even microthrombi. In man, 2 units/kg of Ancrod infused slowly intravenously over six hours generally is considered safe
(Bell et al., 1968; Sharp et al., 1968). Subsequent defibrination may be
maintained by an intravenous injection of two units of Ancrod/kg over a
period of 10 min repeated every 12 h. No decrease in other clotting
factors were noted in animals or in man. A sharp rise in fibrin degradation
products appeared in the circulation in association with the fall in
fibrinogen level. The plasminogen level in blood decreased along with the
fall in the circulating fibrinogen. The reason for this is not clearly understood. We have shown that Ancrod or Reptilase may have an additional
proteolytic action on plasminogen activation, although they are not direct
fibrinolytic agents themselves (Kwaan and Grumet, 1973). This
potentiation of plasminogen activation has obvious therapeutic implications. It forms the rationale for a combined use of urokinase or
streptokinase with Ancrod or Reptilase as a new approach to thrombolytic therapy.

No change occurs in the platelet count or in the platelet turnover.
However, studies on platelet aggregation revealed impaired ADP-induced
aggregation (Prentice et al., 1969). This effect is due to the presence of
fibrin degradation products of low molecular weight and could be reproduced in vitro by the plasmin-digestion products of Ancrod-induced
fibrin clots (Kwaan and Barlow, 1971a; 1971b).

Postulated mechanism for therapeutic effects
Although the clinical results can only be evaluated by more extensive

trials, the available findings are sufficient to form the basis for the rationale of Ancrod and Reptilase therapy. The possible mechanisms of action are illustrated diagramatically in Figure 18.1.

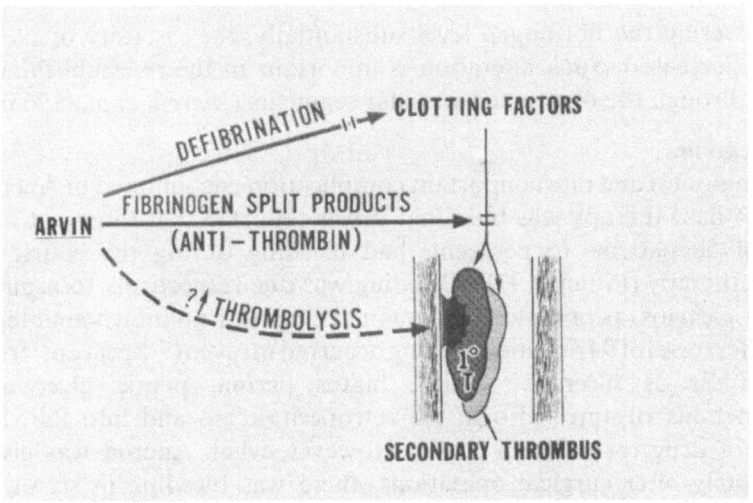

Figure 18.1 Diagram for the possible mechanism of action of Ancrod and Reptilase

If a thrombus is considered a dynamic structure where continuous thrombolysis is occurring simultaneously with a continuous deposition of platelets and fibrin, then an effective prevention of the latter (secondary thrombus formation) will result in reduction of thrombus size (Pitney *et al.*, 1969). The degree of fibrinolytic activity at the site of thrombosis is substantial and can be particularly strong when the intimal lining of the involved vessel is not significantly damaged as, for example, in the case of embolism (Kwaan, 1969). Ancrod would theoretically be a more effective agent than heparin and dicoumarol in preventing the secondary clot formation, because by removing fibrinogen from the circulation it is taking away the 'powder-keg' rather than merely 'stepping on the fuse' (Reid and Chan, 1968). In addition, further deposition of platelets on the primary thrombus is impaired due to the inhibition of platelet aggregation by fibrin degradation products. As a result, the primary thrombus is allowed to resolve more rapidly by lysis.

Although neither Ancrod nor Reptilase possess fibrinolytic activity by themselves, their presence may enhance the activation of plasminogen in the clot or plasminogen in the circulation. This will increase the resolution of the thrombus by lysis.

261

Production of fibrin degradation products (FDP) may contribute also to the prevention of secondary clot formation through their anticoagulant activity and their inhibition of polymerisation of fibrin and platelet aggregation.

By lowering the fibrinogen level substantially, the viscosity of blood may be decreased. Such alteration is important in the re-establishment of flow through the obstructed vascular segments (Merrill *et al.*, 1965).

Complications

The commonest and most important complication encountered in Ancrod and Reptilase therapy was bleeding. It was reported that three out of a series of 58 patients (5 per cent) had bleeding during the course of Ancrod therapy (Pitney, 1971). Bleeding was due respectively to aspirin-induced gastritis, peptic ulcer and vaginal origin of unknown aetiology. In another series of 94 patients bleeding occurred in seven (7·5 per cent) from such causes as ulcerative colitis, hiatus hernia, peptic ulcer and gastrocnemius rupture; also in the retroperitoneum and into the skin at sites of drug rash (Sharp, 1971). However, when Ancrod was given immediately after surgical operations, there was bleeding in six of 11 patients (55 per cent), in three of such severity that therapy had to be stopped (Sharp, 1971). It was felt that Ancrod is contraindicated within 48 h of surgical operations.

It has been reported that tolerance to the defibrinating action of Ancrod may develop rapidly in some patients after intramuscular administration (Pitney *et al.*, 1969). However, with the intravenous route, such resistance to the drug rarely occurs. When refractoriness develops, it can be detected by the failure of large doses of Ancrod to clot the patient's blood *in vitro* and by positive precipitin reaction.

Evidence of impaired tissue repair has been observed in experimental animals after Ancrod therapy (Holt *et al.*, 1970; Silberman and Kwaan, 1971), but not in man.

Clinical results

There was an initial enthusiasm for both Ancrod and Reptilase in the early clinical trials. Some of these are summarised in Table 18.5. However, these therapeutic responses were assessed by clinical observations. If more rigid venographic criteria and stricter controls that include comparison with heparin are used, the results might well be very different. Until we have more extensive data from further clinical trials at multicentre level, we shall not be able to produce a meaningful clinical assessment.

Table 18.5 Clinical results of Ancrod and Reptilase treatment

Author	Disease	No. of patients	Criteria	Response C*	P*	N*
Ancrod						
Bell *et al.*, 1968	Deep venous thrombosis	7	Clinical	6	1	–
Sharp *et al.*, 1968	Deep venous thrombosis	9	Clinical	9	–	–
Kakkar *et al.*, 1969	Deep venous thrombosis	10	(a) Clinical	10	–	–
			(b) Radiological and isotopic	1	3	6
Pitney, 1969	Deep venous thrombosis	18	Clinical	11	–	7
Bell *et al.*, 1969	Priapism	2	Clinical	2	–	–
Pitney, 1969	Priapism	1	Clinical			1
Sharp *et al.*, 1968	Art. thromb.	5	Combined surgery	4	1	
Gilles *et al.*, 1968	Sickle cell crisis	11	Clinical (7 with bone pain) (1 hemiplegia)	9	2	–
Reid *et al.*, 1969	Sickle cell crisis	8	Clinical (7 with bone pain) (1 hemiplegia)	5	3	1
Bowell *et al.*, 1970	Central ret. vein thrombosis	8	Ret. photography	6	1	1
Pitney, 1969	Prosth. valve with embolism	8	Clinical			8
Pitney, 1969	Chr. pulmonary hypertension	7	Clinical			7
Reptilase						
Blomback *et al.*, 1970	Deep venous thrombosis	10	Radiological	3		5
	Central retinal thrombosis	3	Retinal circulation time	2		
	'Old' arterial occlusion	5				
Straub *et al.*, 1970	Venous thrombosis	1	Radiological			1

*C = complete; P = partial; N = none

What then are the results we expect from such trials? Perhaps the most important question is whether there is an added advantage of Ancrod or Reptilase when compared to the conventional heparin treatment. An attempt to list the comparative data on the two forms of anticoagulant therapy is seen in Table 18.6. Ancrod or Reptilase therapy is relatively simple to administer and to control with little fluctuation in its pharmacological effects. Bleeding is surprisingly less common than with heparin therapy (Pitney, 1971). On the other hand, the defibrinating effect of Ancrod or Reptilase can be established safely only after a period of four to six hours while the anticoagulant action of heparin is immediate. Lastly, in the early postoperative period, heparin, and not Ancrod or Reptilase, should be given.

Table 18.6 Comparative merits of Ancrod/Reptilase and heparin

	Ancrod	*Heparin*
Dosage	Simple; no fluctuation	Individual variation occasional resistance
Laboratory control	Fibrinogen	Clotting time, partial thromboplastin time
Bleeding	5 per cent	10 per cent
Safety	Yes	Yes
Rapidity of onset	4–6 h	Immediate
Surgery	After 48 h	Safe

Other uses

The fibrinogen degradation products may be detected by a number of laboratory tests of fibrinogen clotting based on their anticoagulant activity. Ancrod and Reptilase may be used in such tests as well as thrombin. They have an advantage over thrombin in not being affected by heparin. The Ancrod time and the Reptilase time are therefore used instead of the thrombin time for the detection of FDP in patients treated with heparin.

Fibrin is involved in many disease conditions. It is conceivable that by prolonged defibrination such disease processes may be altered. For example, we have shown in our laboratory that fibrin deposits will not form in the neurological lesions of experimental allergic encephalomyelitis and the expected paralysis will not occur when Ancrod treatment is given. Other examples are the delay in transplantation rejection and temporary regression of tumours following Ancrod treatment. Further

Thromboembolism

studies along these lines may open up new and exciting applications for these two agents (Williams and Maughan, 1972).

References

Bell, W. R., Bolton, G. and Pitney, W. R. (1968). The effect of Arvin on blood coagulation factors. *Brit. J. Haematol.*, **15**, 689

Bell, W. R., Pitney, W. R. and Goodwin, J. F. (1968). Therapeutic defibrination in the treatment of thrombotic disease. *Lancet,* **ii**, 490

Bell, W. R. and Pitney, W. R. (1969). Management of priapism by therapeutic defibrination. *New Engl. J. Med.*, **280**, 649

Blombäck, M., Egberg, N., Gruder, E., Johansson, A. A., Johnsson, H., Nilsson, S. E. G. and Blombäck, B. (1971). Treatment of thrombotic disorders with Reptilase. *Thromb. Diath. Haemorrh. (Stuttg.)*, **Suppl. 45**, 51

Bowell, R. E., Marmion, V. J. and McCarthy, C. F. (1970). Treatment of central retinal vein thrombosis with Ancrod. *Lancet,* **ii**, 173

Cross, R. S. and Mowlem, A. (1967). A survey of the current status of pulmonary embolectomy for massive pulmonary embolism. *Circ.*, **35, Suppl. 86,**

Dodman, B., Cunliffe, W. J., Roberts, B. E. and Sibbald, R. (1973). Clinical and laboratory double blind investigation on effect of fibrinolytic therapy in patients with cutaneous vasculitis. *Brit. Med. J.*, **2**, 82

Eagle, H. (1937). The coagulation of blood by snake venoms and its physiologic significance. *J. Exp. Med.*, **65**, 613

Esnouf, M. P. and Tunnah, G. W. (1967). The isolation and properties of the thrombin-like activity from ancistrodon rhodostoma venom. *Brit. J. Haematol.*, **13**, 581

Fearnely, G. R. (1964). Physiology and Pharmacology. *Brit. Med. Bull.*, **20**, 185

Pharmacology Society Symposium. The Fibrinolytic System. (1966). *Fed. Proc.*, **25**, 28

Fletcher, A. P. and Sherry, S. (1966). Thrombolytic agents. *Amer. Rev. Pharmacol.*, **6**, 89

Gilles, H. M., Reid, H. A., Odutola, A., Ransome-Kuti, O., Lesi, F. and Ransome-Kuti, S. (1968). Arvin treatment for sickle-cell crisis. *Lancet,* **ii**, 542

Holt, P. J. L., Holloway, V., Raghupati, N. and Calnan, J. S. (1970). Effect of a fibrinolytic agent (Arvin) on wound healing and collagen formation. *Clin. Sci.*, **38**, 9P

Hyers, T. M. (1971). Urokinase in the treatment of pulmonary embolism. *Thromb. Diath. Hemorrh.*, **Suppl. 47**, 165

Kakkar, V. V., Flanc, C., Howe, C. T., O'Shea, M. and Flute, P. T. (1969). Treatment of deep vein thrombosis. A trial of heparin, streptokinase and Arvin. *Brit. Med. J.*, **1**, 806

Kakkar, V. V., Howe, C. T., Laws, J. W. and Flanc, C. (1969). Late results of treatment of deep vein thrombosis. *Brit. Med. J.*, **1**, 810

Kakkar, V. V. (1970). Treatment of deep vein thrombosis. *Proc. Roy. Soc. Med.*, **63**, 133

Kwaan, H. C., Lo, R. and McFadzean, A. J. S. (1957). On the production of plasma fibrinolytic activity within veins. *Clinc. Sci.*, **16**, 241

Kwaan, H. C. (1969). Endothelial fibrinolytic activity in the prevention and resolution of thrombosis. In: *Dynamics of Thrombus Formation and Dissolution*, 114 (S. A. Johnson and M. M. Guest, editors) (Philadelphia: J. B. Lippincott Co.)

Thromboembolism

Kwaan, H. C. (1969). Endothelial fibrinolytic activity in the prevention and resolution of thrombis In: *Dynamics of Thrombus Formation and Dissolution*, 340 (S. A. Johnson and M. M. Guest, editors) (Philadelphia: J. B. Lippincott)

Kwaan, H. C. and Barlow, G. H. (1971a). The mechanism of action of a coagulant fraction of Malayan pit viper venom, Arvin and of Reptilase. *Thromb. Diath. Haemorrh. (Stuttg.)*, **Suppl. 45**, 63

Kwaan, H. C. and Barlow, G. H. (1971b). The mechanism of action of Arvin and Reptilase. *Thromb. Diath. Haemorrh. (Stuttg.)*, **Suppl. 47**, 361

Kwaan, H. C. and Suwanwela, N. (1971). Inhibitors of fibrinolysis in platelets in polycythaemia vera and thrombocytosis. *Brit. J. Haematol.*, **21**, 313

Kwaan, H. C. (1972). Disorders of fibrinolysis. *Med. Clin. N. Amer.*, **56**, 163

Kwaan, H. C. (1973). Status of 'Arvin' and 'Reptilase' therapy in thromboembolism. In: *Pulmonary Thromboembolism* (K. M. Moser and M. Stein, editors) (Chicago: Yearbook Medical Publishers, Inc.)

Kwaan, H. C. and Grumet, G. N. (1973). Potentiation of plasminogen activation by Ancrod and Reptilase. *Fed. Proc.*, **Vol. 32**, 427 (Abstract)

Kwaan, H. C. (1974). Use of defibrinating agents Ancrod and Reptilase in the treatment of thromboembolism. *Thromb. Diath. Haemorrh.* (In press)

Lesuk, A., Terminellor, L. and Traver, J. H. (1965). Crystalline human urokinase: some properties. *Science*, **149**, 880

Mattock, P. and Esnouf, M. P. (1971). Difference in the subunit structure of human fibrin formed by the action of Arvin, Reptilase and thrombin. *Nature, New Biol.*, **233**, 277

Merrill, E. W., Benis, A. M., Gilliland, E. R., Sherwood, T. K. and Salzman, E. W. (1965). Pressure flow relations of human blood in hollow fibres at low flow rates. *J. Appl. Physiol.*, **20**, 954

Pitney, W. R. (1969). Clinical experience with 'Arvin'. *Thromb. Diath. Haemorrh.*, **Suppl. 38**, 81

Pitney, W. R., Bell, W. R. and Bolton, G. (1969). Blood fibrinolytic activity during Arvin therapy. *Brit. J. Haematol.*, **16**, 165

Pitney, W. R., Bray, C., Holt, P. J. L. and Bolton, G. (1969). Acquired resistance to treatment with Arvin. *Lancet*, **i**, 79

Pitney, W. R. (1971). An appraisal of therapeutic defibrination. *Thromb. Diath. Haemorrh.*, **Suppl. 45**, 43

Pizzo, S. V., Schwartz, M. L., Hill, R. L. and McKee, P. A. (1971). A direct proteolytic effect on soluble fibrin by Arvin. *Clin. Res.*, **19**, 667

Prentice, C. R. M., Hassanein, A. A., Turpie, G. G. G., McNicol, G. P. and Douglas, A. S. (1969). Changes in platelet behaviour during Arvin Therapy. *Lancet*, **i**, 644

Reid, H. A. and Chan, K. E. (1968). The paradox in therapeutic defibrination. *Lancet*, **I**, 485

Reig, H. A. and Gilles, H. M. (1969). Arvin treatment in sickle-cell crisis. *Trans. Roy. Soc. Trop. Med. & Hyg.*, **63**, 22

Robbins, K. C. and Summaria, L. (1971). Biochemistry and fibrinolysis. *Thromb. Diath. Haemorrh.*, **Suppl. 47**, 9

Sharp, A. A., Warren, B. A., Pacton, A. M. and Allington, M. J. (1968). Anticoagulant therapy with a purified fraction of Malayan pit viper venom. *Lancet*, **i**, 493

Sharp, A. A., Warren, B. A., Paxton, A. M. and Allington, M. J. (1968). Anticoagulant therapy with a purified fraction of Malayan pit viper venom. *Lancet*, **i**, 493

Thromboembolism

Snarp, A. A. (1971). Clinical use of Arvin. *Thromb. Diath. Haemorrh.* (*Stuttg.*), **Suppl. 45,** 69

Sherry, S., Fletcher, A. P. and Alkjaersig, N. (1959). Fibrinolysis and fibrinolytic activity in man. *Physiol. Rev.*, **39,** 343

Sherry, S. (1968). Fibrinolysis. *Ann. Rev.ʹMed.*, **18,** 247

Silberman, S. and Kwaan, H. C. (1971). The effect of 'Arvin' on wound healing in the rat. *Fed. Proc.*, **30,** 424

Silberman, S., Potter, E. V. and Kwaan, H. C. (1971). Effects of Arvin in mice. Immunofluorescent and histochemical studies. *Exp. Molec. Pathol.*, **14,** 67

Straub, P. W. and Harder, A. (personal communication)

The Urokinase Pulmonary Embolism Trial. (April 1973). A National Cooperative Study. *Circ.*, **47, Suppl. 2**

Todd, A. S. (1959). The histological localisation of fibrinolysin activator. *J. Pathol. Bacterol.*, **78,** 281

Warren, B. A. (1964). Fibrinolytic activators of vascular endothelium. *Brit. Med. Bull.*, **20,** 213

White, W. F., Barlow, G. H. and Mozen, M. M. (1966). The isolation and characterisation of plasminogen activators (urokinase) from human urine. *Biochem.*, **5,** 2160

Wiener, M., Edisch, W. and Steele, J. M. (1958). Occurrence of fibrinolytic activity following administration of nicotinic acid. *Proc. Soc. Exp. Biol. Med.*, **98,** 755

Williams, J. R. B. and Maughan, E. (1972). Treatment of tumor metastases by defibrination. *Brit. Med. J.*, **II,** 172

Virchow, R. (1871). *Die cellularpathologie,* 194 (4th Ed. Berlin)

19

The management of deep venous thrombosis

A. N. Nicolaides and J. D. Lewis

The management of deep venous thrombosis is directed towards the prevention of pulmonary embolism, the limitation of local venous damage and to the relief of symptoms. The policy presented in this chapter is based on the results of published studies and our own experience gained from the investigation and treatment of 400 patients. It is conveniently summarised in a dichotomous flowchart (Figure 19.1).

There are five main advantages in documenting a procedure such as the management of deep venous thrombosis in the form of a flowchart:

1. It defines the policy which can be seen at a glance and challenges one to justify its steps.

2. It provides uniformity and consistency in the treatment offered by all members of a department.

3. It facilitates documentation (The patient's path can be traced in colour and the flowchart can be kept in the patient's file).

4. It allows easy updating of one's experience. The physician or surgeon must not be a 'slave' of the flowchart. If a situation presents that is not provided for or evidence becomes available that a new approach or therapy is better than the ones in use then the flowchart should be altered. It is by numerous alterations that the present flowchart has been developed.

5. It allows junior members of a team to formulate a plan of management which their lack of experience would otherwise have prevented.

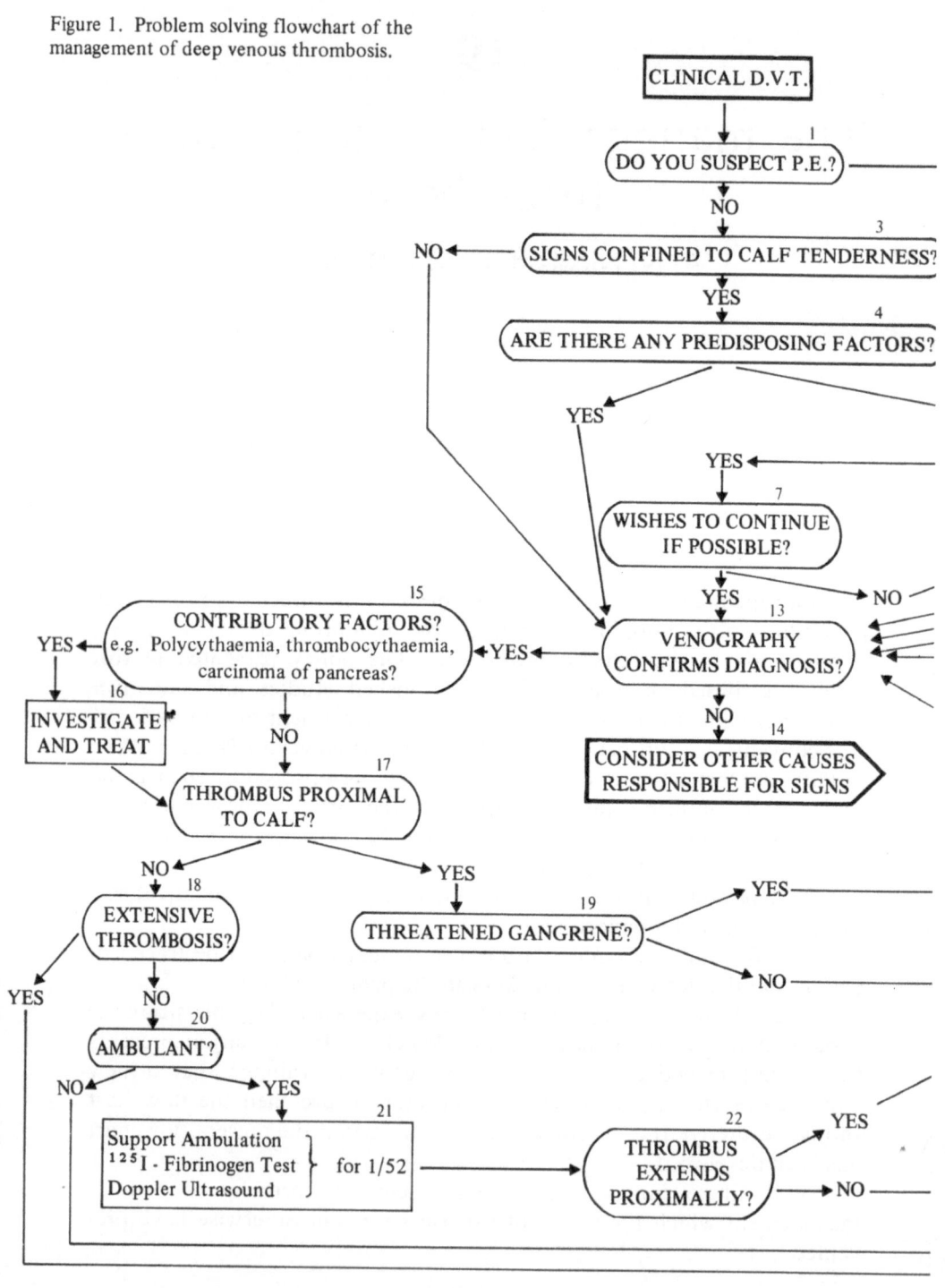

Figure 1. Problem solving flowchart of the management of deep venous thrombosis.

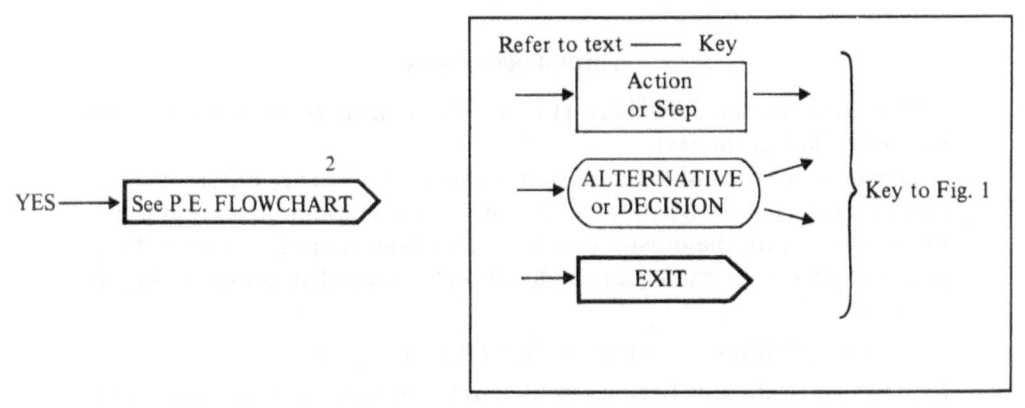

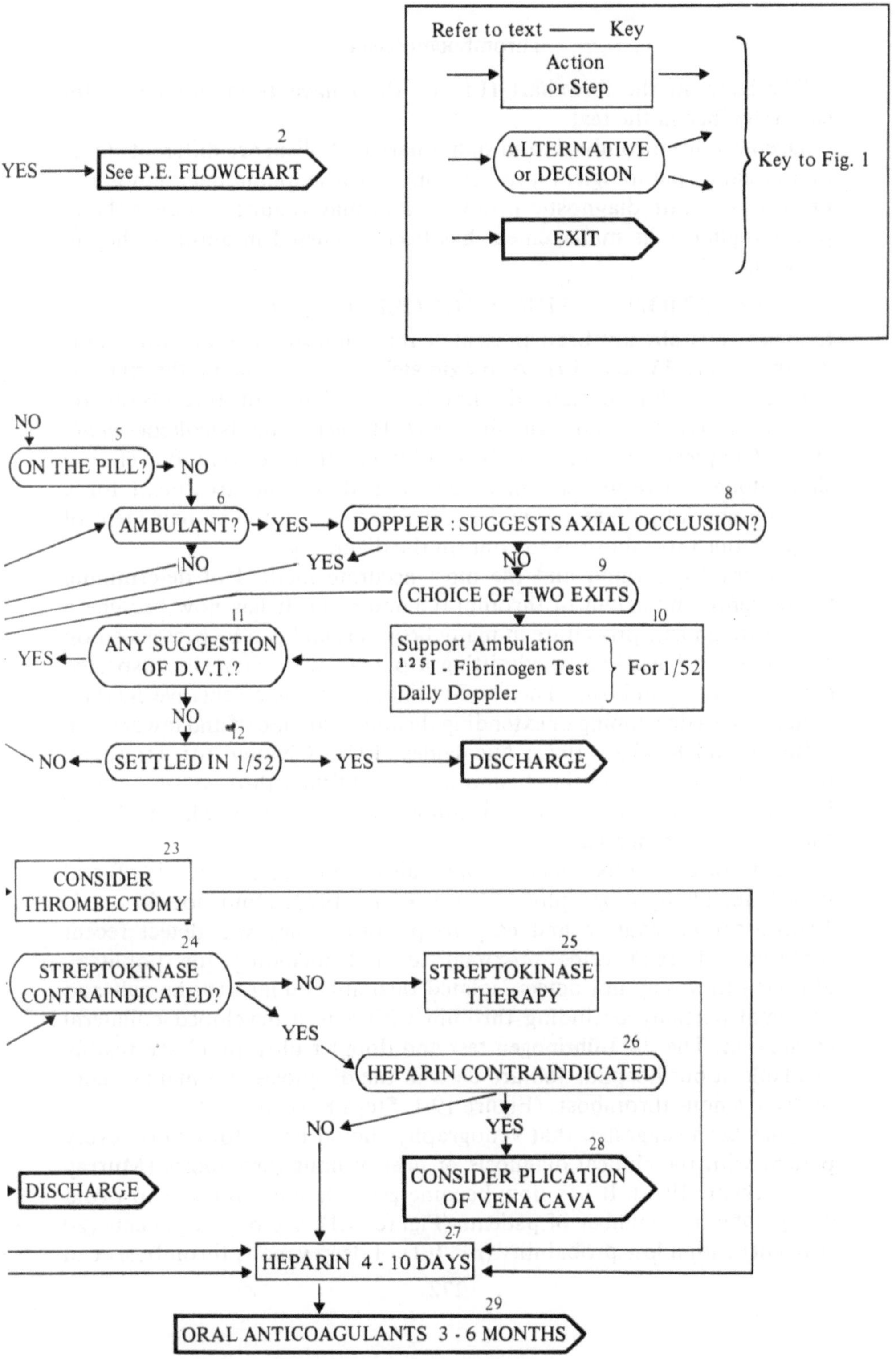

YES ──→ See P.E. FLOWCHART ⟩ 2

Refer to text ──── Key

Action or Step ──→

ALTERNATIVE or DECISION

EXIT ⟩

Key to Fig. 1

NO
↓
(ON THE PILL?) ──→ NO   5
↓
NO
↓
(AMBULANT?) ──→ YES ──→ (DOPPLER : SUGGESTS AXIAL OCCLUSION?)   6   8
↓ NO   ↑ YES   NO
                                              ↓   9
                              (CHOICE OF TWO EXITS)

(ANY SUGGESTION OF D.V.T.?) ←──── Support Ambulation   11   10
YES ←   125I - Fibrinogen Test } For 1/52
↓ NO   Daily Doppler
NO ←── (SETTLED IN 1/52) ──→ YES ──────→ DISCHARGE ⟩   12

CONSIDER THROMBECTOMY   23

(STREPTOKINASE CONTRAINDICATED?) ──→ NO ──→ STREPTOKINASE THERAPY   24   25
↓ YES
(HEPARIN CONTRAINDICATED)   26
NO ←   YES
                      ↓
DISCHARGE ⟩   CONSIDER PLICATION OF VENA CAVA ⟩   28

HEPARIN 4 - 10 DAYS   27
↓
ORAL ANTICOAGULANTS 3 - 6 MONTHS ⟩   29

The steps in the flowchart (Figure 19.1) have been numbered for easy reference in the text.

Deep venous thrombosis and pulmonary embolism are different stages of the same pathological process, but because pulmonary embolism presents separate diagnostic problems and may require different therapeutic regimens its management has been discussed in another chapter (Chapter 20).

CONFIRMATION OF THE DIAGNOSIS (Steps 3–13)

Evidence has already been presented that clinical signs are unreliable (Chapters 11, 13 and 17). Approximately 50 per cent of the patients with positive clinical signs do not have evidence of thrombosis on venography (Haeger and Nylander, 1967; Haeger, 1969; Nicolaides et al., 1971; Chapters 11 and 17). It is obvious that to rely on clinical signs alone will result in unnecessary and dangerous treatment for a large number of patients. Therefore, the first step in the management of deep venous thrombosis is to confirm the diagnosis.

Venography is rapid and the most accurate method of determining the presence and extent of thrombi (Chapter 11). It has now become a routine diagnostic procedure in many hospitals and can be performed on an outpatient basis before admitting a patient with clinically suspected deep venous thrombosis. The ^{125}I-fibrinogen test is a sensitive method of detecting a developing or extending thrombus in the calf and lower thigh (Murray and Kakkar, 1972; Nicolaides, 1972; Chapter 14). However, it is of limited value in the diagnosis of established thrombosis because it takes 48 hours to detect thrombosis and relatively old or lysing thrombi may be missed.

Other objective tests such as doppler ultrasound (Sigel et al., 1972) and impedance plethysmography (Wheeler et al., 1972; Dmochowski et al., 1972) are non invasive and easy to perform. They will detect recent occlusion of axial veins proximal to and including the popliteal, although they may not detect isolated thrombi confined to the calf and proximal partially occluding thrombi with a well developed collateral circulation. The ^{125}I-fibrinogen test and doppler ultrasound are readily available at our hospital and are used in the diagnosis and management of deep venous thrombosis (Figure 19.1, Steps 8, 10 and 21).

It has been suggested that venography should be performed on every patient with the clinical diagnosis of deep venous thrombosis (Murray and Kakkar, 1972). It has now become possible and practical to avoid venography in a number of patients (Figure 19.1). A group of patients (20 per cent) with a low probability ($p < 0.1$) of deep venous thrombosis can be selected (Chapter 17). The majority of these patients have calf tenderness only and no other clinical signs or factors predisposing to thrombosis such as a recently performed operation, recent bedrest, chest infection or a period of hypotension (Nicolaides *et al.*, 1974; Chapter 17).

'LOW RISK' PATIENTS

In patients with calf tenderness only and without clinical factors predisposing to deep venous thrombosis the probability of thrombosis is considered very low ($p < 0.1$) provided they are not taking oral contraceptives and are ambulant. If doppler ultrasound examination does not detect any evidence of occlusion of the axial veins (axial occlusion), a choice between venography and investigation with the ^{125}I-fibrinogen test and ultrasound for one week is possible (Figure 19.1, Step 9). The option may be given to the patient. Doppler ultrasound will exclude axial occlusion and the ^{125}I-fibrinogen test will exlude extension of a small thrombus. Venography is indicated whenever a suggestion of axial occlusion by the doppler ultrasound examination or thrombosis by the ^{125}I-fibrinogen test is found (Figure 19.1, Step 11).

Ultrasonic and isotopic studies take relatively little time to perform and are practical in patients who live near the hospital and can attend daily. When the patients are not ambulant or when there are medical or social indications to continue taking oral contraceptives, venography is indicated. Only when the deep veins are demonstrated to be normal can the patients be allowed to continue oral contraceptive therapy.

'HIGH RISK' PATIENTS (Figure 19.1, Step 3 and 4)

In the presence of signs other than calf tenderness or clinical factors predisposing to deep venous thrombosis the probability of thrombosis is relatively high ($p > 0.1$) and venography is indicated (Chapter 17). Venography will provide an immediate answer about the presence and extent of thrombosis.

THROMBOSIS CONFINED TO THE CALF
(Figure 19.1, Steps 17, 18, 20–22)

It has recently been demonstrated that thrombi confined to the calf are responsible for small silent pulmonary emboli (Browse *et al.*, 1974) and for serious postthrombotic sequelae (Browse and Clemenson, 1974), although the risk of large clinical pulmonary embolism is negligible (Kakkar *et al.*, 1969). It is therefore advisable to treat extensive thrombosis confined to the calf (thrombi longer than 10 cm involving 2 or more tibial veins) with conventional anticoagulant therapy (intravenous heparin for 48 hours followed by oral anticoagulants for 4 to 6 weeks). Thrombi which are smaller and isolated to the tibial or muscular veins of the calf tend to lyse spontaneously. It has been demonstrated by the [125] I-fibrinogen test that the lysis of small thrombi in the calf is particularly rapid if the patients are ambulant, wear elastic stockings and are not allowed to keep their limbs immobile in a dependent position (Flanc et al., 1969; Kakkar et al., 1969). Anticoagulant therapy can be avoided in these patients. However, because 20 per cent of thrombi in the calf extend proximally (Kakkar et al., 1969) the above policy is only safe if the [125] I-fibrinogen test is performed. It does not matter if the existing thrombus is not labelled. Any subsequent proximal extension will contain radioactive fibrin and therefore should be detected (Figure 19.1, step 22).

Patients who are not ambulant (Figure 19.1, Step 20) and have thrombi confined to the calf should be treated with conventional anticoagulant therapy because the risk of proximal extension in immobile limbs is very high. This applies particularly to patients with limbs in plaster of paris in which the [125] I-fibrinogen test cannot be performed with any accuracy.

THROMBOSIS PROXIMAL TO THE CALF
(Figure 19.1, Step 17, 18–29)
When thrombosis involves the popliteal and more proximal veins, the risk of pulmonary embolism and postphlebitic sequelae is high. When the pelvic veins are involved the incidence of pulmonary embolism is 50 per cent (Kakkar et al., 1969). Prompt treatment of these patients is therefore essential. The place of thrombectomy, thrombolytic therapy and anti-coagulants in the management of proximal thrombosis is summarised below. The value of defibrinating agents has not yet been fully evaluated (Chapter 18).

(a) Thrombectomy (Figure 19.1, Step 23)
Thrombectomy has been advoated since the late thirties (Lawen, 1937). The modern operative technique has been described by Mahoner (Mahoner, 1966) and more recently by Beebe (Beebe, 1973). The use of Fogarty's embolectomy catheters allows better clearance of the proximal venous system, diminished risk of pulmonary embolism (Fogarty |et al., 1965) and less blood loss than the use of suction catheters. Radiological control during thrombectomy (Mavor and Galloway, 1967) and the use of radio-opaque medium in the baloon of the Fogarty catheter (Mansfield, 1972 have been advocated as aids to obtaining complete clearance. Passage of the Fogarty catheter distally in the leg destroys the valves and should

be avoided. Distal thrombus can be expressed by elastic and manual compression. By introducing a small catheter into the iliac segment through the superficial circumflex iliac vein serial postoperative venography and the administration of heparin and fibrinolytic agents is possible (Mavor, 1971).

Most surgeons feel that the best results are obtained if thrombectomy is performed within three days from the onset of thrombosis. Complete clearance is difficult to achieve if the thrombus is more than five days old and rethrombosis is then very common (Haller and Abrams, 1963).

Pulmonary embolism during thrombectomy has been reported (Cooley and Beall, 1961; Julian and Hunter, 1965; Salem et al., 1968) but it is uncommon (Haller, 1967; Mavor and Galloway, 1969; Hulme et al., 1970). The technique of using two Fogarty balloon catheters (Mansfield et al., 1971; Mansfield, 1972) reduces the risk of pulmonary embolism, although most surgeons rely on a valsalva manoeuver performed during extraction of the iliac clot (Beebe, 1973).

Despite meticulous technique and careful postoperative management the incidence of recurrence is high (Mavor and Galloway, 1967; Mavor et al., 1973). In some series, repeated venography has demonstrated that early thrombosis and later recanalisation with destruction of valvular function occurs in almost all patients (Barner et al., 1969). It seems that thrombectomy neither reduces early morbidity, nor prevents valvular damage and the postthrombic sequelae (Lansing and Davis, 1968).

Because of these results thrombectomy has not been generally accepted for patients with proximal thrombosis except in the presence of impending or established venous gangrene. Most patients with phlegmasia cerulea dolens will respond to consevative therapy provided the limbs are not so tense that the arterial supply is impaired. (Haimovici, 1971). In a series of 337 patients with phlegmasia cerulea dolens the overall mortality rate was 27 per cent. In 158 of these who had venous gangrene the mortality rate was 42 per cent. Thrombectomy produced a recovery in 39 and out of 44 patients with phlegmasia cerulea dolens and in 6 out of 9 with venous gangrene (Haimovici, 1967). These results demonstrate the place of thrombectomy as an adjunct to anticoagulants in a selected group of patients. Anticoagulant therapy with heparin for several days and subsequent oral anticoagulants for several months should follow thrombectomy (Figure 19.1, Steps 27 and 29), (see Anticoagulant therapy).

Superficial thrombophlebitis with pulmonary embolism is rare, but the authors have treated three patients with thrombophlebitis of the long saphenous vein in the thigh presenting with shortness of breath. In all

275

three patients there was a small partially occluding thrombus projecting into the femoral vein causing repeated pulmonary emboli. There was rapid and complete relief of symptoms after thrombectomy with ligation of the saphenofemoral junction.

(b) Fibrinolytic and defibrinating agents (Figure 19.1, Steps 24 and 25)
The method of action, administration and control of fibrinolytic and defibrinating agents has been discussed in Chapter 18. Complete lysis may require systemic fibrinolytic therapy for several days and the high cost of urokinase is prohibitive. Streptokinase which is less expensive is therefore the drug of choice. The results of the few studies in which repeated venography has been performed indicate that partial to complete lysis of thrombi up to 3 days old may occur in two-thirds of patients provided they are treated for three to five days (Hiemeyer, 1967; Browse et al., 1968; Mavor et al., 1969; Kakkar et al., 1969; Schmutzler, 1969; Olow et al., 1970; Robertson et al., 1970; Diaz and Le Veen, 1971). In controlled trials lysis was observed in only one-fifth of patients treated with anticoagulants (Gormsen, 1967; Browse et al., 1968; Kakkar, Flanc et al., 1969; Robertson et al., 1970).

The presence of valves after successfullysis of thrombi with streptokinase has been reported (Olow et al.,1970; Robertson, 1971), but their function has not been studied. In a clinical trial (Kakkar, Flanc et al., 1969) 30 patients with deep venous thrombosis of less than four days duration were allocated at random to treatment with heparin, streptokinase or ancrod. Assessment of the fate of the thrombi by venography and the ^{125}I-fibrinogen test revealed complete thrombolysis in 7 of the 10 patients treated with streptokinase. Complete clearance occurred in 3 of the 10 patients treated with heparin and in only 1 of the 10 patients treated with ancrod. Bleeding complications occurred in all the groups but were least with ancrod. This study also revealed that complete disappearance of symptoms and signs did not always mean disappearance of the thrombi. In a follow up study (Kakkar, Howe, Laws et al., 1969), ascending functional venography was used to determine valvular function. It was found that the valves were more often normal after streptokinase therapy than with heparin or ancrod.

Bleeding is the commonsest complication of streptolinase therapy. Its incidence varies from 15 per cent to 40 per cent in different series (Brogden, Speight and Avery, 1973). In most patients bleeding has occurred at sites of previous venous or arterial punctures (Mavor et al., 1969; Verstraete et al., 1971) and at sites of operations performed within 8 days before the start of therapy (chesterman et al., 1969; Mavor et al.,

1969; Timmes *et al.*, 1971). However, in some patients severe bleeding occurred without obvious reason. Other complications include rigors and fever (Mavor *et al.*, 1969; Brogden *et al.*, 1973) anaphylactic reactions (Kakkar, Flanc *et al.*, 1969) and embolic episodes. In one study pulmonary embolism has occurred in 4 per cent and was fatal in 1·1 per cent of patients during thrombolytic therapy for deep venous thrombosis (Hess, 1969). It has also been reported by others (Robertson *et al.*, 1970; Hume *et al.*, 1971).

The evidence available so far suggests that thrombolytic therapy will produce rapid clearance of the veins with preservation of valves in patients with recent deep venous thrombosis. Further studies are still required to confirm its therapeutic effects and define its exact place in the management of venous thrombosis. Because of its high rate of complications it is suggested that at the moment its use should be confined to young patients with proximal thrombosis of less than 3 days duration. It is contraindicated in patients who have a history of asthma or allergic diathesis, sensitisation by previous administration of the drug, a wound which is less than 10 days old, hypertension (diastolic greater than 100 mmHg) any bleeding diathesis or history of peptic ulceration. Streptokinase therapy should always be followed by conventional anticoagulants in order to prevent rethrombosis (Figure 19.1).

Ancrod is as effective as heparin (Bell *et al.*, 1968, Sharp *et al.*, 1968; Kakkar *et al.*, 1969) and the incidence of bleeding (5 per cent) is less than with heparin (Chapter 18). Its main disadvantage is that its defibrinating effect can be established safely only after 4 to 6 hours while the anticoagulant effect of heparin is immediate. Further clinical trials are required before this drug is fully assessed (Chapter 18).

(c) Heparin therapy (Figure 19.1, Steps 26 and 27)

Heparin interferes with blood coagulation by inactivating factors XIa, IXa, Xa and thrombin. Its complications are haemorrhage which is uncommon in the absence of a wound and severe thrombocytopenia which is rare (Gollup and Ulin, 1962). The latter has been reported only in patients receiving heparin by the subcutaneous or intramuscular routes. The presence of large wounds, peptic ulceration, and thrombocytopenia are contraindications to its administration. Because heparin is eliminated in the urine it must be given with caution when glomerular filtration is impaired.

Soon after heparin was discovered it was found to be effective in the treatment of deep venous thrombosis (Zilliacus, 1946; Jorpes, 1947; Murray, 1947; Bauer, 1964; Sawyer *et al.*, 1964) and lifesaving after pulmonary embolism (Barvitt and Jordan, 1960; Kernolan and Todd, 1966; O'Sullivan *et al.*, 1968). It is now realised that the beneficial clinical effect of heparin is not always accompanied by clearance of thrombi as determined by venography (Kakkar, Flanc *et al.*, 1969).

Heparin may be administered by intermittent intravenous injections (Morris and Balk, 1965; Gurewich *et al.*, 1967), continuous intravenous infusion (O'Sullivan *et al.*, 1968) or by subcutaneous injections (Chapter 21). Intermittent intravenous injections avoid the use of a continuous infusion, but blood levels of heparin fluctuate from dangerously high to below the therapeutic range. Continuous intravenous infusion produces more constant blood levels, but the risk of bleeding is higher. The subcutaneous route produces more sustained blood levels, but may make neutralisation by protamine sulphate more difficult. It is the method of choice in treating patients outside the hospital (Chapter 21).

The amount of heparin required to produce an adequate therapeutic level depends on the patient's weight and on the amount of circulating antiheparin substances which are extremely variable. Usually 30000 to 60000 units of intravenous heparin over 24 hours are required to prolong the whole blood clotting time to between 2 and 3 times the normal, a level which is effective and safe.

It is safer to start with a high dose and then reduce it than to start with a low dose and gradually increase it to the required level (Gurewich *et al.*, 1967). Effective therapy during the early hours will arrest thrombosis (Carey and Williams, 1960; Gurewich and Thomas, 1965; Hunt *et al.*, 1966) and eliminate thromboembolic recurrences (Kernohan and Todd, 1966).

The optimum duration of heparin therapy has not been established. There is general agreement that a minimum period of 48 hours is required, provided the administration of oral anticoagulants is commenced at the same time as heparin. This may be adequate for thrombi distal to the popliteal vein but in patients with proximal thrombosis heparin administration may be required for 8 to 10 days before oral anticoagulants are commenced. After this period most thrombi are firmly attached to the venous wall (Wessler *et al.*, 1961).

(d) Supportive treatment

Bed rest with leg elevation during the first few days of anticoagulant therapy helps to reduce oedema and theoretically prevents dislodgement of thrombi which are not firmly adherent to the vessel. Analgesics may also be required during the same period. Salicilates should be avoided because of the risk of gastrointestinal erosions and the potentiation of oral anticoagulants. Active exercises are encouraged in bed and most patients are allowed up after they have been on anticoagulants for one week. The study of the fate of thrombi labelled with ^{125}I-fibrinogen suggests that active leg exercises and ambulation encourages early lysis (Flanc et al., 1969). Elastic stockings or leg bandages are indicated when oedema persists or tends to recur when the patient is ambulant. Elastic stockings with graded compression decreasing proximally should be used.

VENOUS INTERRUPTION (Figure 19.1, Step 28)

Prophylactic interruption of the superficial femoral vein was first introduced by Homans (Homans, 1934). Subsequent studies demonstrated that superficial femoral ligation is accompanied by a high mortality from pulmonary embolism arising in the iliofemoral segment (Homans, 1949; Mozes et al., 1964) and a high incidence of postphlebitic sequelae (Coon, 1974). Caval interruption has now been accepted as more effective because it controls the source of the majority of emboli (Crane, 1964).

(a) Indications for interruption of the vena cava

In patients with deep venous thrombosis proximal to the knee interruption of the vena cava is indicated when there is failure of anticoagulants to prevent embolism or when anticoagulants are contraindicated. The efficacy of anticoagulants particularly heparin in preventing pulmonary embolism has now been demonstrated (Barritt and Jordan, 1960; Kernolan and Todd, 1966; O'Sullivan et al., 1968). The operative mortality from pulmonary embolism and other complications after caval interruption is several times higher than that from embolic and haemorrhagic deaths during treatment with anticoagulants (Coon, 1974). However, when anticoagulants have failed or are contraindicated caval interruption is a practical alternative.

Failure of anticoagulants is the commonest indication for surgical interruption of the vena cava (Beebe, 1973). It is said to occur when one or more episodes of pulmonary embolism confirmed by lung scans and possibly pulmonary angiography have occurred during *adequate* heparin therapy administered by a continuous intravenous infusion. When heparin therapy is not well managed or when the patient is on oral anticoagulants adequate heparin therapy is indicated before interruption of the vena cava is considered.

Caval interruption is also indicated in patients with proximal thrombosis in whom anticoagulants are contraindicated because of any of the following conditions: Active bleeding before or during anticoagulant therapy; the presence of a haemostatic defect; when even a small haematoma is unacceptable, e.g. in operations on the nervous system; when extensive surgery is urgent and essential; and when the risk of bleeding from a coexisting lesion is high, e.g. from an active peptic ulcer, a large gastric tumour or ulcerative colitis.

(b) Method

The retroperitoneal route through a transverse incision at the level of the umbilicus is the commonest method of approach to the inferior vena cava (Madden, 1954; Murray and Kakkar, 1972). A variety of techniques of interruption have been practiced: They include ligation (Crane, 1964), flattening of the cava to a lumen of 3 mm using a stainless steel or Teflon clip (Moretz et al., 1954) temporary ligation using catgut (Dale et al., 1956), plication using multiple sutures (De Weese and Hunter, 1963), a toothed plastic clip (Miles et al., 1964) or a mechanical stapler (Ravitch et al., 1966). In recent years an umbrella filter for interruption of the inferior vena cava which can be inserted via the internal jugular vein under local anaesthesia has been developed (Mobin-Uddin et al., 1971; Orvald et al., 1973).

Comparisons of caval ligation with partial interruption involve too few patients to demonstrate a definite difference in mortality, but after partial interruption severe postphlebitic sequelae are fewer and proved recurrent pulmonary embolism slightly higher although fatal ones are rare (Schowengerdt and Schreiber, 1971). Late sequelae are related to whether the plicated segment remains patent (Wheeler et al., 1966; De Meester et al., 1967). Hospital mortality after ligation or plication of the inferior vena cava in patients without severe heart disease in various studies ranges from 3 per cent to 12 per cent; after ligation in patients with heart failure it ranges from 20 per cent to 40 per cent (Nasbeth and Moran, 1965; Crane, 1966; Mozes et al., 1966; De Meester et al., 1967; Coon, 1974). The high mortality associated with caval ligation in patients with cardiac failure (Nasbeth and Moran, 1965; Crane, 1966; Mozes et al., 1966) is the result of a sudden decrease in the cardiac output after ligation (Gazzaniga et al., 1967). Reduction in the cardiac output is less after plication (Benarides and Noon, 1967) although a chronic reduction of 20 to 50 per cent in the rate of venous return does occur.

In patients with suppurative thrombophlebitis who continue to have showers of septic pulmonary emboli inspite of specific antibiotic and heparin therapy and in patients with thromboembolic pulmonary hypertension ligation is more effective than plication because the latter will not prevent microemboli (Collins et al., 1951; Sautter et al., 1966).

The haemodynamic changes that occur after ligation or plication of the vena cava are avoided by the transvenous caval interruption with the 'umbrella' filter (Mobin-Uddin et al., 1971). The filter is inserted via the internal jugular vein and in most patients it results in a gradual caval thrombosis. The frequency of recurrent embolism is 2 per cent. Although complications such as retroperitoneal haemorrhage from the spokes of the filter, dislodgement and embolisation of the filter, misplacement in iliac and renal veins have been reported, the operative mortality is less than with other caval interruption procedures, particularly in patients with heart disease (Mobin-Uddin et al., 1971).

It cannot be overemphasised that there is no place for any caval interruption procedure without venographic evidence of the presence and extent of thrombosis.

ORAL ANTICOAGULANTS (Figure 19.1, Step 29)

Oral anticoagulants act by inhibiting the production of Factors VII, IX, X and prothombin by the liver. Their action is antagonised and slowly reversed by the administration of vitamin K_1 (Poller, 1962; Douglas, 1962). Chemically they are classified into coumarin (e.g. warfarin) and indanedione (e.g. phenindione) derivatives. Certain side effects are related to chemical structure. More than a hundred agents have been synthesised: Short-acting, intermediate and long-acting, the latter having a potentially cumulative effect. Sodium warfarin and phenindione belong to the intermediate-acting group and have become the most popular because they are suitable for both short-term and long-term therapy. Toxic and sensitivity reactions are relatively infrequent with warfarin and it is therefore the drug of choice in most centres.

Reliable laboratory control is essential for effective and safe therapy. Without it either ineffective therapy or severe haemorrhage will occur. Many tests have been used to measure the effect of oral anticoagulants. The one-stage prothrombin time (Quick, 1935) is used in most laboratories. Using this test the patient's prothrombin time is compared with a normal control and therapy is aimed to maintain an effect between certain limits. It is imperative that the therapeutic range which is effective against venous thrombosis and which will avoid haemorrhage is defined for each laboratory. In recent years, efforts to standardise reagents and techniques (Biggs, 1965; Biggs and Denson, 1967; Poller, 1969) have produced a standard thromboplastin available to all laboratories in England, but as yet there is no international standard. Using the British standard thromboplastin, the therapeutic range of the prothrombin time lies between 1.8 and 3 times the control value.

Thromboembolism

Certain drugs are contraindicated during anticoagulation therapy. Salicylates broad spectrum antibiotics, ACTH, quinidine, alcohol. phenylbutzaone and clofibrate may cause haemorrhage. Barbituarates, aminophylline, chloral hydrate and certain tranquilisers such as diazepam antagonise the effect of therapy. Drug resistance is rare (Souler and Blatrix, 1966) and is an indication for changing to an oral anticoagulant of a different chemical group.

The contraindications to oral anticoagulants are the same as the ones for heparin (see p 276) but inadequate laboratory facilities, hypertension, severe anaemia, hepatic disease, pregnancy (Chapter 21) and insufficient cooperation by the patient are additional contraindications.

The duration of therapy with oral anticoagulants is controversial. In patients with thrombi extending to the veins proximal to the knee, oral anticoagulants are recommended for 6 weeks provided that the patient is ambulant and symptom free (O'Sullivan *et al.*, 1968; Hume *et al.*, 1970). In patients with clinical pulmonary embolism, therapy for 3 to 6 months is recommended and in patients with thromboembolic pulmonary hypertension therapy should be permanent (Hume *et al.*, 1970).

There is now some evidence that therapy for more than 6 weeks in patients with deep venous thrombosis might be beneficial though the optimum time is not known. If anticoagulants are discontinued the risk of rethrombosis is at its maximum immediately after discharge from hospital (Coon and Willis, 1973; Chapter 1). This risk gradually decreases during the subsequent three years. In patients not on anticoagulant therapy who present with rethrombosis within six months from the original episode venography often demonstrates fresh thrombi in the collateral circulation (Nicolaides, 1974). The protection of this collateral circulation is one of the functions of therapy. For these reasons it is recommended that after venous thrombosis proximal to the knee oral anticoagulants should be administered for 3 to 6 months. In patients with pulmonary embolism this period should be even longer.

References

Barner, H. B., Willman, V. L., Kaiser, G. C. and Hanlon, C. R. (1969). Thrombectomy for iliofemoral venous thrombosis. *J. Amer. Med. Ass.*, **208**, 2442

Barritt, D. W. and Jordan, S. C. (1960). Anticoagulant drugs in the treatment of pulmonary embolsim: A controlled trial. *Lancet*, **i**, 1309

Bauer, G. (1964). Clinical experiences of a surgeon in the use of heparin. *Amer. J. Cardiol.*, **14**, 29

Beebe, H. G. (1973). Deep venous thrombosis and complications of peripheral venous procedures. Chapter in: *Complications in Vascular Surgery* (H. G. Beebe, editor) (Philadelphia and Toronto: J. B. Lippincott Company)

Thromboembolism

Bell, W. R., Pitney, W. R., Oakley, C. M. and Goodwin, J. F. (1968). Therapeutic defibrination in the treatment of thrombotic disease. *Lancet,* **i,** 490

Benarides, J. and Noon, R. (1967). Experimental evaluation of inferior vena cava procedures to prevent pulmonary embolsim. *Ann. Surg.,* **166,** 195

Biggs, R. (1965). Report on the standardisation of the one-stage prothrombin-time for the control of anticoagulant therapy. In: *Genetics and the Interaction of Blood Clotting Factors,* p. 303 (Stuttgart; Schattauez-Verlag)

Biggs, R. and Denson, K. W. E. (1967). Standardisation of the one-stage prothombin time for the control of anticoagulant therapy. *Brit. Med. J.,* **i,** 84

Browse, N. L. and Clemenson, G. (1974). Sequelae of an [125] I-fibrinogen detected thrombus. *Brit. Med. J.,* **2,** 468

Browse, N. L., Clemenson, G. and Croft, D. N. (1974). Fibrinogen-detectable thrombosis in the legs and pulmonary embolism. *Brit. Med. J.,* **1,** 603

Browse, N. L., Thomas, M. L. and Pim, H. P. (1968). Streptokinase and deep vein thrombosis. *Brit. Med. J.,* **3,** 717

Carey, L. C. and Williams, R. D. (1960). Comparative effects of dicoumarol, tromexan and heparin on thrombus propagation. *Ann. Surg.,* **152,** 919

Chesterman, C. N., Biggs, J. C., Morgan, J. and Hickie, J. B. (1969). Streptokinase therapy in acute major pulmonary embolism. *Med. J. Austral.,* **2,** 1096

Collins, C. G., MacCallum, E. A., Nelson, E. W., Weinstein, B. B., Collins, J. H. (1951). Suppurative Pelvic Thrombophlebitis. *Surgery,* **30,** 298, 311

Cooley, D. A. and Beall, A. C. (1961). A technic of pulmonary embolectomy using temporary cardio-pulmonary bypass: Clinical and experimental considerations. *J. Thorac. Cardior. Surg.,* **2,** 469

Coon, W. W. (1974). Operative therapy of venous thromboembolism. *Med. Conc. Cardior. Dis.,* **43,** 71

Coon, W. W. and Willis, P. W. (1973). Recurrence of venous thromboembolism. *Surgery,* **73,** 823

Crane, C. (1964). Femoral vs. caval interruption for venous thromboembolism. *New Engl. J. Med.,* **270,** 819

Crane, C. (1966). The diagnosis and treatment of pulmonary embolism. *Surg. Clin. N. Amer.,* **46,** 551

Dale, W. A., Pualawan, F. and Bauer, F. M. (1956). Ligation of inferior vena cava with absorbable gut. *Surg. Gynec. Obstet.,* **102,** 517

De Meester, T. R., Rutherford, R. B., Blazek, J. V. and Zuidema, G. D. (1967). Plication of the inferior vena cava for thromboembolism. *Surgery,* **62,** 56

De Weese, M. S. and Hunter, D. C., Jr. (1963). Vena cava filter for the prevention of pulmonary embolism. *Arch. Surg.,* **86,** 852

Diaz, C. and Le Veen, H. H. (1971). Enzymatic clot lysis in the treatment of venous and arterial occlusive disease. *Thrombosis et diathesis haemorrhagica* **(Suppl. 47),** 179

Dmochowski, J. R., Douglas, F. A. and Couch, N. P. (1972). Impedance measurement in the diagnosis of deep venous thrombosis. *Arch. Surg.,* **104,** 170

Douglas, A. S. (1962). Anticoagulant therapy (Oxford: Blackwell Scientific Publications)

Flanc, C., Kakkar, V. V. and Clarke, M. B. (1969). Postoperative deep-vein thrombosis: Effects of intensive prophylaxis. *Lancet,* **i,** 477

Fogarty, T. J. and Krippaehne, W. W. (1965). Catheter technique for venous thrombectomy. *Surg. Gynec. Obstet.,* **121,** 362

Gazzaniga, A. B., Cahill, J. L., Repogle, R. L. and Tilney, N. L. (1967). Changes in blood

Thromboembolism

volume and renal function following ligation of the inferior vena cava. *Surgery,* **62,** 417

Gollup, S. and Ulin, A. W. (1962). Heparin induced thrombocytopenia in man. *J. Lab. Clin. Med.,* **59,** 430

Gormsen, J. (1967). Streptase treatment of acute phleuothrombosis. *Symposium on thrombolytic therapy with streptokinase,* Munich, p. 41

Gurewich, V. and Thomas, D. P. (1965). Pathogenesis of venous thrombosis in relation to its prevention by dextran and heparin. *J. Lab. Clin. Med.,* **66,** 604

Gurewich, V., Thomas, D. P. and Stuart, R. K. (1967). Some guidelines for heparin therapy of venous thromboembolic disease. *J. Amer. Med. Ass.,* **199,** 116

Haeger, K. (1969). Problems of acute deep venous thrombosis. *Angiology,* **20,** 219

Haeger, K. and Nylander, G. (1967). Acute phlebography. *Triangle,* **8,** 18

Haimovici, H. (1967). Ischemic forms of venous thrombosis: Phlegmasia cerulea dolens and venous gangrene. *Heart Bull.,* **16,** 101

Haimovici, H. (1971). Ischemic forms of venous thrombosis. (Springfield: Charles C. Thomas)

Haller, J. A., Jr. (1967). Deep thrombophlebitis: Pathophysiology and treatment, vol. VI of Major Problems in Clinical Surgery, (Philadelphia: Saunders)

Haller, J. A., Jr. and Abrams, B. L. (1963). Use of thrombectomy in the treatment of acute iliofemoral venous thrombosis in forty-five patients. *Ann. Surg.,* **158,** 249

Hess, H. (1969). Zur Streptokinase-therapie akuter verschlüsse von gliedmassengefässen. *Thrombosis et diathesis haemorrhagica,* **Suppl. 32,** 275

Hiemeyer, V. (1967). Thrombolytic therapy in acute vascular occlusion. *German Medical Monthly,* **12,** 461

Homans, J. (1934). Thrombosis of the deep veins of the leg, causing pulmonary embolism. *New Engl. J. Med.,* **211,** 993

Homans, J. (1949). Management of recovery from venous thrombosis in the lower limb. *Surgery,* **26,** 8

Hume, M., Gurewich, J. B., Dealy, J. B. and Gaewski, J. (1971). Streptokinase for chronic arterial disease. Effective lysis and thromboembolic complications, *Thrombosis et diathesis haemorrhagica,* **Suppl. 47,** 229

Hume, M., Sevitt, S. and Thomas, D. P. (1970). Venous thrombosis and pulmonary embolism. (Cambridge, Massachusetts: Harvard University Press)

Hunt, P. S., Reeve, T. E. and Holling, R. M. A. (1966). Standard experimental thrombus: Observations on its production, pathology, response to heparin and thrombectomy. *Surgery,* **59,** 812

Jorpes, J. E. (1947). Anticoagulant therapy in thrombosis. *Surg. Gynec. Obstet.,* **84,** 677

Julian, O. C. and Hunter, J. A. (1965). Vascular emergencies in the lower extremity. *Surg. Clin. N. Amer.,* **45,** 135

Kakkar, V. V., Flanc, C., Howe, C. T., O'Shea, M. and Flute, P. T. (1969). Treatment of deep vein thrombosis. Atrial of heparin, streptokinase and arvin. *Brit. Med. J.,* **1,** 806

Kakkar, V. V., Howe, C. T., Flanc, C. and Clarke, M. B. (1969). Natural history of postoperative deep-vein thrombosis. *Lancet,* **ii,** 230

Kakkar, V. V., Howe, C. T., Laws, J. W. and Flanc, C. (1969). Late results of treatment of deep-vein thrombosis. *Brit. Med. J.,* **1,** 810

Kernolan, R. J. and Todd, C. (1966). Heparin therapy in thromboembolic disease. *Lancet,* **i,** 621

Lansing, A. M. and Davis, W. M. (1968). Five-year follow-up study of iliofemoral venous thrombectomy. *Ann. Surg.,* **168,** 620

Thromboembolism

Lawen, A. (1937). Uber thrombectomie bei venenthrombose und arteriospasmus. *Arch. Klin. Chia.*, **189**, 53

Madden, J. (1954). Ligation of the inferior vena cava. *Ann. Surg.*, **140**, 200

Mahorner, H. (1966). Technique of thrombectomy for massive venous thrombosis. *Surgery*, **60**, 773

Mansfield, A. O. (1972). Control of pulmonary embolism. *Ann. Roy.' Coll. Surg. Engl.*, **51**, 373

Mansfield, A. O., Carmichael, J. H. E. and Parry, E. W. (1971). Thrombectomy employing continuous radiological control. *Brit. J. Surg.*, **58**, 119

Mavor, G. E. (1971). Surgery of deep vein thrombosis. *Brit. J. Hosp. Med.*, **6**, 755

Mavor, G. E. and Galloway, J. M. D. (1967). Radiographic control of iliofemoral venous thrombectomy. *Brit. J. Surg.*, **54**, 1019

Mavor, G. E. and Galloway, J. M. D. (1969). Iliofemoral venous thrombosis: Pathological considerations and surgical management. *Brit. J. Surg.*, **56**, 45

Mavor, G. E., Dhall, D. P., Dawson, A. A., Duthie, J. S., Walker, M. G., Mahaffy, R. G. and Allardyce, A. (1973). Streptokinase therapy and deep vein thrombosis. *Brit. J. Surg.*, **60**, 468

Mavor, G. E., Bennett, B., Galloway, J. M. D. and Karmody, A. M. (1969). Streptokinase in iliofemoral venous thrombosis. *Brit. J. Surg.*, **56**, 564

Miles, R. M., Chappel, F. and Renner, R. (1964). Partially occluding vena caval clip for prevention of pulmonary emboli. *Amer. Surg.*, **30**, 40

Mobin-Uddin, K., Trinkle, J. K. and Bryant, L. R. (1971). Present status of the inferior vena cava umbrella filter. *Surgery*, **70**, 914

Moretz, W. H., Nesbitt, P. F. and Stevenson, G. P. (1954). Experimental studies on temporary occlusion of the inferior vena cava. *Surgery*, **36**, 384

Mouris, L. E. and Balk, P. (1965). The management or mismanagement of acute venous thrombosis (thrombophlebitis) of the extremities. *Angiology*, **16**, 339

Mozes, M., Adar, R., Bogokowsky, H. and Agmon, M. (1964). Vein ligation in the treatment of pulmonary embolism. *Surgery*, **55**, 621

Mozes, M., Bogokowski, H., Antebi, E., Tzur, N. and Penchas, S. (1966). Inferior vena cava ligation for pulmonary embolism: Review of 118 cases. *Surgery*, **60**, 790

Murray, G. (1947). Anticoagulants in venous thrombosis and the prevention of pulmonary embolism. *Surg. Gynec. Obstet.*, **84**, 665

Murray, J. G. and Kakkar, V. V. (1972). Deep vein thrombosis. In: *Scientific Basis of Surgery*. (W. T. Irvine, editor) (Edinburgh and London: Churchill Livingstone)

Nabseth, D. C. and Moran, J. M. (1965). Reassessment of the role of inferior vena cava ligation in venous thromboembolism. *New Engl. J. Med.*, **273**, 1250

Nicolaides, A. N. (1972). The prevention of postoperative deep venous thrombosis. Jacksonian Prize Essay.

Nicolaides, A. N. (1974). Unpublished data.

Nicolaides, A. N., Kakkar, V. V., Field, E. S. and Renney, J. T. G. (1971). The origin of deep vein thrombosis: a venographic study. *Brit. J. Radiol.*, **44**, 653

Nicolaides, A. N., Meadway, J., Irving, D. and Dupont, P. A. (1974). Clinical factors in the diagnosis of deep venous thrombosis. *Brit. J. Surg.*, (In press).

Olow, B., Johanson, C., Anderson, J. and Eklöf, B. (1970). Deep venous thrombosis treated with a standard dosage of streptokinase. *Acta. Chir. Scand.*, **136**, 181

Orvald, T. O., Callard, G. M. and Jude, J. R. (1973). Prevention of pulmonary embolus with vena caval umbrella. Results in 150 patients. *Ann. Thorac. Surg.*, **15**, 196

Thromboembolism

O'Sullivan, E. F., Hirsh, J., McCarthy, R. A. and de Gruchy, G. C. (1968). Heparin in the treatment of venous thromboembolic disease: Administration, control and results. *Med. J. Aust.*, **2,** 153

Poller, L. (1962). The theory and practice of anticoagulant treatment. (Bristol: Wright and Sons)

Poller, L. (1969). Progress in laboratory control of anticoagulant treatment. In Recent Advances in Blood Coagulation (London: Churchill)

Quick, A. J. (1935). Prothrombin in haemophilia and obstructive jaundice. *J. Biol. Chem.*, **109,** 73˙

Ravitch, M. M., Snodgran, E. and Rivarola, A. (1966). Compartmentation of the vena cava with the mechanical stapler. *Surg. Gynec. Obstet.*, **122,** 561

Robertson, B. R. (1971). On thrombosis, thrombolysis and fibrinolysis. *Acta Chir. Scand.*, **Suppl. 421**

Robertson, B. R., Nilsson, I. M. and Nylander, G. (1970). Thrombolytic effect of streptokinase as evaluated by phlebography of deep venous thrombi of the leg. *Acta Chir. Scand.*, **136,** 137

Salem, M. R., Baraka, A., Rattenborg, C. C. and Holaday, D. A. (1968). Bronchospasm: An early manifestation of pulmonary embolism during and after anesthesia. *Anesth. Analg. Govr. Res.*, **47,** 103

Sautter, R. D., Fletcher, F. W., Lewis, R. F. and Wengel, F. J. (19). Inferior rena caval and ovarian vein ligation for antepartum pulmonary thromboembolism. *J. Amer. Med. Assoc.*, **196,** 290

Sawyer, P. N., Schaefor, H. C., Domingo, R. T. and Wesolowski, S. A. (1964). Comparative therapy of thrombophlebitis. *Surgery*, **55,** 113

Schmutzler, R. (1969). Observations on thrombolytic treatment. *Intermist.*, **10,** 21

Schowengerdt, C. G. and Schreiber, J. T. (1971). Interruption of the vena cava in the treatment of pulmonary embolism. *Surg. Gynec. Obstet.*, **132,** 645

Sharp, A. A., Warren, B. A. and Paxton, A. M. (1968). Anticoagulant therapy with a purified fraction of Malayan pit viper venom. *Lancet*, **i,** 493

Sigel, B., Felix, W. R., Jr., Popky, G. L. and Ipsen, J. (1972). Diagnosis of Lower limb venous thrombosis by doppler ultrasound technique. *Arch. Surg.*, **104,** 174

Soulier, J. P. and Blatrix, C. (1966). Resistance to coumarin anticoagulant drugs in man. In: *Pathogenesis and Treatment of Thromboembolic Diseases.* (Stuttgart: Schattauer-Verlag)

Timmes, J. J., Demos, N. J., Chong, S. I. and Müller-Ehrenberg, K. (1971). Thrombolysis in acute arterial and venous occlusions. *Thromb. Diath. Haem.*, **Suppl. 47,** 193

Verstraete, M., Vermylen, J. and Donati, M. B. (1971). The effect of streptokinase infusion on chronic arterial occlusions and stenoses. *Annals Intern. Med.*, **74,** 377

Wessler, S., Freiman, D. G., Ballon, J. D., Katz, J. H., Wolff, R. and Wolf, E. (1961). Experimental pulmonary embolism with serum-induced thrombi. *Amer. J. Path.*, **38,** 89

Wheeler, H. B., Pearson, D., O'Connell, D. and Mullick, S. C. (1972). Impedance plethysmography: Technique, interpretation and results. *Arch. Surg.*, **104,** 164

Zilliacus, H. (1946). On specific treatment of thrombosis and pulmonary embolism with anticoagulants, with particular reference to post-thrombotic sequelae: Results of five years treatment of thrombosis and pulmonary embolism at a series of Swedish hospitals during years 1940–45. *Acta. Med. Scand.*, **Suppl. 171**

20

The management of pulmonary embolism

George C. Sutton

INTRODUCTION

When a thrombus becomes detached from the veins of the leg or pelvis, passes through the vena cava and right side of the heart and lodges in the pulmonary circulation, pulmonary embolism is said to have occurred. Such an event commonly follows surgery or trauma (Sevitt and Gallagher, 1961). It may occur as a complication of many illnesses, when bedrest is enforced, or during the course of therapy with oestrogens (Inman and Vessey, 1968).

The effect of such a sudden obstruction to the pulmonary circulation depends largely on its size, although an additional disturbance due to pulmonary vasoconstriction, independent of the magnitude of the mechanical obstruction, has been postulated to occur. If the individual survives the initial impact of pulmonary embolism, adaptive processes occur within the heart and circulation which gradually overcome the haemodynamic derangement caused by the obstruction. At the same time, processes occur within the lungs which initiate lysis of the thrombus.

The clinical presentation of the patient with pulmonary embolism will depend not only on the magnitude of embolism but also on the time that has elapsed from the initial impact. In addition, the state of the cardiac and respiratory systems prior to embolism will modify the effect in the individual patient. For example, a patient who has severe heart or lung disease with a resultant abnormality of the pulmonary circulation and an elevation of pulmonary artery pressure will tolerate a small amount of embolic material less well than the patient who has a previously normal pulmonary circulation. If there is failure of resolution of pulmonary embolism and particularly if repeated episodes of pulmonary embolism occur, then permanent obstruction of the pulmonary circulation results and chronic thromboembolic pulmonary hypertension may develop.

It becomes apparent that the clinical spectrum of pulmonary embolic disease is wide and management has to be considered in the light of the precise clinical condition of the patient. Fortunately, with the increasing use of cardiac catheterisation and pulmonary arteriography it has become possible to difine more precisely the severity of pulmonary embolism both with respect to the magnitude of obstruction and to the resultant haemodynamic effect. Such investigation taken in conjunction with the clinical assessment of the patient enables the clinician to place an individual patient with pulmonary embolic disease into one of three main groups, acute massive embolism, acute minor embolism and chronic thromboembolic pulmonary hypertension, any one of which may in addition be complicated by pre-existing cardio-respiratory disease.

In the discussion that follows each of these groups will be considered separately, indicating how the diagnosis can be made clinically and by the use of special investigations. The typical natural history of each group will be described and how this may be modified by specific treatment.

ACUTE MASSIVE PULMONARY EMBOLISM

Diagnosis

When more than 50 per cent of the major pulmonary arteries suddenly become occluded, the pulmonary embolism is defined as massive. The effect of sudden massive obstruction to the pulmonary circulation is to reduce cardiac output, to cause right ventricular failure and to disturb the normal balance of ventilation and perfusion in the lungs. As a consequence of sudden reduction in cardiac output, the patient may 'collapse' because cerebral perfusion is reduced. 'Collapse' may range from transient syncope to circulatory arrest (Dalen and Dexter, 1969; Sutton et al., 1969; Miller and Sutton, 1970; Oakley, 1970), the latter probably reflecting grossly reduced coronary artery perfusion. Central chest pain, which mimics the pain of myocardial infarction, may be due to reduced coronary perfusion, although right ventricular distension is another possible mechanism. The sudden onset of dyspnoea, and the clinical observation of tachypnoea and hypernoea presumably reflects the compensatory mechanism for the increase in dead space resulting from malperfusion of areas of lung which are normally ventilated (Robin, 1965). An increase in airway resistance has been found in pulmonary embolism (Gurewich *et al.*, 1965) and this may contribute to the dyspnoea. However, clinically detectable bronchospasm is usually not observed in acute massive pulmonary embolism. Pleurisy and haemoptysis are not usual features of massive embolism, but may have occurred as premonitory episodes from minor pulmonary emboli causing infarction. The physical signs of a low cardiac output include a sinus tachycardia with a small, sharp arterial pulse. Ectopic tachycardias are rare, apart from patients in whom there is pre-existing cardiac disease. There may be evidence of poor tissue perfusion with a cold, constricted periphery, reduced urinary output, or mental confusion. The physical signs of right ventricular failure include a raised jugular venous pressure and a gallop rhythm at the left sternal edge. The gallop rhythm may be the result of an increased right atrial contraction (fourth heart sound), reduced right ventricular compliance (third heart sound), or a combination of both factors in the presence of a shortened diastole due to the sinus tachycardia (Sutton, 1970). Neither palpable right ventricular hypertrophy nor a loud pulmonary valve closure sound are to be found in the acute phase of massive pulmonary embolism. Central cyanosis is frequently observed and is more likely to be the result of venous admixture of underventilated and malperfused areas of lung than right-to-left intracardiac shunting at atrial level due to patency of the foramen ovale (Elliott and Beamish, 1953).

Support for the clinical diagnosis of acute massive pulmonary embolism comes from the electrocardiogram, the plain chest radiograph and measurement of arterial blood gases. The electrocardiogram (Figure 20.1) usually reflects the acute strain placed on the right ventricle: an $S_1 Q_3 T_3$ pattern may be seen (McGinn and White, 1935), or T wave inversion over the right ventricle, or right bundle branch block (Cutforth and Oram, 1958; Sutton *et al.*, 1969). These electrocardiographic features may be transient. The plain chest radiograph (Figure 20.2) shows diminished vascular markings in the areas where embolism has lodged (Westermark, 1938; Kerr *et al.*, 1971). Occasionally, compensatory increased markings in other zones reflecting hyperaemia may be seen (Torrance, 1963). These abnormalities of vascular markings may be difficult to detect. Easier to recognise on plain chest radiographs is evidence of premonitory pulmonary infarction which includes infarct shadows, elevation of the dome of the diaphragm and pleural effusion. A 'plump' hilar shadow is frequently seen in massive pulmonary embolism (Kerr *et al.*, 1971) and is probably the result of a slightly

Thromboembolism

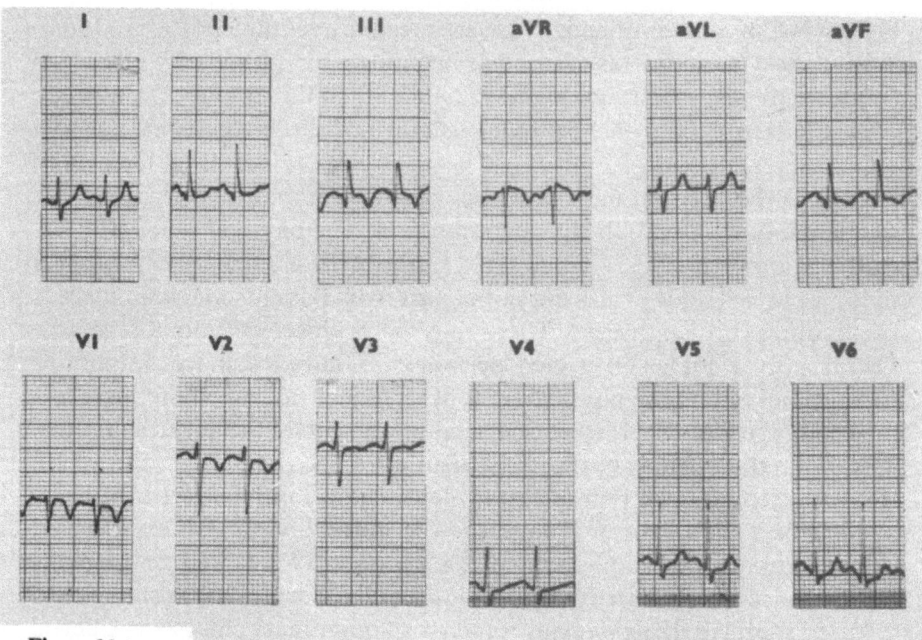

Figure 20.1

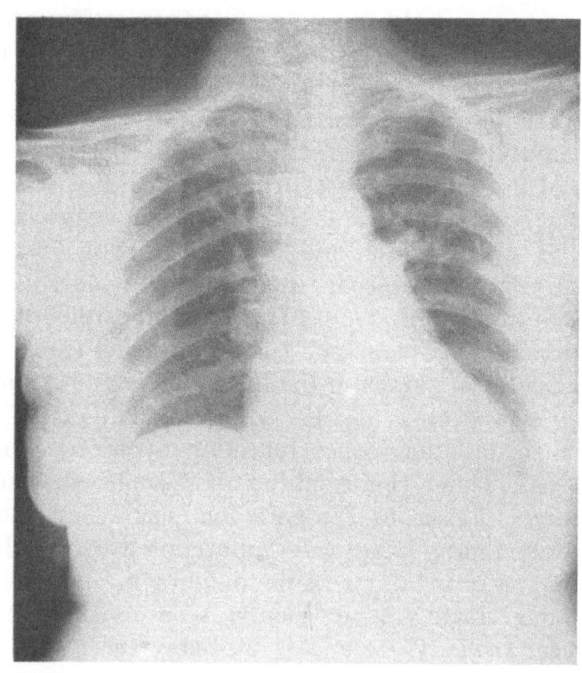

Figure 20.2

dilated major pulmonary artery proximal to the obstruction by embolism. The arterial blood gases characteristically show an arterial oxygen tension which is markedly reduced (30–50 mmHg) (Sutton, 1970) and an abnormally low carbon dioxide tension reflecting the hyperventilation. However, such abnormalities of arterial blood gases are not specific for pulmonary embolism, and may be seen in many other disorders.

Special investigations which may provide important evidence of pulmonary embolism are cardiac catheterisation, pulmonary arteriography and lung scans. The pulmonary arteriogram (Figure 20.3) is the most specific diagnostic proof of massive pulmonary embolism as it reveals the presence of filling defects in the major pulmonary arteries (Miller and Sutton, 1970; Raphael, 1970). In addition, visualisation of variations of flow of contrast medium in different areas of the lungs is obtained. These appearances in conjunction provide the best available assessment of the anatomical severity of embolism. The age of the emboli can also be deduced to a certain extent from the arteriographic appearances in that recent emboli bulge into the contrast-filled pulmonary arteries, whereas with time, the embolism recedes forming a concave border to the contrast medium.

At the time of pulmonary arteriography measurements of intracardiac pressures can be made which reveal the severity of the haemodynamic disturbance (Figure 20.4). There is a moderate degree of pulmonary hypertension (35–50 mmHg pulmonary artery systolic pressure), a raised right ventricular end-diastolic pressure and consequently right atrial pressure and a reduction in cardiac output with a wide arterio-venous oxygen difference. Arterial oxygen desaturation is usually present (Miller and Sutton, 1970; Sutton, 1970; McIntyre and Sasahara, 1971). These findings are characteristic of acute massive pulmonary embolism without preexisting cardiorespiratory disease, but variations will occur if additional cardiorespiratory disease is present (Sasahara et al., 1966), or the duration of embolism is not recent (Sutton, 1970).

Lung scanning is a relatively safe and simple technique which may provide important information in patients with pulmonary embolism (Wagner et al., 1964). Although abnormalities of perfusion revealed by the scan can be due to lung pathology other than pulmonary embolism

Figure 20.1 Electrocardiogram of patient with acute massive pulmonary embolism showing S1, Q3, T3, TAVF with T wave inversion in V1 – V3

Figure 20.2 Plain chest X-Ray of patient with acute massive pulmonary embolism showing oligaemia of right mid and lower zones and left lower zone, with a plump right hilar shadow

Thromboembolism

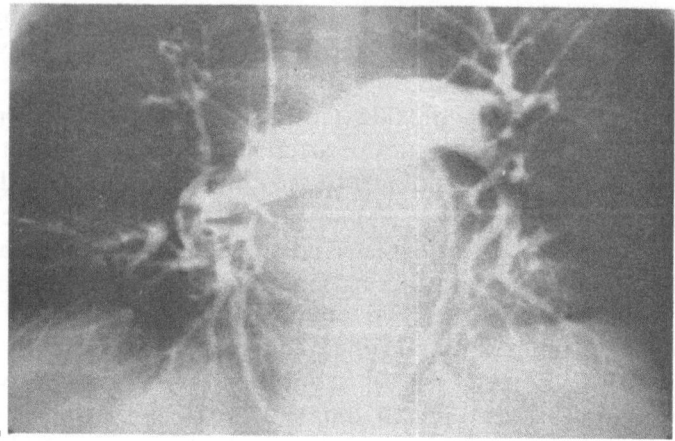

Figure 20.3.

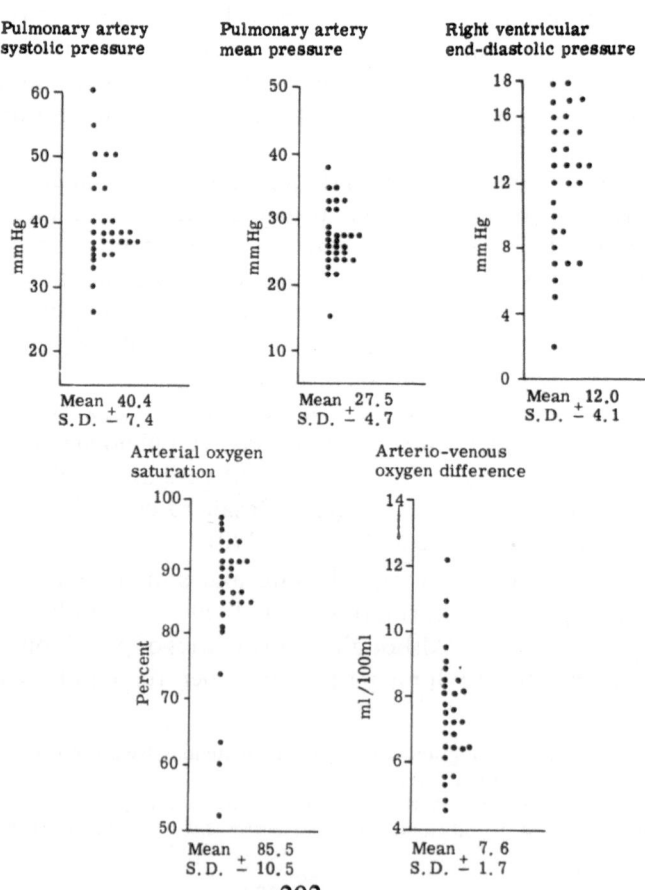

Figure 20.4.

(Secker-Walker, 1968), once the diagnosis of pulmonary embolism is established by other means, the lung scan is particularly valuable in following the progress of an individual patient with pulmonary embolism (Tow and Wagner, 1967). The correlation between lung scans and pulmonary arteriograms is particularly high in patients who have negative scans and arteriograms (Poulouse *et al.*, 1970), so that a normal scan makes pulmonary embolism very unlikely.

Management

The combination of clinical judgement and these special investigations enables an accurate diagnosis of massive pulmonary embolism to be made and this is the first requirement in the rational management of the patient with this disorder. The management of the individual patient depends largely on the severity of the disturbance.

The patient who presents with circulatory arrest demands immediate resuscitation. Analysis of autopsies has shown that the highest mortality from pulmonary embolism occurs in the period shortly following the event (Gorham, 1961; Donaldson *et al.*, 1963). Immediate resuscitation is mandatory with external cardiac massage being continued until the cardiac rhythm is established from the electrocardiogram. Ventricular asystole is probably more common than ventricular fibrillation so that D.C. countershock may only be of value in a few cases. External cardiac massage may effect propulsion of the embolism away from the central pulmonary artery thereby reducing the obstruction to overall pulmonary flow; given an adequate pulmonary flow, the normal left ventricle can maintain an adequate systemic blood flow. Oxygen administration by mask or endotracheal tube improves oxygenation of tissues suffering from a reduced cardiac output. Correction of the metabolic acidosis, inevitable during circulatory arrest of any duration, is achieved by the infusion of sodium bicarbonate. Right ventricular function may be improved by drugs which have a positive inotropic effect on the heart such as isoprenaline. Peripheral vasoconstrictor drugs are theoretically of less value, but may have a particular use during the induction of anaesthesia to compensate for the vasodilatory effect of this procedure prior to pul-

Figure 20.3 Pulmonary arteriogram of patient with acute massive pulmonary embolism showing major filling defects in right and left pulmonary arteries with resultant reduction in filling of distal vessels in all areas

Figure 20.4 Individual values of pulmonary artery systolic pressure, mean pulmonary artery pressure, right ventricular end-diastolic pressure, arterial oxygen saturation, and arterio-venous oxygen difference in 30 patients with acute massive pulmonary embolism. The mean values and standard deviations (SD) for each measurement are shown.

monary embolectomy (Paneth, 1970). The suggestion has been made that a single intravenous injection of heparin (15 000 units) may be of immediate benefit: the basis for this would be that heparin blocks serotonin release from platelets in the thrombus and consequently may abolish broncho-constriction and possibly pulmonary vasoconstriction (Comroe *et al.*, 1953; Gurewich *et al.*, 1965; Gurewich *et al.*, 1967). Although the evidence for such phenomena in man is lacking, the administration of heparin does not prejudice other treatment and perhaps should be part of the immediate resuscitative measures.

As a result of these resuscitative measures, the patient with acute massive pulmonary embolism may either maintain an adequate circulation spontaneously while remaining critically ill, or fail to respond. The patient who fails to respond can only be treated with immediate pulmonary embolectomy. Without cardiopulmonary bypass the operation can be carried out using outflow occlusion as described by Trendelenburg (Trendelenburg, 1908) or inflow occlusion (Pisko-Dubienski, 1968). More recently, special suckers have been described for the removal of pulmonary emboli without opening the chest, but by introducing suction cup-ended catheters through the femoral vein (Greenfield *et al.*, 1971). Pulmonary embolectomy without cardiopulmonary bypass carries as high a mortality as 87 per cent (Cross and Mowlem, 1967). In centres where cardio-pulmonary bypass is available the mortality for pulmonary embolectomy is lower but still unacceptably high varying from 25–57 per cent (Cross and Mowlem, 1967; Miller, 1972).

The patient who fails to maintain a circulation demands pulmonary embolectomy because immediate relief of pulmonary obstruction is the only way to establish a systemic cardiac output. In such a patient, the diagnosis may have to be made clinically without resort to special investigations. The availability of a portable pump oxygenator as a means of partial cardiopulmonary bypass for immediate resuscitation and for support during pulmonary angiography will allow a definitive preoperative diagnosis to be made (Beall, 1974). The patient who is able to maintain an adequate circulation following initial resuscitation may also require confirmation of the diagnosis in a difficult case. This also is best achieved by pulmonary arteriography. Although this investigation carries an obvious risk in a critically ill patient, it is usually well-tolerated apart from the short period following the injection of contrast medium when peripheral vasodilatation occurs with resultant hypotension. External cardiac massage may be required to combat this short-lived effect (Miller and Sutton, 1970).

When the diagnosis has been confirmed, the alternative methods of treatment available to the patient with acute massive pulmonary embolism are anticoagulant therapy, thrombolytic therapy or pulmonary embolectomy. Before discussing these, it is important to recognise that the natural history of pulmonary embolism is variable and there are few objective data which enable a prognosis to be made in the individual patient. The most dramatic sequel to massive pulmonary embolism is sudden death. Other patients may remain critically ill, making a gradual clinical recovery over a period of about 10 days: such patients if examined and investigated six months or a year later may not have any evidence of abnormality in the pulmonary circulation irrespective of the initial treatment, the embolism having resolved spontaneously. (Sautter *et al.*, 1964; Fred *et al.*, 1966; Paraskos *et al.*, 1973).

A third group of patients remain critically ill following the acute event and instead of making a gradual improvement over several days, deteriorate slowly over a period of one to two weeks and die. Whether these late deaths represent the development of further pulmonary thromboembolism or inability of the heart to overcome the initial sever haemodynamic disturbance may vary from patient to patient. Finally, there may exist a small group of patients who having suffered a massive pulmonary embolism initially recover, but ultimately fail to lyse the embolism spontaneously. With the passage of time, such patients could develop chronic thromboembolic pulmonary hypertension. Having recognised that the natural history is variable and that there is no method available for predicting the prognosis in the individual patient, let us examine the possible roles of the three methods of definitive treatment of pulmonary embolism.

Anticoagulant therapy
Sevitt and Gallagher demonstrated the value of oral anticoagulants in the prophylaxis of venous thromboembolism in elderly patients with fractured necks of femur (Sevitt and Gallagher, 1959). In 1960, a significant reduction in the mortality of patients with pulmonary embolism treated by heparin was demonstrated (Barritt and Jordan, 1960). These results with heparin and oral anticoagulants have been confirmed by subsequent trials, (Kernohan and Todd, 1966; Salzman *et al.*, 1966). Heparin has no thrombolytic activity, but is a potent antithrombin agent which exerts its therapeutic potential by preventing the propagation of an embolus which is the result of the conversion of fibrinogen to fibrin under the influence of thrombin absorbed to the embolus. Not only is ex-

tension of pulmonary embolism controlled, but also extension of the venous thrombosis which gave rise to it. At the same time, heparin prevents the release of serotonin from platelets and this may prevent harmful bronchoconstriction (Thomas *et al.*, 1964; Thomas *et al.*, 1966). It has been suggested that very large doses (100 000 units in 24 h) of heparin are required to combat this latter effect (Morris and Balk, 1965; Crane *et al.*, 1969). It would seem that 60 000 units of heparin in the first 24 h are a minimum both to prevent propagation of embolism and platelet accretion on an embolus. Thereafter, a smaller dose of heparin may be given. The dose should be sufficient to keep the clotting time prolonged to at least twice the control level. After 48 hours oral anticoagulants can be begun and should overlap treatment with heparin.

If anticoagulant therapy with heparin and oral agents is adopted, then the assumption is being made that the resolution of embolism will occur as a result of spontaneous thrombolysis. There is no doubt that such an assumption is frequently valid, but at the same time it is known that spontaneous resolution of massive embolism takes weeks or months to occur and the patient will remain clinically unwell for at least several days. The rate of resolution can be more readily assessed by lung scans than by pulmonary arteriograms as this technique is less traumatic for the patient, readily repeatable and more sensitive in demonstrating per-fusion deficits due to pulmonary emboli than the pulmonary arteriogram. A patient may continue to show abnormalities of the scan at a time when a pulmonary arteriogram would be judged as normal.

Although there are haemorrhagic complications from anticoagulant therapy, these are usually slight and less significant than with throm-olytic agents. With a clear therapeutic effect and few disadvantages, anti-coagulants are indicated in any patient with pulmonary embolic disease to prevent further extension of thromboembolism. Heparin and oral anticoagulants would also be the treatment of choice in the patient who is either first seen several days following massive embolism, or judged not to be critically ill.

Whether pulmonary embolectomy, thrombolytic therapy or anti-coagulant therapy has been used initially in the treatment of massive pulmonary embolism, following surgery, trauma or bed-rest, oral anti-coagulants should be continued until the patient is fully recovered and returned to his normal activities. If there has not been an obvious pre-cipitating factor for the development of thromboembolism, the duration of anticoagulant therapy remains controversial. A minimum period of six months may be advised and some believe that anticoagulation should be maintained indefinitely, particularly if additional cardiorespiratory disease is present.

Thrombolytic therapy

Two main thrombolytic agents, urokinase and streptokinase have been used in the treatment of pulmonary embolism (Chapter 18). Following initial reports on the use of urokinase (Sasahara *et al.*, 1967; Sautter *et al.*, 1967; Tow *et al.*, 1967; Genton and Wolf, 1968). the Urokinase Pulmonary Embolism Trial was conducted in the USA (The Urokinase Pulmonary Embolism Trial, 1973). Much smaller series have been reported on the use of streptokinase (Browse and James, 1964; Hirsh *et al.*, 1968; Miller *et al.*, 1971) and in both urokinase and streptokinase studies the control group of patients was treated with heparin. A further study is being carried out in the USA comparing patients treated with urokinase and with streptokinase.

The main conclusions of these studies are that although thrombolytic agents significantly accelerate the rate of resolution of pulmonary embolism by comparison with heparin, there is no evidence that mortality rates are altered by using these drugs. There is no evidence that the incidence of further embolism is more effectively reduced or that there is any difference in the state of the pulmonary circulation at six months or one year following the embolism in patients treated initially with thrombolytic agents (The Urokinase Pulmonary Embolism Trial, 1973). Moreover, the studies indicated an increased risk of haemorrhagic complications in patients treated with thrombolytic agents compared with those treated with heparin. The techniques of treating pulmonary embolism with thrombolytic agents have already been described (Chapter 18).

Following pulmonary arteriography, an initial dose of 250 000 to 600 000 units of streptokinase in dextrose or physiological saline have been infused over a 30 min period followed by a dose of 100 000 units/h for a 24–72 h period (Hirsh *et al.*, 1968; Miller *et al.*, 1971). The infusion has been into the main pulmonary artery through the catheter used for obtaining the pulmonary arteriogram. This technique has enabled the clinician to repeat the pulmonary arteriogram in order to assess the arteriographic effect of treatment in the least traumatic way for the patient. The above dosage schedule is usually adequate both to overcome any initial antistreptokinase antibodies present and to maintain an adequate fibrinolytic state*. The Urokinase Pulmonary Embolism trial

*Hydrocortisone 100 mg intravenously 6-hourly has been given to present possible hypersensitivity reactions.

employed a loading dose of 2000 CTA units/lb body weight followed by a 12 h intravenous infusion of 2000 CTA units/lb/h: the pulmonary arteriogram was repeated 24 h following the initiation of urokinase therapy. Whether differences might be observed by direct infusion of thrombolytic agents into the pulmonary artery in contrast to intravenous infusion has not been resolved.

At the end of therapy with urokinase or streptokinase the improvements in the right atrial and right ventricular end-diastolic pressures and in the total pulmonary resistance were greater than at the end of heparin therapy. There were also striking differences in the appearances of the pulmonary arteriogram after treatment with thrombolytic agents and heparin (Figure 20.5). Usually there was little change following

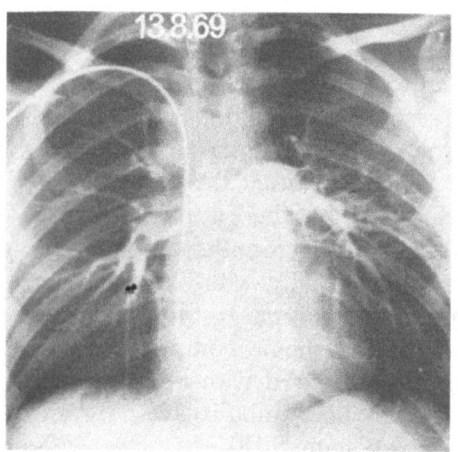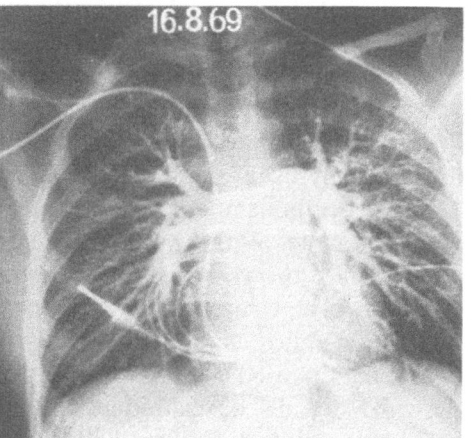

Figure 20.5 *Left panel:* shows pulmonary arteriogram of a patient with acute massive pulmonary embolism involving right pulmonary artery with reduction in flow to right lung, and left upper lobe and left lower lobe arteries with severe reduction in flow to the left upper and lower zones
Right panel: shows a repeat pulmonary arteriogram in the same patient following a 72 hour infusion of streptokinase. The arteriogram is near normal

heparin and striking 'resolution' following thrombolytic agents. Accompanying such measured indices of the rate of resolution was the clinical impression of improvement in the state of the patient with relief of tachypnoea, disappearance of right ventricular failure and improvement in cardiac output. In the urokinase trial, which included both minor and massive pulmonary emboli, it was observed that the most striking improvements were in patients with massive embolism. Most of the patients in the streptokinase trials also had massive embolism. However, there were some patients who deteriorated while receiving thrombolytic therapy and many of these were treated with pulmonary embolectomy. The impression was that a higher number of patients deteriorated while receiving heparin therapy than while receiving thrombolytic drugs. Bleeding was always seen more frequently in patients receiving thrombolytic therapy than heparin. This was particularly common at cutdown sites and other sites of trauma, as well as spontaneous bleeding. The longer-term result was assessed in the urokinase study. There was no significant difference in the recurrence rate of pulmonary embolism in the urokinase or heparin groups; the lung scan improvement was the same after one week and at one year in the two groups.

The above data suggest that if rapid resolution of pulmonary embolism is desired, then urokinase or streptokinase will usually achieve this whereas heparin will not. In the long term, there is no obvious benefit to the patient by the initial use of thrombolytic agents, nor do they prevent the mortality observed from pulmonary embolism. Under what circumstances should thrombolytic agents then be used? One answer should lie in the known mortality of patients with massive pulmonary embolism who die at a period varying from several hours to several days following the acute event (Gorham, 1961; Donaldson et al., 1963). Such patients survive the immediate impact, remain critically ill and deteriorate in a more gradual manner with eventual death presumably due to inability to overcome the prolonged, severe haemodynamic disturbance. If it is possible to reverse this disturbance rapidly by the use of thrombolytic agents, the patient must benefit and the need for pulmonary embolectomy (the only available alternative) will be averted. Alternatively, delayed deterioration of the patient may be the result of further or repeated emboli, although evidence for this complication is seldom obvious clinically. If further emboli were to occur then it would seem advantageous to lyse the initial massive embolism as rapidly as possible so that further embolism would occur at a time when the haemodynamic disturbance had either been totally or partially reversed. Such rationalisation for the use of thrombolytic agents in the management of acute massive pulmonary embolism still demands justification, as statistically acceptable evidence for an improvement in the mortality of these patients is lacking. Even if such evidence does become available, there will remain a proportion of patients in whom the high risk of haemorrhagic complications will constitute a contraindication to the use of thrombolytic agents. Such contraindications include recent surgery to sites where excessive bleeding is dangerous, systemic hypertension, known previous cerebrovascular accident, active peptic ulceration and a known bleeding state.

If both urokinase and streptokinase were readily available, there are a number of known and unknown problems concerning these drugs which would influence a choice between them. Urokinase has the disadvantage of very high cost, but the advantage of non-antigenicity and consequently may be used more than once. Both the substances have been shown to accelerate lysis of emboli, but it may be that one has a greater risk of haemorrhagic complications than the other. The Urokinase – Streptokinase Pulmonary Embolism Trial currently in progress in the USA may answer some of these questions.

Pulmonary embolectomy

This operation, proposed by Trendelenburg in 1908 (Trendelenburg, 1908), was the only operation carried out until the early 1960s when successful embolectomy using cardiopulmonary bypass was reported (Cooley *et al.*, 1961; Sharp, 1962). Cross and Mowlem (Cross and Mowlem, 1967) surveyed the results of pulmonary embolectomy carried out in a large number of centres in the USA: the immediate mortality with cardiopulmonary bypass was 57 per cent (rising to 68 per cent with late deaths). Only 2 out of 15 patients with bilateral pulmonary emboli operated without cardiopulmonary bypass survived (although the outcome was favourable in seven others with unilateral emboli). A large individual series using cardiopulmonary bypass has a mortality of less than 25 per cent (Paneth, 1973).

Whereas pulmonary embolectomy appears to afford the only chance of survival for the patient with massive pulmonary embolism who is unable to maintain an adequate circulation without assistance such as external cardiac massage, other indications for pulmonary embolectomy are much more difficult to define. Objective measurements such as a high mean right ventricular pressure and low cardiac output have been proposed as indications that the patient is likely to die (Del Guercio *et al.*, 1966). Others suggested that a mean pulmonary artery pressure in excess of 30 per cent of mean systemic pressure was an indication for operation (Diacoff, 1966). In patients in whom pulmonary arteriograms were obtained, a systemic pressure below 100 mmHg (systolic) in conjunction with a high arteriographic index of severity of pulmonary embolism was associated with either a 70 per cent chance of death or the deterioration

300

of the patient on medical (streptokinase or heparin) therapy and resultant pulmonary embolectomy (Tibbutt *et al.*, 1974). A simpler clinical assessment as an indication for pulmonary embolectomy is the patient who has an unacceptably low systemic pressure despite the use of vasopressor agents (Crane *et al.*, 1969).

The use of thrombolytic agents in the treatment of acute massive pulmonary embolism has modified the indications for pulmonary embolectomy. The immediate removal of major emboli from the pulmonary arteries by embolectomy can now be matched in only a slightly longer time by the use of thrombolytic agents in most patients. Thus the rapid improvement on haemodynamic disturbance can no longer be a valid reason for pulmonary embolectomy. On the other hand, there will be patients who are started on thrombolytic therapy and who either fail to improve or deteriorate while receiving this treatment. At present, it is not known what determines the success of thrombolytic therapy, but if it fails and the patient deteriorates then most clinicians would agree with Paneth that pulmonary embolectomy should be carried out (Paneth, 1970).

Another group of patients in whom embolectomy might be considered are those who have survived the initial impact of pulmonary embolism, who are critically ill, but not requiring circulatory support and in whom thrombolytic drugs are contraindicated. A direct comparison between the results of embolectomy or heparin in reducing mortality under these circumstances is not available, but the Urokinase Pulmonary Embolism Trial (The Urokinase Pulmonary Embolism Trial, 1973) questions the value of embolectomy in such patients. Eleven patients with massive embolism and sustained hypotension were not included in the trial, but had embolectomy performed with a 63 per cent mortality. This high mortality contrasts with one of 18 per cent in a similar number of similar patients included in the study and treated medically.

Summary of treatment of acute massive pulmonary embolism
Immediate resuscitative measures consequent on the collapse of the patient are designed to maintain an adequate circulatory state. These include external cardiac massage, oxygen and the use of positive inotropic and vasopressor drugs. An immediate intravenous dose of heparin has, at any rate, theoretical justification. Such measures are designed to propel the embolism into more distal pulmonary arteries, improve tissue oxygenation, assist the severely stressed right ventricle and counteract any additional pulmonary vasoconstriction. If such measures

fail to achieve a satisfactory circulatory state, then pulmonary embolectomy is the only available treatment recognising that the diagnosis must be correct for any chance of success and that although the mortality will inevitably be high, patients' lives may be saved.

If a stable circulatory state is achieved by immediate resuscitation, the critically-ill patient with an established diagnosis and who has no contra-indications to the use of thrombolytic agents will benefit most from urokinase or streptokinase in the early postembolism period. If the patient deteriorates while receiving thrombolytic agents, then pulmonary embolectomy with cardiopulmonary bypass is indicated. When thrombolytic therapy is contraindicated then heparin may be used unless the patient deteriorates when embolectomy again is indicated. Patients who are not critically ill (and this group will consist mainly of those seen many hours or days after the incident), can be managed with heparin and oral anticoagulant drugs to prevent further extension of thromboembolism while spontaneous lysis is permitted to occur.

ACUTE MINOR PULMONARY EMBOLISM

Diagnosis

The clinical presentation of a patient with minor pulmonary embolism is usually dependent on the development of a resultant pulmonary infarct. The patient complains of pleurisy or haemoptysis with other symptoms being rare in the patient without previous cardiorespiratory disease (Sutton, 1970). The presentation may be more dramatic if there is pre-existing cardiac or respiratory disease. Under such circumstances, a minor embolism will present in a similar way to that of a patient with a massive embolism and a previously normal cardio-respiratory system. The reason is that the haemodynamic disturbance may be identical in spite of differences in the size of pulmonary embolism. The disturbance will consist of reduction in cardiac output, right ventricular failure, moderate pulmonary hypertension and hypoxaemia.

The patient with an uncomplicated minor embolism may have the physical signs of pleurisy and pulmonary infarction, signs confined to the respiratory system. Because the obstruction to the pulmonary circulation is small, pulmonary hypertension, reduction in cardiac output and right ventricular failure do not occur and consequently physical examination of the circulation and the heart is normal.

For similar reasons, the electrocardiogram remains normal. By contrast the plain chest X-Ray is a valuable aid to the diagnosis (Figure 20.6) for it may reveal an infarct shadow, a pleural effusion, elevation of the

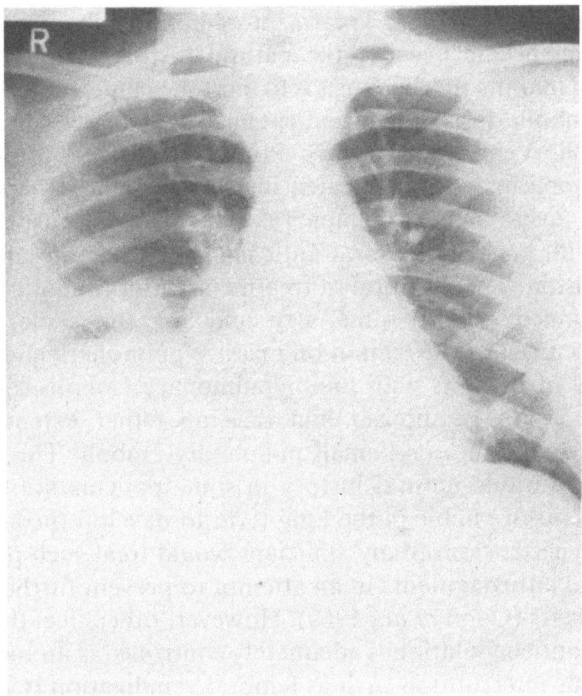

Figure 20.6 Plain chest X-Ray of a patient with pulmonary embolism showing an infarct shadow at the right base, elevation of the right dome of the diaphragm and a plump right hilar shadow

diaphragm, linear atelectases or a reduction in vascular markings. A lung scan will show areas of reduced pulmonary perfusion, but does not reveal whether such abnormal perfusion is due to embolism, infarction or other conditions affecting uniform lung perfusion. A ventilation scan revealing a ventilation – perfusion discrepancy will improve the diagnostic accuracy. Pulmonary arteriography is the ultimate diagnostic aid and this investigation will be particularly useful in distinguishing between massive and minor embolism in a patient with a previously abnormal cardiorespiratory system.

Management
The natural history of minor pulmonary embolism is usually spontaneous lysis and complete recovery. Sometimes, pulmonary infarction gives rise to a large pleural effusion which may persist and occasionally the infarcted area of lung breaks down to form a cavity which may

become secondarily infected. Treatment of minor pulmonary embolism usually is non-specific because the natural history is favourable. The importance of making the diagnosis is to alert the clinician to the existence of thromboembolic disease in the patient and to introduce steps to prevent further emboli. Venous thrombosis in the pelvis or legs which is the source of embolism must be treated in its own right (Chapter 19). The patient with overt minor pulmonary embolism will usually be anti-coagulated with heparin and oral anticoagulant drugs in an attempt to prevent extension. The duration of treatment with oral anticoagulants is usually continued in the same way and for the same reasons as have been discussed in the section on massive pulmonary embolism.

A minority of patients with minor pulmonary embolism may fail to achieve lysis of the embolism and develop either extension of the embolism *in situ* or repeated small pulmonary emboli. The reasons for such an unfavourable natural history in some patients are not known, but such patients are liable in the long-term to develop thromboembolic pulmonary hypertension. Many clinicians would treat such patients with long-term oral anticoagulants in an attempt to prevent further thrombo-embolic incidents (Coon *et al.*, 1969). However, others feel that repeated emboli while anticoagulation is adequately controlled is an indication for surgical venous interruption such as femoral vein ligation (Crane, 1964), inferior vena caval ligation (O'Neill, 1945), plication (De Weese and Hunter, 1958) or insertion of intraluminal devices (Eichelter and Schenk, 1968) in an attempt to prevent further pulmonary emboli (Chapter 19). Unfortunately, such surgery carries an operative mortality, recurrence of emboli is not totally eliminated and sometimes fatal pulmonary emboli occur (Bernstein, 1973).

CHRONIC THROMBOEMBOLIC PULMONARY HYPERTENSION
Diagnosis
Within the spectrum of pulmonary embolic disease there are patients with subacute or chronic thromboembolic pulmonary hypertension. This situation may have resulted from a failure of spontaneous lysis or recurrent pulmonary emboli, usually minor in severity, and as a result of repeated episodes of massive obstruction to the pulmonary circulation develops. This complication may take several years to develop.

An alternative pathogenesis which would produce the same end-result is that the patient who has had massive pulmonary embolism although recovering from the initial impact, fails to lyse the embolism. With time, such a patient may develop extension of embolism and severe pulmonary hypertension will finally result.

The patient with established pulmonary hypertension from chronic pulmonary thromboembolism will complain of exertional dyspnoea and syncope (Goodwin *et al.*, 1963; Fowler, *et al.*, 1966). He may complain of repeated attacks of pleurisy or haemoptysis as a result of further emboli or thrombosis *in situ* causing fresh pulmonary infarction.

The physical signs in a patient with chronic thromboembolic pulmonary hypertension differ from those found in acute massive or minor pulmonary embolism. They are the signs of severe pulmonary hypertension with accentuation of the pulmonary valve closure sound. Sometimes, there is an abnormally wide splitting of the second heart sound on expiration (although respiratory variation of splitting remains normal) and a pulmonary ejection sound may be heard. These auscultatory features may be accompanied by right ventricular hypertrophy on palpation of the praecordium and a dominant 'a' wave in the jugular venous pulse. There may be an ejection systolic murmur, a right atrial sound (S4) and a right ventricular filling sound (S3) if the patient is in overt right heart failure. The electrocardiogram may show right ventricular hypertrophy, while the chest X-Ray shows dilatation of the main pulmonary artery and asymmetrical areas of oligaemia in the lung fields.

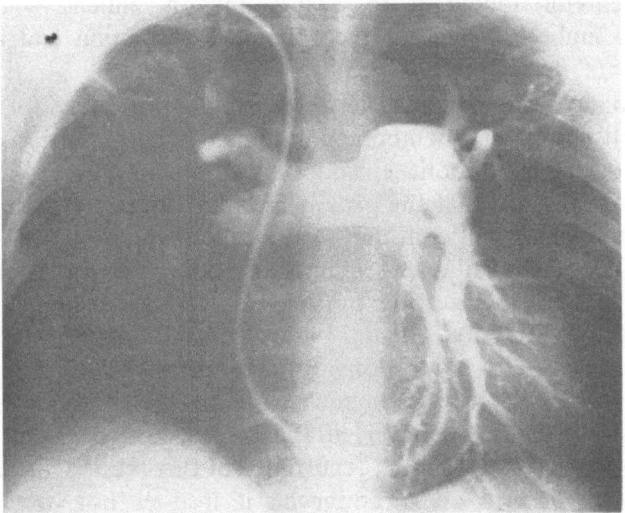

Figure 20.7 Pulmonary artriogram of a patient with chronic thromboembolic pulmonary hypertension. The central pulmonary arteries are dilated; there is convex tapering of the right descending pulmonary artery; the left lower pulmonary artery is dilated and tortuous. There is severe reduction in filling of distal vessels in many zones

Thromboembolism

Cardiac catheterisation confirms the presence of a very high pulmonary artery pressure, while pulmonary arteriography (a procedure which carries a high risk in patients with severe pulmonary hypertension) demonstrates asymmetrical occlusions of the pulmonary arteries and marked dilatation of the central pulmonary arteries (Chrispin *et al.*, 1963) (Figure 20.7). Whereas the arteriographic appearances of recent pulmonary emboli are of occlusive lesions bulging with a convex-leading border to the contrast-filled vessel, chronic embolism has a characteristic concave border.

Although abnormalities of respiratory function occur in patients with chronic thromboembolic pulmonary hypertension, (Jones and Goodwin, 1965) these do not contribute towards making the diagnosis. Non-specific abnormalities of perfusion may be demonstrated by lung scans (Wilson *et al.*, 1973).

Treatment

When thromboembolic pulmonary hypertension has developed, treatment has not been shown to be effective in either reversing the disease, or in altering its natural history which tends to be gradual deterioration and eventual death of the patient (Owen *et al.*, 1953). Prevention of the disease is important and measures outlined in the treatment of acute pulmonary embolism, particularly adequate anticoagulant therapy, careful follow-up to ensure that a patient who has had pulmonary embolism has achieved complete resolution and attention to the source of the embolism should all be considered.

Maintenance anticoagulant therapy is usually prescribed for the patient with established thromboembolic pulmonary hypertension in an attempt to prevent further embolic episodes or extension of existing disease. There is no evidence that the prognosis is improved by such treatment, but most clinicians will continue to use anticoagulants until alternative treatment becomes available. Attempts to produce rapid lysis of embolism of more than recent duration by thrombolytic agents have not so far proved successful (Hirsh *et al.*, 1968; Miller *et al.*, 1969). There are reports of successful operations for the removal of clot from the proximal pulmonary arteries in such patients (Brock *et al.*, 1967; Moor and Sabiston, 1970). However, if the disease has been present for a long period, it seems likely that recurrence of thrombosis at the site of its removal will tend to occur and even if it does not, the underlying process which has resulted in sufficient pulmonary vascular obliteration to cause severe pulmonary hypertension will not be halted by removal of surgically accessible thrombi.

Thromboembolism

References

Barritt, D. W. and Jordan, S. C. (1960). Anticoagulant drugs in treatment of pulmonary embolism: controlled trial. *Lancet*, **1,** 1309

Beall, A. C. (1974). Pulmonary embolectomy. In: *Venous Diseases – Medical and Surgical Management* (American European Symposium on venous diseases, Montreux).

Bernstein, E. F. (1973). The place of venous interruption in the treatment of pulmonary thromboembolism. In: *Pulmonary Thromboembolism*, 312 (K. M. Moser, and M. Stein, editors) (Chicago: Year Book Medical Publishers Inc.)

Brock, Lord, Nabil, N. and Gibson, R. V. (1967). Case of late pulmonary embolectomy. *Brit. Med. J.* **4,** 598

Browse, W. L. and James, D. C. O. (1964). Streptokinase and pulmonary embolism. *Lancet*, **2,** 1039

Chrispin, A. R., Goodwin, J. F. and Steiner, R. E. (1963). The radiology of obliterative pulmonary hypertension and thromboembolism. *Brit. J. Radiol.*, **36,** 705

Comroe, J. H., Van Lingen, B., Stroud, R. C. and Roncoroni, A. (1953). Reflex and direct cardiopulmonary effects of 5-OH tryptamine (Serotonin); their possible role in pulmonary embolism and coronary thrombosis. *Amer. J. Physiol.*, **173,** 379

Cooley, D. A., Beall, A. C. Jr and Alexander, J. K. (1961). Acute massive pulmonary embolism. *J. Amer. Med. Assoc.*, **177,** 283

Coon, W. W., Willis, P. W. and Symons, M. J. (1969). Assessment of anticoagulant treatment of venous thromboembolism. *Ann. Surg.*, **170,** 559

Crane, C. (1964). Femoral vs caval interruption for venous thromboembolism. *New Eng. J. Med.*, **270,** 819

Crane, C., Hartsuck, J., Birtch, A., Couch, N. P., Zollinger, R., Matloff, J., Dalen, J. and Dexter, L. (1969). The management of major pulmonary embolism. *Surg. Gynaecol. Obstet.* **128,** 27

Cross, F. S. and Mowlem, A. (1967). A survey of the current status of pulmonary embolectomy for massive pulmonary embolism. *Circulation*, **35, Suppl. 1,** 86

Cutforth, R. H. and Oram, S. (1958). The electrocardiogram in pulmonary embolism. *Brit. Heart J.*, **20,** 41

Dalen, J. E. and Dexter, L. (1969). Pulmonary embolism. *J. Amer. Med. Assoc.*, **207,** 1505

De Weese, M. S. and Hunter, D. C. (1958). A vena caval filter for the prevention of pulmonary emboli. *Bull. Soc. Int. Chir.*, **17,** 17

Del Guercio, L. R. M., Cohn, J. D., Feins, N. R., Coomaraswamy, R. P. and Mantle, L. (1966). Pulmonary embolism shock. *J. Amer. Med. Assoc.*, **196,** 751

Diacoff, G. R., Rams, J. J. and Moulder, P. V. (1966). Pulmonary embolectomy. *Surg. Clin. N. Amer.*, **46,** 27

Donaldson, G. A., Williams, C. Scannell, J. G. and Shaw, R. S. (1963). Reappraisal of application of Trendelenburg operation to massive fatal embolism: report of successful pulmonary artery thrombectomy using cardiopulmonary bypass. *New Eng. J. Med.*, **268,** 171

Eichelter, P. and Schenk, W. G. Jr (1968). Prophylaxis of pulmonary embolism: a new experimental approach with initial results. *Arch. Surg.*, **97,** 348

Elliott, G. B. and Beamish, R. E. (1953). Embolic occlusion of patent foramen ovale. *Circulation*, **8,** 394

Fowler, N. O., Black-Shaffer, B., Scott, R. C. and Gueron, M. (1966). Idiopathic and thromboembolic pulmonary hypertension. *Amer. J. Med.*, **40,** 331

Fred, H. L., Axelrad, M. A., Lewis, J. M. and Alexander, J. K. (1966). Rapid resolution

Thromboembolism

of pulmonary thromboemboli in man: angiographic study. *J. Amer. Med. Assoc.*, **196**, 1137

Genton, E. and Wolf, P. S., (1968). Urokinase therapy in pulmonary thromboembolism. *Amer. Heart J.*, **76**, 628

Goodwin, J. F., Harrison, C. V. and Wilcken, D. E. L. (1963). Obliterative pulmonary hypertension and thrombo-embolism. *Brit. Med. J.*, **1**, 701

Gorham, L. W. (1961). A study of pulmonary embolism. *Arch. Int. Med.*, **108**, 8

Greenfield, L. J., Reif, M. E. and Guenter, C. E., (1971). Hemodynamic and respiratory responses to transvenous pulmonary embolectomy. *J. Thorac. Cardiovasc. Surg.*, **62**, 890

Gurewich, V., Sasahara, A. A. and Stein, M. (1965). Pulmonary embolism, broncho-constriction and response to Heparin. In: *Pulmonary Embolic Disease*, 162 (A. A. Sasahara and M. Stein, editors) (New York: Grune and Stratton)

Gurewich, V., Thomas, D. P. and Stuart, R. K. (1967). Some guidelines for Heparin therapy of venous thromboembolic disease. *J. Amer. Med. Assoc.*, **199**, 116

Hampton, A. D. and Castleman, B. (1940). Correlation of post-mortem chest teleroentgenograms with autopsy findings with special reference to pulmonary embolism and infarction. *Amer. J. Roentgen.*, **43**, 305

Hirsh, J., Hale, G. S., McDonald, I. G., McCarthy, R. A. and Pitt, A. (1968). Streptokinase therapy in acute major pulmonary embolism: effectiveness and problems. *Brit. Med. J.*, **4**, 729

Inman, W. H. W. and Vessey, M. P. (1968). Investigations of deaths from pulmonary, coronary and cerebral thrombosis and embolism in women of childbearing age. *Brit. Med. J.*, **2**, 193

Jones, N. L. and Goodwin, J. F. (1965). Respiratory function in pulmonary thromboembolic disorders. *Brit. Med. J.*, **1**, 1089

Kernohan, R. S. and Todd, C. (1966). Heparin therapy in thromboembolic disease. *Lancet*, **1**, 621

Kerr, I. H., Simon, G. and Sutton G. C. (1971). The value of the plain radiograph in acute massive pulmonary embolism. *Brit. J. Radiol.*, **44**, 751

McGinn, S. and White, P. D. (1935). Acute cor pulmonale resulting from pulmonary embolism; its clinical recognition. *J. Amer. Med. Assoc.*, **104**, 1473

McIntyre, K. M. and Sasahara, A. A. (1971). The haemodynamic response to pulmonary embolism in patients without prior cardiopulmonary disease. *Amer. J. Cardiol.*, **28**, 288

Miller, G. A. H., Gilbson, R. V., Honey, M. and Sutton, G. C. (1969). Treatment of pulmonary embolism with streptokinase: a preliminary report. *Brit. Med. J.*, **1**, 812

Miller, G. A. H. and Sutton, G. C. (1970). Acute massive pulmonary embolism. Clinical and haemodynamic findings in 23 patients studied by cardiac catheterisation and pulmonary arteriography. *Brit. Heart J.*, **32**, 518

Miller, G. A. H., Sutton, G. C., Kerr, I. H., Gibson, R. V. and Honey, M. (1971). Comparison of streptokinase and heparin in treatment of isolated acute massive pulmonary embolism. *Brit. Med. J.*, **2**, 681

Miller, G. A. H., (1972). The diagnosis and management of massive pulmonary embolism. *Brit. J. Surg.*, **59**, 837

Moor, G. F. and Sabiston, D. C. Jr (1970). Embolectomy for chronic pulmonary embolism and hypertension. Case report and review of the problem. *Circulation*, **41**, 701

Morris, L. E., and Balk, P. (1965). The management and mismanagement of acute venous thrombosis. *Angiology*, **16**, 339

Oakley, C. M. (1970). Diagnosis of pulmonary embolism. *Brit. Med. J.*, **2**, 773

Thromboembolism

O'Neill, E. E. (1945). Vena caval ligation for phlebo-thrombosis. *New Eng. J. Med.,* **232,** 641

Owen, W. R., Thomas, W. A., Castleman, B. and Bland, E. F. (1953). Unrecognised emboli to the lungs with subsequent cor pulmonale. *New Eng. J. Med.,* **249,** 919

Paneth, M. (1970). Surgical management of massive pulmonary embolism. *Brit. Med. J.,* **2,** 778

Paneth, M. (1973) (personal communication)

Paraskos, J. A., Adelstein, S. J., Smith, R. T., Rickman, F. D., Grossman, W., Dexter, L. and Dalen, J. S. (1973). Late prognosis of acute pulmonary embolism. *New Eng. J. Med.,* **289,** 55

Pisko-Dubienski, Z. A. (1968). A new approach to pulmonary embolism. *Brit. J. Surg.,* **55,** 138

Poulouse, K. P. Reba, R. C., Gilday, D. L., Deland, F. H. and Wagner, H. N. (1970). Diagnosis of pulmonary embolism. A correlative study of the clinical, scan and angiographic findings. *Brit. Med. J.,* **3,** 67

Raphael, M. J. (1970). Pulmonary angiography. *Brit. J. Hosp. Med.,* 377

Robin, E. D. (1965). Ventilation – perfusion abnormalities in pulmonary embolism. In: *Pulmonary Embolic Disease,* 149 (A. A. Sasahara, and M. Stein, editors) (New York: Grune and Stratton)

Salzman, E. W., Harris, W. H. and De Sanctis, R. W. (1966). Anticoagulation for prevention of thromboembolism following fractures of the hip. *New Eng. J. Med.,* **275,** 122

Sasahara, A. A., Sidd, J. J., Tremblay, G. and Leland, O. S. (1966). Cardiopulmonary consequences of acute pulmonary embolic disease. *Prog. Cardiovasc. Dis.,* **9,** 259

Sasahara, A. A., Cannilla, J. E., Belko, J. S., Morse, R. L. and Criss, A. J. (1967). Urokinase therapy in clinical pulmonary thromboembolism. *New Eng. J. Med.,* **277,** 1168

Sautter, R. D., Fletcher, F. W., Emanuel, D. A. Lawton., B. R. and Olsen, T. G. (1964). Clinical notes: complete resolution of massive pulmonary thromboembolism. *J. Amer. Med. Assoc.,* **189,** 948

Sautter, R. D., Emanuel, D. A., Fletcher, F. W., Wenzel, F. J. and Matson, J. I. (1967). Urokinase for the treatment of acute pulmonary thromboembolism. *J. Amer. Med. Assoc.,* **202,** 215

Secker-Walker, R. H. (1968). Scintillation scanning of lungs in diagnosis of pulmonary embolism. *Brit. Med. J.,* **2,** 206

Sevitt, S. and Gallagher, N. G. (1959). Prevention of venous thrombosis and pulmonary embolism in injured patients. *Lancet,* **2,** 981

Sevitt, S. and Gallagher, N. G. (1961). Venous thrombosis and pulmonary embolism. A clinico-pathological study in injured and burned patients. *Brit. J. Surg.,* **48,** 475

Sharp, E. H. (1962). Pulmonary embolectomy: Successful removal of a massive pulmonary embolus with the support of cardiopulmonary bypass. A case report. *Ann. Surg.,* **156,** 1

Sutton, G. C., Honey, M. and Gibson, R. V. (1969). Clinical diagnosis of acute massive pulmonary embolism. *Lancet,* **1,** 271

Sutton, G. C. (1970). *Cardiovascular Consequences of Acute Massive Pulmonary Embolism and the effect of Treatment* (M.D. Thesis, Cambridge University)

The Urokinase Pulmonary Embolism Trial. (1973). Amer. Heart Assoc. Monograph No. 39, *Circulation,* **47,** No. 4, Suppl. 2

Thromboembolism

Thomas, D. P., Stein, M., Tanabe, G., Rege, V. and Wessler, S. (1964). Mechanism of bronchoconstriction produced by thromboemboli in dogs. *Amer. J. Physiol.*, **206**, 1207

Thomas, D. P., Gurewich, V. and Ashford, T. P. (1966). Platelet adherence to thromboemboli in relation to the pathogenesis and treatment of pulmonary embolism. *New Eng. J. Med.*, **274**, 953

Tibbutt, D. A., Davies, J. A., Anderson, J. A., Fletcher, E. W. L., Hamill, J., Holt, J. M., Lea Thomas, M., Lee, G., De, J., Miller, G. A. H., Sharp, A. A. and Sutton, G. C. (1974). Comparison by controlled clinical trial of streptokinase and heparin in treatment of life-threatening pulmonary embolism. *Brit. Med. J.*, **1**, 343

Torrance, D. J. (1963). In: *The Chest Film in Massive Pulmonary Embolism* (Springfield, Illinois: Charles C. Thomas)

Tow, D. E. and Wagner, H. N. (1967). Recovery of pulmonary arterial blood flow in patients with pulmonary embolism. *New Eng. J. Med.*, **276**, 1053

Tow, D. E., Wagner, H. N. and Holmes, R. A. (1967). Urokinase in pulmonary embolism. *J. Amer. Med. Assoc.*, **277**, 1161

Trendelenburg, F. 1908). Uber die operative behandlung der embolie der lungenarterie. *Arch. Klin. Chir.*, **86**, 686

Wagner, H. N., Sabiston, D. C., McAfee, J. G., Tow, D. and Stern, H. S. (1964). Diagnosis of Massive pulmonary embolism in man by radio-isotope scanning. *New Eng. J. Med.*, **271**, 377

Westermark, N. (1938). On the roentgen diagnosis of Lung embolism. *Acta. Radiol. (Stockholm)*, **19**, 357

Wilson, A. G., Harris, C. N., Lavender, J. P. and Oakley, C. M. (1973). Perfusion lung scanning in obliterative pulmonary hypertension. *Brit. Heart J.* **35**, 917

21

Thromboembolism in obstetric and gynaecological patients

John Bonnar

INTRODUCTION

In recent years a striking and continuing rise has occurred in the mortality and morbidity from venous thrombosis and pulmonary embolism in England and Wales. During the period 1961–1967 the death rates in men and women were similar except in women in the age group 35–44 years. Morbidity data for venous thrombosis and pulmonary embolism show a similar pattern but there is a sharp increase in non-pregnant women of child bearing age. The most likely explanation of this increase of fatal and non-fatal pulmonary embolism in women in the age group 35–44 years over this period is the thrombogenic effects of oral contraceptives which were introduced into the United Kingdom in 1960 (Vessey 1973).

In marked contrast to the trend in the general population, the mortality from venous thromboembolism during pregnancy and particularly the puerperium has declined. Nonetheless, if deaths from abortion were excluded, the commonest cause of death related to pregnancy in England and Wales would be pulmonary embolism (Reports on Confidential Enquiries into Maternal Deaths in England and Wales, 1967–1969).

Detailed information concerning deaths from thromboembolism during pregnancy and the puerperium for the period 1952–1969 has been collected in England and Wales and published in triennial reports

*Unpublished work reported in this chapter has been supported by the Medical Research Council (Grant G971/755/C).

by the Confidential Enquiry into Maternal Deaths. The data show that in the eighteen years 1952–1969, 757 women in England and Wales died of thromboembolism associated with pregnancy. Table 21.1 shows that the number of deaths following all forms of vaginal delivery has

Table 21.1 Maternal deaths due to pulmonary embolism in England and Wales (1952–1969)

	During pregnancy	After vaginal delivery	After Caesarean section	Total
1952–54	4	104	30	138
1955–57	24	114	26	164
1958–60	36	80	22	138
1961–63	47	66	27	140
1964–66	27	43	25	95
1967–69	28	36	18	82

Figures taken from the Reports on Confidential Enquiries into Maternal Deaths in England and Wales (HMSO) for the years 1952–1969 inclusive

fallen steadily while that following Caesarean section has remained constant. During the last twenty years the proportion of women being delivered by Caesarean section has increased and now averages 5 per cent of all hospital deliveries. Therefore, the risk of fatal pulmonary embolism after Caesarean section has probably fallen. However, in recent years the proportion of deaths from thromboembolism taking place during pregnancy has sharply increased (Henderson *et al.*, 1972). Thrombo-embolism was previously regarded as a disease of the puerperium. Table 21.1 shows that only four of the 138 women who died in the period 1952–1954, died during pregnancy. Since 1961 25 per cent of the deaths have occurred during the antenatal period and have been distributed throughout pregnancy. The decline in mortality from puerperal pulmonary embolism could be attributed to a number of factors. These include the trend towards younger mothers and smaller families; the virtual disappearance of traumatic operative delivery, early ambulation and better diagnosis and treatment. The rise in the proportion of deaths during the antenatal period could be the result of the increased hospital admission and bed rest for complications of pregnancy such as hypertension and antepartum haemorrhage.

PHYSIOLOGICAL CHANGES IN THE COAGULATION AND FIBRINOLYTIC SYSTEMS DURING PREGNANCY

The blood coagulation and fibrinolytic systems have a key role in maintaining the integrity of the vascular compartment and the physiological changes in these mechanisms which occur during pregnancy are relevant to the prevention and treatment of thromboembolic disease. Normal pregnancy is accompanied by major changes in the coagulation system, particularly an increase in the level of plasma fibrinogen, and Factors VII, VIII and X (Strauss and Diamond, 1963; Rutherford *et al.*, 1964; Todd *et al.*, 1965; Bonnar, 1973). The increase in these factors occurs mainly in the second half of pregnancy and the extent of the changes is shown in Figure 21.1. A marked decrease in plasma fibrinolytic activity as measured by the level of plasminogen activator in the circulation and also by the amount of activator which can be released from venous endothelium takes place in the third trimester (Astedt, ·1972; Bonnar, 1973).

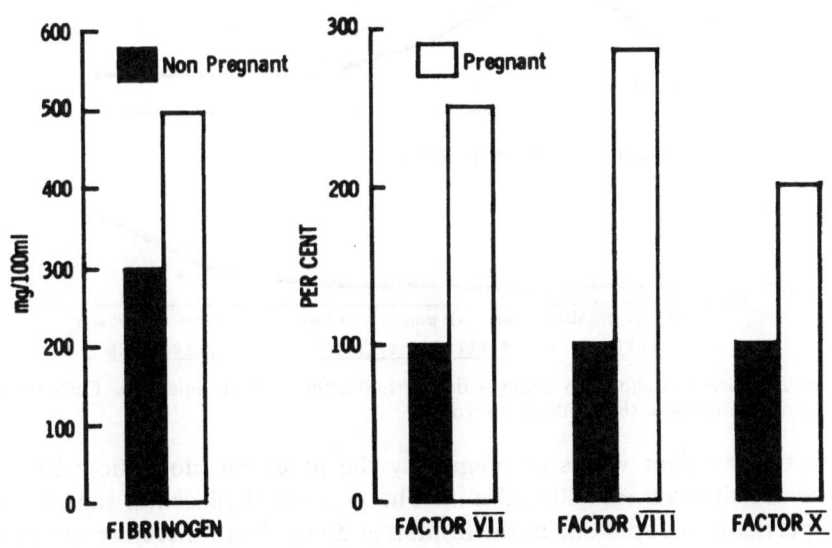

Figure 21.1 Changes in the levels of coagulation factors by the third trimester of normal pregnancy. Mean values from 15 normal pregnancies and age-matched non-pregnant women

Thromboembolism

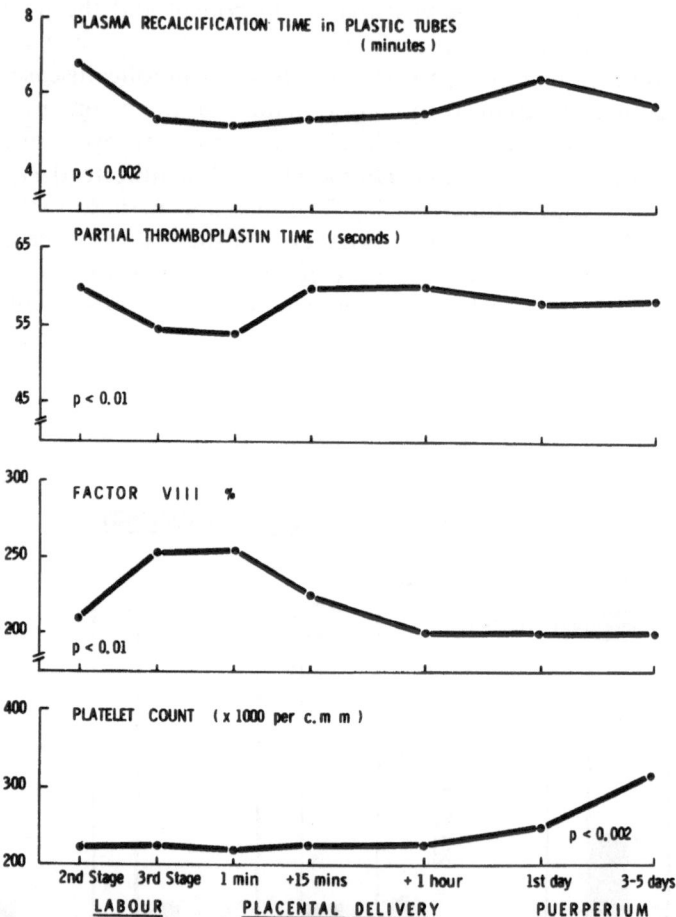

Figure 21.2 Serial coagulation changes during and after normal childbirth. Each point represents the mean of the results in 15 women

In the last four weeks of pregnancy the maternal blood flow to the placental site averages 600 ml/min. The process of placental separation is a particularly rapid one in the human and childbirth therefore presents a hazard of serious haemorrhage. Parturition is accompanied by the unique mechanism of myometrial contraction which reduces the blood flow to the placental site by extravascular compression. Simultaneously a local activation of the coagulation mechanism plays a vital role in controlling uterine bleeding (Bonnar *et al.*, 1970a; Bonnar *et al.*, 1970b). Figure 21.2

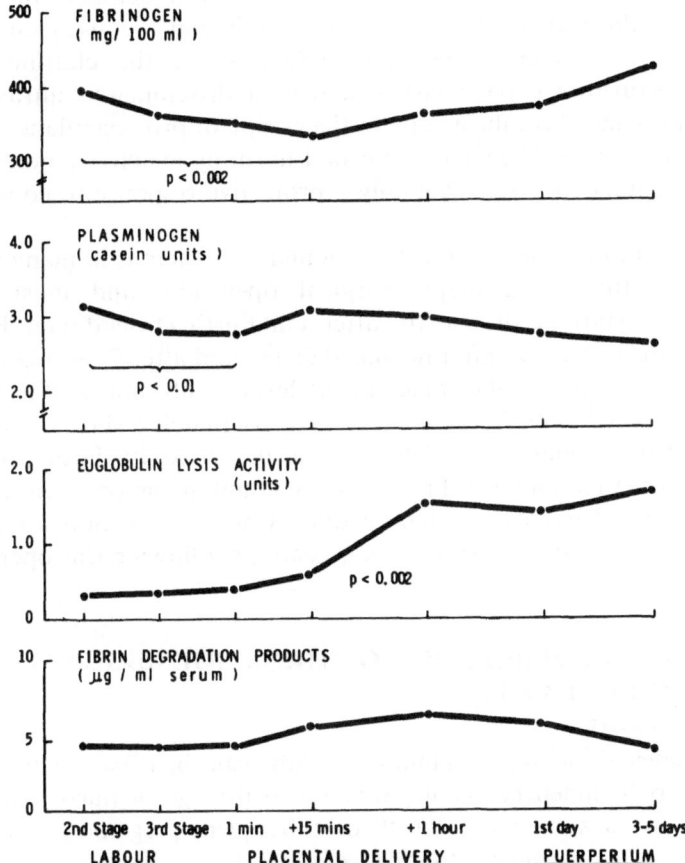

Figure 21.3 Plasma fibrinogen levels and the components of the fibrinolytic enzyme system during and after normal childbirth. Same subjects as Figure 21.2

shows changes in the circulating plasma which reflect the activation of coagulation in the uterus during and after childbirth. The depressed fibrinolysis of late pregnancy disappears rapidly after delivery of the placenta. The level of circulating plasminogen activator returns to normal within a half to one hour (Figure 21.3).

The changes in the coagulation and fibrinolytic systems which take place during pregnancy, together with the increased blood volume, combat the hazard of haemorrhage during and after placental separation. If reserves of haemostatic components were not available, a situation that can occur in patients with congenital coagulation defects such as von Willebrand's disease, the utilisation of coagulation factors at the time of delivery could lead to dangerously low levels and a consequent risk of severe uterine haemorrhage. The activation of the clotting system during parturition carries with it a risk of disseminated intravascular coagulation and thrombosis due to the escape of pro-coagulants into the circulation; the rapid reutrn of normal fibrinolytic activity immediately after placental delivery is probably a protective response to combat this hazard.

The effect of parturition on the coagulation system is in many respects similar to that of a major surgical operation, and most of the thromboses start at or shortly after childbirth (Friend and Kakkar, 1972). In the two weeks after normal delivery and after Caesarean section a secondary increase takes place in the level of fibrinogen; Factor VIII remains elevated and the number of adhesive platelets shows a steep rise (Ygge 1969, Bonnar et al., 1970b). The increased levels of fibrinogen and Factor VIII and the high platelet count in association with the limited physical activity which may follow Caesarean section, are possible explanations of the thrombotic complications following this operation.

FACTORS PREDISPOSING TO THROMBOEMBOLISM IN OBSTERIC PATIENTS
Age and parity
The incidence of fatal pulmonary embolism increases with age but appears to be independent of parity up to the age of thirty years. After this age, women having a fourth or subsequent pregnancy have a high incidence of embolism (Arthure et al., 1972).

Obesity
Obesity is accepted as an important factor in the development of thromboembolism (Barker et al., 1941; Turnbull, 1960) and approximately one out of four patients dying of embolism associated with pregnancy are considerably overweight, exceeding 73 kg. Often obesity is associated with hypertension of pregnancy which in the interest of the foetus necessitates admission to hospital for bedrest in late pregnancy.

Method of delivery
The increased risk of thromboembolism after Caesarean section is well-known and the fatality rate has been estimated at 1 : 2500 operations

(Arthure *et al.*, 1972). As shown in Table 21.2 the risk of fatal pulmonary embolism was increased five to sixfold by Caesarean section.

Table 21.2 Maternal deaths from pulmonary embolism following vaginal delivery and caesarean section

	Death rate per 10 000 vaginal deliveries	*Death rate per 10 000 Caesarean section deliveries*
1955–57	0·9	5·3
1958–60	0·6	3·7
1961–63	0·4	3·6
1964–66	0·2	2·7
1967–69	0·2	1·8

Figures taken from the Reports on Confidential Enquiries into Maternal Deaths in England and Wales (1955–1969)

Suppression of lactation

Oestrogen administration has been shown to predispose to thromboembolism in several clinical situations. An association between suppression of lactation with stilboestrol and thromboembolism was first suggested by Daniel and his colleagues (Daniel *et al.*, 1967). They showed that there was a tenfold increase of non-fatal thromboembolism in low parity women, 25 years of age and over, who were not lactating,compared with those who were. The evidence suggests that suppression of lactation with oestrogens is likely to be a precipitating factor, particularly in patients already at risk as the result of age and operative delivery (Tindall, 1971). In particular women over 35 years of age having Caesarean section should not be given oestrogen to inhibit lactation. Indeed the value of oestrogens for this purpose is in considerable doubt and in nearly 90 per cent of patients suppression of lactation can be achieved by the use of a breast binder alone; in the other 10 per cent analgesics will be required because of breast discomfort.

Hospitalisation

It has been reported that one-third of the cases of antenatal thromboembolism were in patients admitted to hospital during the antenatal period for rest (Jeffcoate and Tindall, 1965). Women admitted to hospital on account of obstetric complications such as pre-eclampsia, hypertension, heart disease and placental insufficiency should be regarded as at increased risk particularly if obese. Certainly, in any such patient who has a history of thrombosis, prophylactic therapy is advised. Women with a previous episode of thromboembolism seem particularly prone to a repetition of this complication during pregnancy.

Association with ABO blood grouping

It appears that patients of blood group O are much less likely to develop thromboembolic disease during pregnancy and the puerperium (Jick *et al.*, 1969; Allan and Stewart, 1971; Westerholm *et al.*, 1971).

DIAGNOSIS OF DEEP VENOUS THROMBOSIS DURING PREGNANCY

Clinical features

Before the introduction of biophysical methods of diagnosis the local signs in the legs, unexplained tachycardia or pyrexia, clinical evidence of pulmonary embolism or the postmortem examination were the only ways of diagnosing venous thrombosis. When physical signs such as marked local leg tenderness and extensive oedema are present, the diagnosis of deep venous thrombosis is very likely (Chapter 17). The acute massive venous occlusion of the iliac and femoral veins with progressive ischaemia of the lower limb is the most life threatening, but this florid type of venous thrombosis is now rare. In most patients the clinical signs are often minor or equivocal and venographic studies have shown that the deep veins are in fact normal in 40–50 per cent of patients with positive clinical signs confined to the calf (Chapters 11 and 17).

Venography in pregnancy

Because of the dangers of anticoagulant therapy in pregnancy and the puerperium, especially following operative delivery, the clinical diagnosis of deep venous thrombosis should be confirmed if possible by venography. Many obstetricians have the wrong impression that this procedure is technically difficult, time-consuming and dangerous for the patient. In fact venography can usually be carried out rapidly, causes little or no discomfort to the patient and is free of serious complications. Venography will provide information not only about the presence of a thrombus but also about its exact position, size and whether it is loose or adherent to the vein wall.

Venography has been rarely employed during pregnancy because of the associated radiation hazard to the foetus. However, it is possible to provide a large measure of protection to the pregnant uterus by the use of a lead apron. Certainly the hazard of thromboembolism to the mother and the risks of unnecessary anticoagulants to the foetus are such that if facilities are available venography with the uterus suitably protected should be carried out. In the puerperium a venographic diagnosis is also recommended before deciding as to the necessity of anticoagulant therapy (Chapter 19).

Ultrasound

Doppler ultrasound examination may also be used in the diagnosis of deep venous thrombosis but is much less precise than venography. The apparatus is similar to that employed for listening to the foetal heart. It can detect complete occlusion in the potentially hazardous sites, namely the popliteal or more proximal veins. Because of the presence of collateral venous channels in the calf the method will not detect minor calf thrombosis (Chapter 19).

Radioactive fibrinogen

The use of the ^{125}I-fibrinogen test is not acceptable as a screening procedure during pregnancy or in breastfeeding mothers because of radiation hazards. Jackson investigated one hundred obstetric patients who were in a 'high risk' category because of age or operative intervention and detected deep venous thrombosis in one patient only. Negative isotope scans were found in thirteen women with positive clinical signs, confirming the unreliability of the clinical diagnosis in the puerperium (Jackson, 1973).

DIAGNOSIS OF PULMONARY EMBOLISM

The symptoms and signs of pulmonary embolism are predominantly associated with the cardiovascular and respiratory systems (Chapter 20) and are similar in the pregnant and non-pregnant patient. The presence of the symptoms suggestive of pulmonary embolism in a patient who has deep venous thrombosis confirmed by venography is practically diagnostic of embolism. Because of the potentially fatal outcome of antepartum thromboembolism any pain in the leg or chest in pregnancy should be considered to be due to deep venous thrombosis or pulmonary embolism respectively and treated as such until the diagnosis is confirmed or disproved by venography, radio-isotope lung scanning or pulmonary angiography.

When less than 50 per cent of the pulmonary arterial tree is involved the embolism is unlikely to be fatal if the patient survives the immediate vasomotor and respiratory effects. If more than 50 per cent of the pulmonary tree is involved the likelihood of survival is much less and such

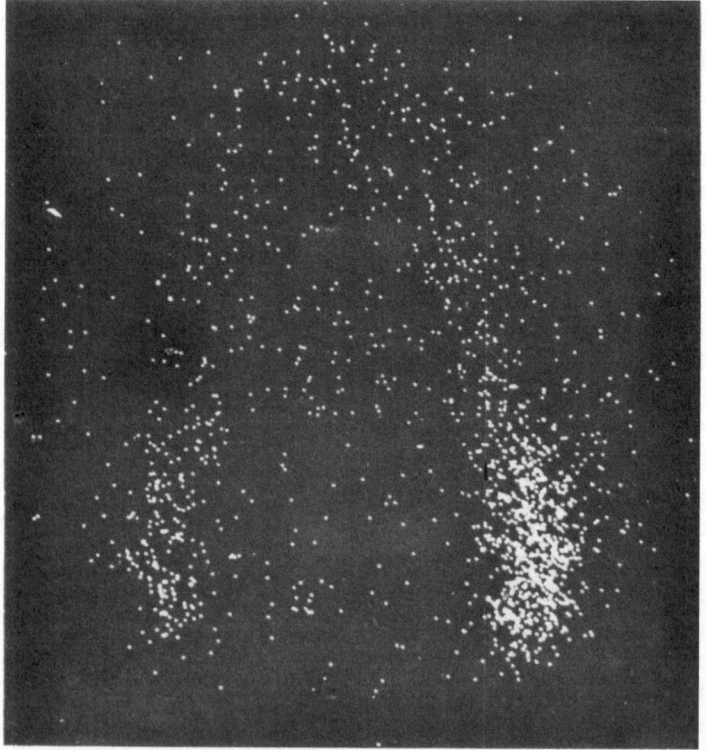

Figure 21.4 Left ilio-femoral vein thrombosis demonstrated by albumen macroaggregate labelled with technetium 99m

patients may become candidates for thrombolytic therapy or embolectomy on a cardiopulmonary by-pass (Chapter 20). In less extensive pulmonary embolism and in cases unassociated with hypotension and cyanosis rapid anticoagulation with intravenous heparin is advisable in an attempt to control further thrombus formation and embolism.

Thromboembolism

In the puerperal patient with suspicious symptoms and signs in the legs or the chest, venography has many advantages as it will demonstrate the deep veins from the ankle to the inferior vena cava and the size and fixity of any thrombus. If venography is not available ultrasound doppler examination should be employed. These techniques have to a great extent superseded the time honoured diagnosis from clinical signs. Less than 25 per cent of cases of massive pulmonary embolism are preceded by any warning signs either in the legs or in the chest. The use of radioactive labelled macroaggregates of human albumen is a reliable method of diagnosing low or absent lung perfusion which may be the result of embolism or infarction. The use of technietium labelled macroaggregates for the diagnosis of venous thrombosis during pregnancy has recently been investigated (Bonnar, 1974). The macroaggregates are injected into the dorsal veins of the feet and if a venous channel has a major obstruction the flow of the radioactive material is delayed and the obstruction can be detected as a hot-spot by the gamma camera (Figure 21.4). The method has a particular advantage in allowing examination of the major venous channels and the lung fields as one procedure with minimal radiation hazard.

ANTICOAGULANT THERAPY IN PREGNANCY

Drugs of the coumarin and indanedione group have a molecular weight of approximately 1000 and cross the placenta. In pregnant women taking oral anticoagulants an 18 per cent foetal mortality mainly as a result of haemorrhage in the infant before or during labour has been reported (Villasanta, 1965). It is also possible that the use of these drugs in early pregnancy may carry a small hazard of foetal abnormality (Kerber et al., 1968). The risk of congenital abnormality in any pregnancy approaches one per cent and a cause and effect relationship with anticoagulants is difficult to establish. Nonetheless, the use of oral anticoagulants in both early and late pregnancy must be regarded as a distinct hazard to the foetus. In an analysis of perinatal deaths associated with the use of coumarin derivatives in pregnancy the main hazard of these drugs was found to arise from their administration in early and late pregnancy (Hirsh et al., 1970). The levels of Factors II, VII, IX and X in the healthy newborn are low and contrast with the elevated levels of these factors in the maternal circulation (Figure 21.5) (Bonnar et al., 1971). Coumarin derivatives cross into the foetal circulation and produce a further depletion of the vitamin K-dependent factors. The haemostatic competence of the infant is therefore further impaired and the risk of haemorrhage during and after delivery is consequently increased.

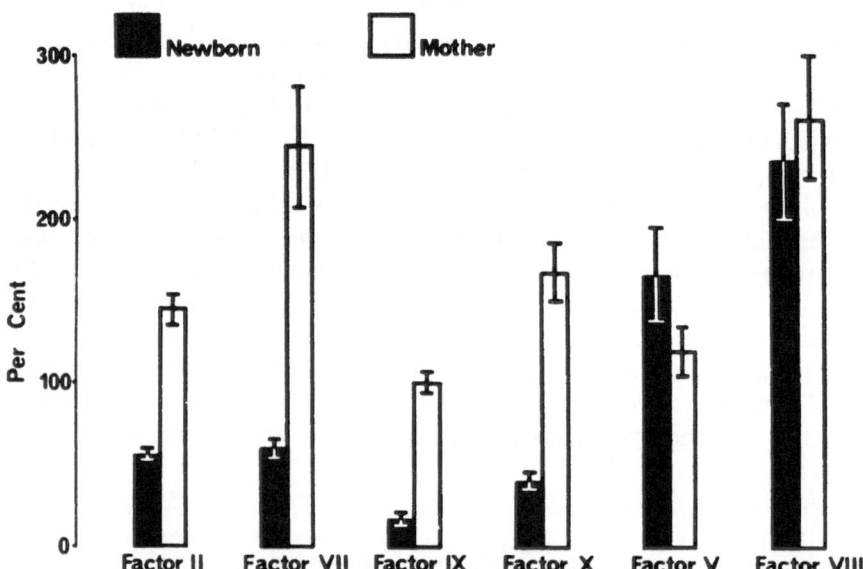

COAGULATION FACTORS IN THE NEWBORN AND THE MOTHER

Figure 21.5 A comparison between the levels of coagulation factors in the maternal blood and cord blood of the healthy newborn infant in full-term pregnancy. Mean and standard error from 10 mothers and their babies (From Bonnar *et al.*, 1971, by courtesy of *J. Obstet. Gynaecol. Brit. Cwlth.*)

Heparin with an average molecular weight of 20 000 does not cross the placenta and is not associated with any known foetal hazard. The action of heparin can be rapidly reversed by intravenous protamine sulphate. Heparin is therefore the safest anticoagulant to use during pregnancy, particularly in the first and last trimester.

Heparin in pregnancy

When administered intravenously heparin is immediately effective as an anticoagulant directly inhibiting various coagulation enzyme systems especially activated Factor X and thrombin (Chapter 19). Heparin is rapidly metabolised in the body and a sustained level in the plasma can be maintained by either continuous intravenous infusion or administration by the subcutaneous route. To maintain an immediate effect 5000 units (50 mg) should be given as an intravenous priming dose followed by an hourly dosage rate of 1500 units. The whole blood clotting time should be checked and maintained at at least 2–3 times the control value. In pregnant women with extensive deep venous thrombosis we have found that initially as high as 3000 units/hour is required to detect free heparin in the plasma. This is most probably the result of high levels of platelet Factor 4 in the circulation arising from the site of the thrombosis.

Heparin is a potent anticoagulant and in any patient who is at risk from haemorrhage from some other cause such as placenta praevia or recent delivery, the risks are considerable and must be clearly understood. In the presence of haemorrhage the action of heparin can be rapidly reversed by intravenous protamine sulphate 1·5 mg for every 100 units (1 mg) of heparin in the circulation.

Heparin may also be given by intermittent intravenous injection – 10 000 units every six hours; when given by this method a small cannula can be introduced into a superficial vein on the forearm or hand to avoid repeated venepuncture. As shown however in Figure 21.6 intravenous injections produce heparin levels in the circulation which fluctuate from a dangerously high level immediately after the injection to barely-

PLASMA HEPARIN LEVELS FOLLOWING INTRAVENOUS AND SUB-CUTANEOUS ADMINISTRATION

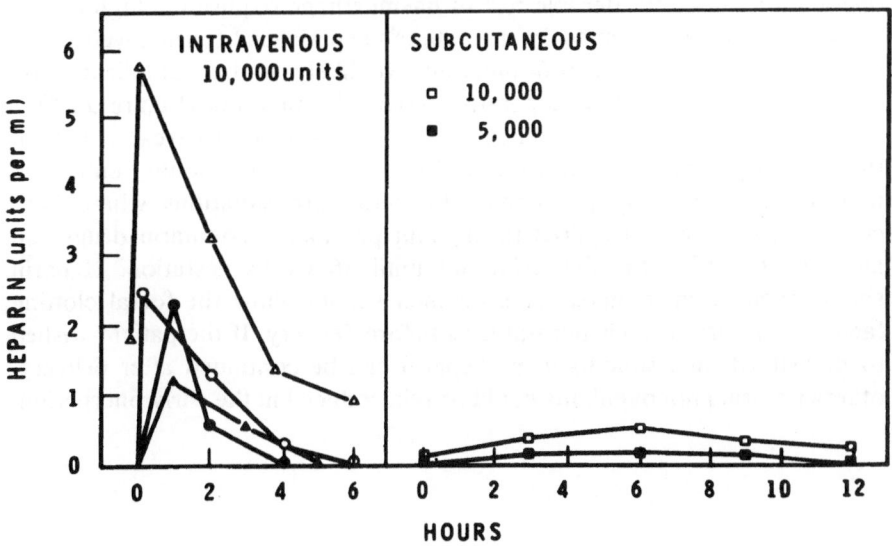

Figure 21.6 Heparin levels in the plasma after intravenous and subcutaneous heparin injections

detectable levels within 4–6 h. The intramuscular injection of heparin should be avoided as the anticoagulant effect is unpredictable and painful haematomas may form at the site of injection.

The use of subcutaneous heparin for long-term therapy in pregnancy has recently been investigated and the results indicate that effective levels of heparin in the circulation can be achieved by self-administered subcutaneous injections (Bonnar, 1974). Figure 21.7 shows the levels of heparin in a patient with extensive ilio-femoral thrombosis at the 29th week of pregnancy treated over a period of four months with self-administered subcutaneous heparin. A major advantage of the regimen is that the patient can be allowed home and effective antithrombotic therapy continued on an out-patient basis. The level of heparin in the circulation should be carefully monitored in the pregnant patient both during pregnancy and after delivery. A not uncommon complication in pregnancy is renal impairment which may be a long-standing condition or the result of conditions such as pre-eclampsia. In these situations the heparin level in the plasma rises to a potentially hazardous level, most probably as the result of reduced renal excretion (Bonnar, 1974). It is therefore vital that the heparin dosage be reduced at delivery to avoid the distinct hazard of severe postpartum haemorrhage in these patients. The increasing levels of heparin found in a patient with renal impairment and fetal growth retardation are shown in Figure 21.8. Caesarean section is an operation with a considerable risk of haemorrhage requiring a high degree of haemostatic competence. In the author's experience heparin levels in the circulation in excess of 0·6 units/ml are likely to be complicated by excessive bleeding and postoperative wound heamatoma (Figure 21.8).

Recent experience does indicate that it is possible to treat a patient throughout pregnancy with heparin, if for example a pulmonary embolism had occurred in early pregnancy. In these rare situations where anti-coagulant therapy is required throughout pregnancy coumarin drugs can also be used after the first trimester until 36 weeks gestation. Heparin should then be introduced. This regimen should allow the foetal clotting factors to return to their normal level before delivery. If the patient wished to breastfeed then subcutaneous heparin can be continued after delivery, otherwise oral anticoagulants could be reintroduced in the early puerperium

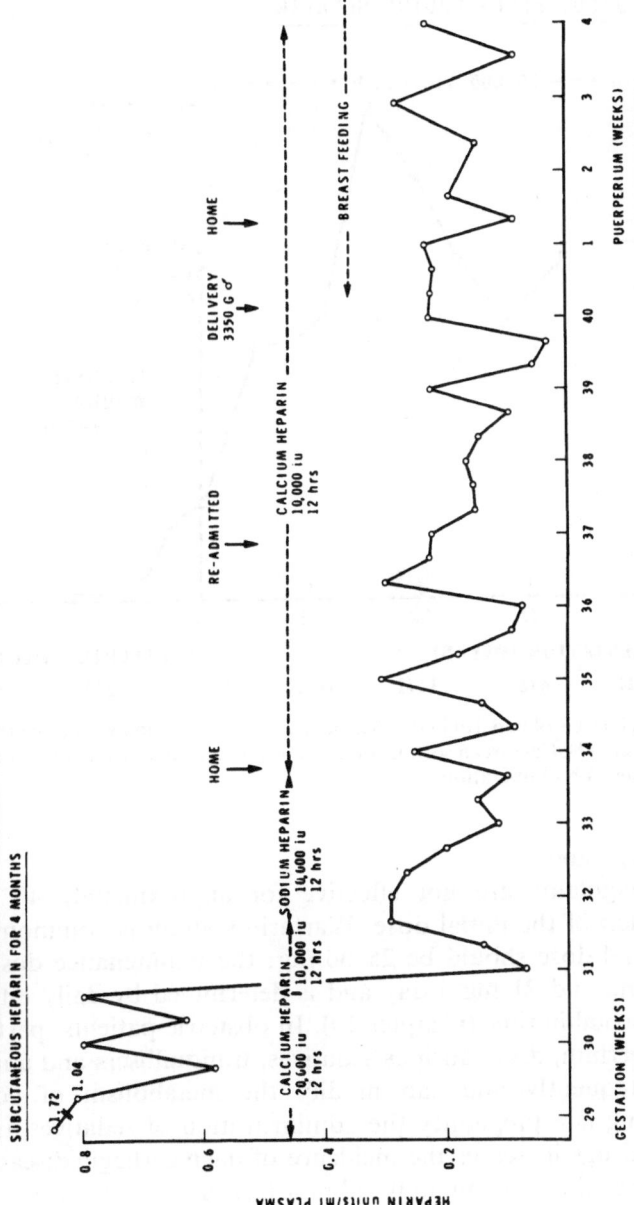

Figure 21.7 Treatment of ilio-femoral thrombosis from 29th week of pregnancy until four weeks after delivery by self-administered subcutaneous heparin

RENAL IMPAIRMENT AND FETAL GROWTH RETARDATION

SUBCUTANEOUS SODIUM HEPARIN

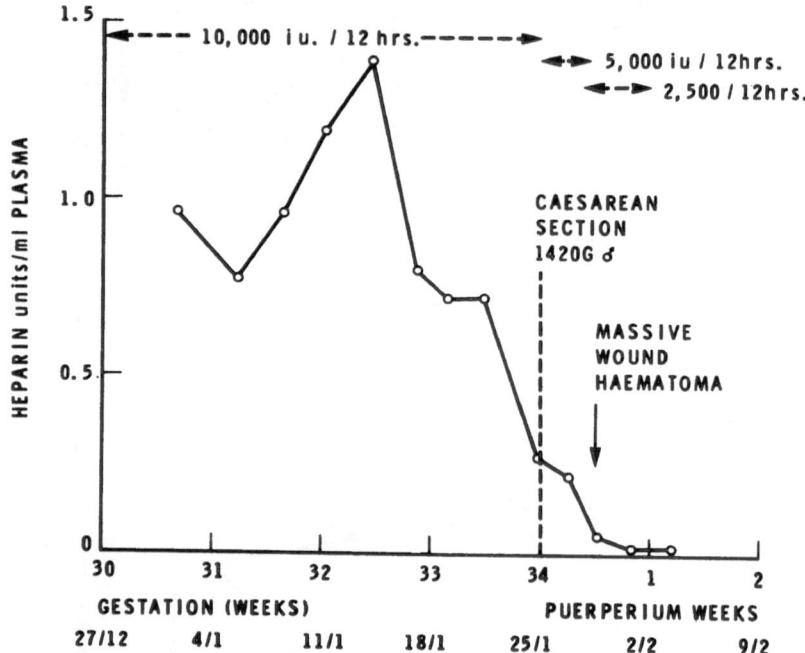

Figure 21.8 High levels of heparin in the plasma found in association with renal impairment in late pregnancy. The Caesarean section wound was complicated by a massive haematoma occurring within 24 h of operation

Oral anticoagulants

Oral anticoagulants are not effective for approximately 48 h after administration of the initial dose. Warfarin sodium is commonly given and the initial dose should be 25–30 mg; the maintenance dose varies between 3 mg and 21 mg a day and is determined by daily estimation of the prothrombin time (Chapter 19). In obstetric patients, particularly in the puerperium, drugs such as sedatives, tranquillisers and antibiotics are used frequently and can modify the metabolism of coumarin drugs. During late pregnancy the administration of sedatives and anti-convulsant drugs increases the incidence of haemorrhagic disease in the newborn and the concomitant administration of oral anticoagulant drugs would therefore aggravate the bleeding hazard in the foetus. Oral anticoagulants are also excreted in the milk and therefore breastfeeding is contraindicated as the drugs may have an effect on the infant at a time when production of vitamin K dependent factors is impaired.

When the anticoagulant effect of coumarin and indanedione drugs requires to be reversed vitamin K_1 should be administered. the dose of vitamin K_1 given orally or intravenously will depend on the clinical situation. If frank haemorrhage is present associated with conditions such as placenta praevia, abruptio placentae, or severe bleeding after a normal or operative delivery and a firm decision is taken that anticoagulant therapy will not be continued, a dose of 25–50 mg should be given. Dosage of this order will render the patient resistant to further anticoagulant therapy for about two weeks. When there is frank haemorrhage but it is intended to continue therapy, 15 mg of vitamin K_1 should be given to reduce the effect of the drug with cancelling it. When the prothrombin time is excessively increased, but the patient is not bleeding, a dose of 5 mg of vitamin K_1 is advisable, particularly when anticoagulant therapy has been employed after surgery. If a patient goes into premature labour while on oral anticoagulant therapy vitamin K_1 (25 mg–50 mg) should be given intravenously in the interests of the baby. It is not known how well the premature baby's liver can utilise vitamin K_1 but it is possible that the administration to the mother before delivery will reduce the risk of haemorrhage in the baby as a consequence of the birth process. When the effect of oral anticoagulant therapy is neutralised by vitamin K_1 and antithrombotic therapy is still indicated heparin should be used. The route of administration and dosage will depend on the clinical circumstances.

The duration of oral anticoagulant therapy in the management of deep venous thrombosis is still controversial (Chapter 19). When a patient suffers from deep venous thrombosis in the puerperium and oral anticoagulant therapy has been instituted our practice is to continue treatment for at least six weeks on an out-patient basis after the patient has become fully ambulant. If a patient had a pulmonary embolism then a much more prolonged period of anticoagulant therapy is indicated.

Defibrinating drugs
Experience with defibrinating agents such as Ancrod (Chapter 18) in pregnancy is limited and their precise effect in the foetal circulation has not been clarified. A serious drawback to their possible use in pregnancy is the fact that the defibrinating effect in the foetus cannot be readily reversed. To neutralise the effect of Ancrod an injection of specific antiserum must be given and a transfusion of fibrinogen. Although

antiserum given to the mother will neutralise the Ancrod in the foetal circulation it is not possible to raise the fibrinogen level in the foetal circulation because it does not cross the placenta. Whether Ancrod would be useful in the puerperium for the treatment of deep venous thrombosis would depend on the incidence of bleeding complications and this aspect has not yet been investigated.

FIBRINOLYTIC DRUGS

These agents have a direct effect on the thrombus and the most widely used at present is streptokinase, a purified fraction of streptococcal exotoxin (Chapter 18). Streptokinase, like heparin, does not pass across the placenta to the foetus. It has been used for the treatment of 22 pregnant women with venous thrombosis of which 17 were clinically successful (Ludwig, 1968). No toxic effects in the foetus were observed. Animal experiments have indicated that, depending on the species, between 0·1 and 1 per cent of doses in the therapeutic range cross the placenta (Ludwig 1966).

Treatment of acute massive pulmonary embolism at the 32nd week of pregnancy with streptokinase has been reported in one patient who had a suspected melanoma excised from her left calf and had a massive pulmonary embolism on the eighth postoperative day (Hall *et al.*, 1972). Pulmonary arteriography confirmed the presence of pulmonary embolism and streptokinase was given (6000 000 units in half an hour followed by 100 000 units hourly). The patient's symptoms were greatly improved eight hours later and she commenced in labour. While still on streptokinase she had a spontaneous vaginal delivery without episiotomy. Despite the administration of ergometrine and oxytocin, severe and persistent uterine haemorrhage occurred. The streptokinase was discontinued three hours after delivery and 8 gm of aminocaprioc acid were administered to reverse the fibrinolysis. This accompanied by continuous oxytocin administration and fundal massage brought the haemorrhage under control but during the 36 h after delivery the patient required transfusion with eleven pints of blood. The baby at birth had no external evidence of haemorrhage and no adverse effect of the streptokinase was detected.

The use of streptokinase in the puerperium is also fraught with the danger of haemorrhage from the uterus. Serious bleeding from the uterus has been encountered when streptokinase has been employed as late as 10–14 days after delivery (Bonnar, 1974). Because of the serious risk of haemorrhage from the uterus after placental separation at delivery and in the early puerperium thrombolytic therapy is not recommended.

The situation is akin to using fibrinolytic agents in a patient during or immediately after operation when the haemorrhagic hazards of thrombolytic therapy could well outweigh their potential benefit.

If a patient in late pregnancy is considered to be at serious risk from a fatal pulmonary embolism and streptokinase is employed the therapy should be discontinued if labour commences and a plentiful supply of fresh blood obtained so that it can be administered in the event of serious haemorrhage. It would seem unwise to use aminocaproic acid or aprotinin (Trasylol) unless serious haemorrhage does occur which is not controlled by the administration of fresh blood. The true value of thrombolytic therapy for the treatment of thromboembolic complications is by no means established and despite intensive efforts in many centres over the last ten years it has not achieved a place in routine treatment of thromboembolic vascular disease (Prentice and McNicol 1973). Experience of thrombolytic therapy during pregnancy is limited and a possible complication which must always be considered is abruptio placentae due to the lysis of the fibrin which is normally present in the uteroplacental circulation.

AFTER-CARE
Too often when a patient is discharged from hospital after deep venous thrombosis the only subsequent supervision concerns her anticoagulant therapy. It is vital to take steps to improve venous return from the leg and thereby reduce the chances of recurrence and the development of the postphlebitic syndrome. In some patients troublesome oedema persists despite anticoagulant therapy and in these cases physiotherapy and elastic stockings or bandages may be of help. The patient should be instructed to take regular exercise and avoid prolonged periods in a sitting position. Until such time as all oedema has subsided she should sleep with the foot of the bed elevated.

PROPHYLAXIS OF THROMBOEMBOLISM IN PREGNANCY
A previous history of thrombosis or pulmonary embolism indicates that the patient is at special risk from a recurrence of this complication (Chapter 13). This applies in particular to women who have sustained an episode of thrombosis while taking oral contraceptives. In certain patients the risk of recurrence of thrombosis in pregnancy may be so high that the patient should be advised against further pregnancy. Women who are obese should be asked to reduce weight before becoming pregnant. During pregnancy the increased hazard of thrombosis when a patient is

admitted to hospital should be appreciated. Where bedrest in hospital is necessary because of an obstetric complication the patient should have supervised leg exercises to avoid prolonged venous stasis.

During Caesarean section the patient's heels should be supported to protect the veins from the pressure of the operating table. Strict asepsis, gentle handling of tissues and good haemostasis are of vital importance as they will affect the recovery and mobility of the patient in the puerperium. Following delivery or operation, early ambulation with active walking beginning on the day of delivery is recommended. If a patient's condition does not permit this activity exercises performed in bed supervised by a physiotherapist are necessary. Those responsible for the supervision of patients in the puerperium must appreciate that early ambulation does not mean sitting at a bedside in a chair with knees and thighs flexed – more aptly termed 'early angulation' – a position which seriously impedes venous return from the legs. An additional precaution in high-risk patients is elevation of the foot of the bed by at least an angle of 15 degrees to improve venous blood flow from the lower limbs.

While it is true that the most convenient time for a sterilisation operation is the immediate puerperium it is nonetheless likely to expose the mother to an additional hazard of thromboembolism, particularly the patient who is already at high risk because of age, obesity and parity. Sometimes, however, these patients will only accept the operation if it can be done during the lying-in period. Where this is so, prophylactic treatment as described below is advisable.

Prophylaxis against thrombosis using low dose subcutaneous heparin can be employed to cover the period of labour and the early puerperium. The author's team is at present evaluating the effect of the administration of 500 ml of Dextran 70, during labour because this agent has been effective in patients undergoing gynaecological surgery (Bonnar and Walsh, 1972). Studies on the use of low doses of heparin (5000 units eight hourly by subcutaneous injections) are also in progress.

PULMONARY EMBOLISM AND DEEP VENOUS THROMBOSIS AFTER GYNAECOLOGICAL OPERATIONS

Patients undergoing major pelvic operations must be regarded as especially at risk of deep venous thrombosis and pulmonary embolism. The absence of premonitory signs in over 50 per cent of patients dying of pulmonary emboli (Sevitt and Gallagher 1959) and of clinical evidence in 50 per cent of patients with deep venous thrombosis (Flanc et al., 1968) has made the study of this condition difficult. Using the ^{125}I-fibrinogen test,

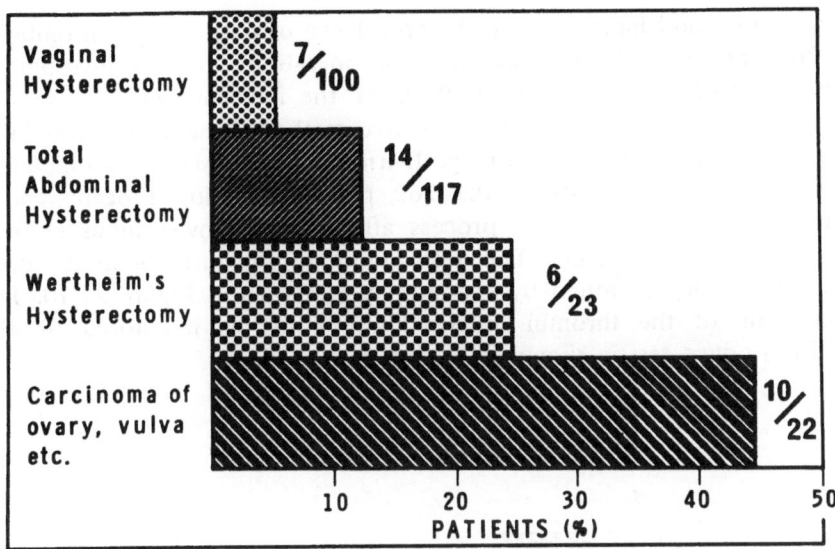

Figure 21.9 Incidence of deep venous thrombosis as found by the [125] I-fibrinogen test and venography in 262 patients after various gynaecological operations. (From Walsh *et al.*, 1974, by courtesy of *J. Obstet. Gynaecol. Brit. Cwlth.*)

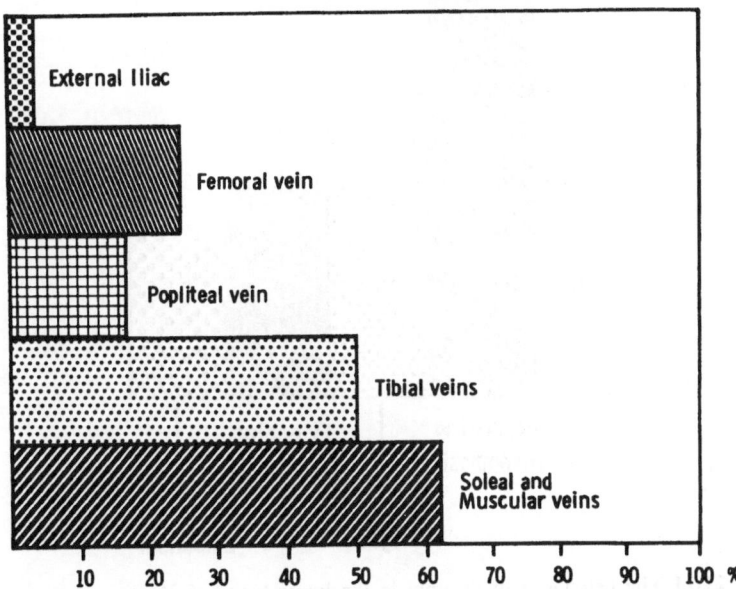

Figure 21.10 Distribution of thrombi as shown by venography in 37 patients with deep venous thrombosis after pelvic surgery. (From Walsh *et al.*, 1974, by courtesy of *J. Obstet. Gynaecol. Brit. Cwlth.*)

venography and lung-scanning the prevalence of deep venous thrombosis in 262 patients undergoing major pelvic operations has been investigated (Walsh *et al.*, 1974). Figure 21.9 shows the incidence of deep venous thrombosis as shown by these objective methods in patients who have various forms of pelvice surgery. During the first seven postoperative days, 37 (14 per cent) of the 262 patients developed deep venous thrombosis. The thrombotic process affected both lower limbs in over one-third of the patients. The distribution of the thrombi in the deep veins in the leg as found by venography is shown in Figure 21.10. The behaviour of the thrombi in the lower limbs as monitored by the ^{125}I-fibrinogen test is shown in Figure 21.11.

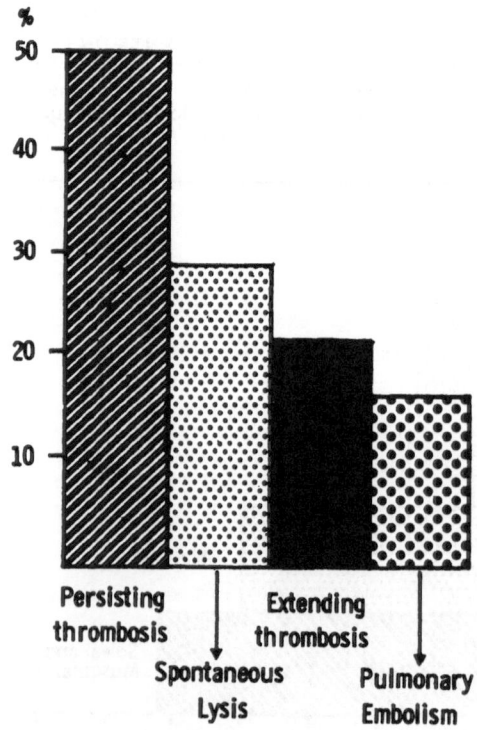

Figure 21.11 The behaviour of thrombi in the lower limbs of 37 patients diagnosed and monitored by the [125] I-fibrinogen test. Pulmonary embolism as shown by lung scanning occurred in 15 per cent of patients with isotopic evidence of leg vein thrombosis. (From Walsh *et al.*, 1974, by courtesy of *J. Obstet. Gynaecol. Brit. Cwlth.*)

Thromboembolism

In general surgical patients the frequency of postoperative deep venous thrombosis as diagnosed by labelled fibrinogen has been reported near 35 per cent (Flanc *et al.*, 1968; Negus *et al.*, 1968). In the study by Walsh the mean age of the patients was 48 years whereas in the study of Negus the mean age was 62 years. As discussed in Chapter 13 the incidence of postoperative thrombosis increases with age and this is the most likely explanation of the lower incidence of postoperative thrombosis between gynaecological patients and general surgical patients. Kemble (1971) reported isotopic evidence of postoperative leg vein thrombosis in 27 per cent of male and 29 per cent of female surgical patients. Other studies reported in this volume (Chapter 13) do not demonstrate any significant sex difference in the incidence of deep venous thrombosis.

The frequency of deep venous thrombosis was low after vaginal hysterectomy (7 per cent) (Friend amd Kakkar, 1972; Walsh *et al.*, 1974). It was expected that the lithotomy position might increase the risk of thrombosis due to the pressure on the calf during the procedure. This position however does allow better drainage of the veins by gravity. The incidence of deep venous thrombosis following abdominal hysterectomy was 12 per cent and it is possible that the opening of the abdominal cavity and packing of the intestines may impede venous flow in the inferior vena cava and thus promote more stasis than occurs in the vaginal procedure. In addition, abdominal hysterectomy produces more extensive coagulation changes in the systemic circulation than vaginal hysterectomy (Bonnar, 1974). In Oxford, carcinoma of the cervix is treated by preoperative radiotherapy and Wertheim's operation combined with lymphadenectomy. The postoperative incidence of deep venous thrombosis after Wertheim's operation was 25 per cent. The highest incidence of thrombosis (45 per cent) was found in patients having operations for carinoma of the ovary and carcinoma of the corpus uteri.

Lymphoedema of the leg following pelvic lymphadenectomy can be mistakenly diagnosed as massive ilio-femoral thrombosis. In this condition the ^{125}I-fibrinogen test reveals high counts over the whole limb. Veonography will demonstrate the absence of thrombosis and as shown in Figure 21.12 a lymphangiogram may show a lymphocyst in the pelvis.

The frequency of deep venous thrombosis following gynaecological operations is therefore considerably higher than that of 2–5 per cent previously reported by clinical studies (Jeffcoate and Tindall, 1965). Symptomless thrombosis which is not detectable by clinical examination of the legs is a frequent occurrence. Less than 50 per cent of patients with isotopic and venographic evidence of deep venous thrombosis have

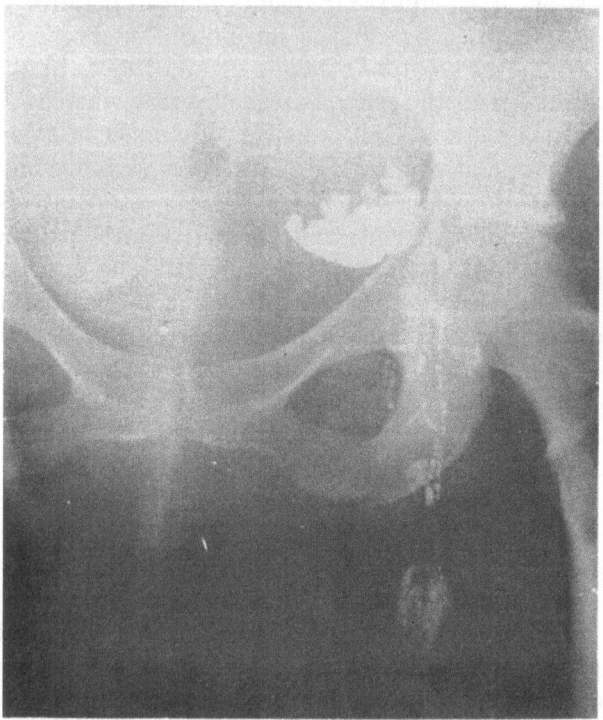

Figure 21.12 Lymphangiogram showing a lymphocyst in a patient who had massive swelling of the left leg three days after Wertheim's operation and pelvic lymphadenectomy for carcinoma of the cervix. No thrombi were seen on phlebographic examination of the legs and ilio-femoral segments

any clinical signs (Walsh *et al.*, 1974). In about 25 per cent of patients with silent thrombosis the condition involves the venous system above the knee and such patients are especially at risk of pulmonary embolism (Chapter 19).

PROPHYLAXIS OF THROMBOSIS AND EMBOLISM AFTER PELVIC SURGERY

General

Prevention of postoperative thrombosis begins when the patient is first seen in the out-patient department. Carcinoma, obesity, pregnancy, previous history of thrombosis or pulmonary embolism, varicose veins, oral contraception and advanced years are considered to be high risk factors. In patients with benign gynaecological conditions requiring

334

surgery, weight reduction and treatment of anaemia prior to operation is advisable. An increased incidence of deep venous thrombosis has been reported in women undergoing surgery who have been taking combined oestrogen progestogen oral contraceptives at the time of operation (Vessey et al., 1970). If discontinued for 4–6 weeks before operation this additional hazard appears to be prevented. Immobolisation in bed before operation can increase the hazard of thrombosis considerably (Gibbs, 1959). All Necessary preoperative investigations and consultations should therefore be completed as out-patient procedures and if possible the patient should be admitted the day before operation.

The full movement of the diaphragm is of physiological importance in maintaining good venous return from the lower limbs and pelvis. Diaphragmatic movement after operation will be influenced adversely by abdominal incisions but much less so by a low transverse incision than a vertical one. In this context vaginal hysterectomy has obvious advantages. During operation certain precautions are also advised to reduce venous pooling in the pelvic veins and lower limbs. The 10–30 degrees tilt of the patient which is commonly employed during gynaecological operations performed via the abdomen, improves venous blood flow from the legs. The patient's heels should be supported during abdominal surgery to protect the calf veins from the pressure of the operating table and possible endothelial damage. Pressure on the inferior vena cava due to an excess of abdominal packing should be avoided, particularly during prolonged operative procedures. Care must be taken to prevent trauma to the iliac vessels with retractors. Good haemostasis is particularly important and suction drains are recommended to prevent haematomas in patients undergoing radical operations for carcinoma of the uterus or vulva. Pelvic haematomas may become infected and prolong the post-operative stay in hospital. Suction drains following Wertheim's operation or radical vulvectomy usually aspirate over 300 ml of bloody serum and lymph.

After operation active walking beginning within 24 h of surgery is recommended. If the patient's condition does not allow this activity exercises performed in bed and supervised by a physiotherapist are necessary. An additional precaution particularly in the elderly patients is elevation of the foot of the bed by at least 15 degrees to improve venous return from the lower limbs. Other methods of preventing venous stasis after operation include intermittent calf compression using a plastic bag inflated with compressed air (Hills et al., 1972). These methods which can be used during surgery create problems by taking up valuable time in the operating theatre and they are impractical in patients in the lithotomy position.

Specific antithrombotic treatment

The methods of counteracting the hypercoagulability of blood which occurs during and after operation include the use of oral anticoagulants, heparin and Dextran 70. Oral anticoagulant therapy has been widely advocated as a prophylactic measure against venous thrombosis and pulmonary embolism in the postoperative period. Turnbull (1961) used anticoagulant prophylaxis from the 1st to 12th postoperative day in women over 45 years, in young obese women and in those with varicose veins or a history of previous thromboembolism: embolism occurred in 1.8 per cent of 222 controls and in none of the 201 treated patients, but haemorrhagic complications occurred in 14 per cent of the latter and in 3 per cent were severe. Oral anticoagulants commenced after operation are not effective until the 3rd or 4th day and hence offer no protection during the critical period of the first three days during which two-thirds of the thrombotic complications commence. Pelvic surgery in patients under effective therapy with oral anticoagulants would be particularly hazardous. Haemostasis at the site of operation would be impaired and the danger of haemorrhage would possibly outweigh the benefit of preventing thrombosis. Indeed, well-controlled oral anticoagulant therapy employed in the postoperative period is so often accompanied by haemorrhage that its overall benefit to the patient must be doubtful.

Recent reports have shown that subcutaneous low dosage heparin effectively reduces the incidence of postoperative deep venous thrombosis as diagnosed by the ^{125}I-fibrinogen test (Kakkar et al., 1971; Nicolaides et al., 1972; Chapters 14-16). The recommended dose is 5000 units of heparin given by subcutaneous injection 8-hourly starting two hours before operation. The method appears to be effective in patients undergoing gynaecological operations (Ballard et al., 1973). Haematoma formation and postoperative haemorrhage may be a particular hazard of pelvic surgery and this aspect requires careful investigation before subcutaneous heparin can be recommended for routine use in gynaecological patients. Accurate monitoring of heparin levels during and after surgery is now possible (Denson and Bonnar, 1973; Yin et al., 1973) and regimens may be modified in the light of future information on heparin levels.

A recent double blind study showed that Dextran 70 was effective in preventing postoperative deep venous thrombosis shown by the ^{125}I-fibrinogen test and venography, in patients undergoing pelvic surgery

(Bonnar and Walsh, 1972). One litre of Dextran 70 was administered during and immediately after operation over a six hour period which started at the initiation of anaesthesia. In the control group of 140 patients 15 developed deep venous thrombosis and in four of these the thrombus extended into the femoral vein. In 120 patients who received Dextran 70 thrombosis occurred in the calf of one patient. No evidence of any significant increase in blood loss during operation was found in the test group. In a study of 62 high risk patients having radical pelvic surgery for malignant disease of the genital tract the incidence of postoperative deep venous thrombosis was also reduced (Bonnar *et al.*, 1973). Of the 42 control patients 14 (33 per cent) developed deep venous thrombosis, while of 20 patients receiving Dextran 70 only one (5 per cent) developed thrombosis. The infusion of one litre of Dextran 70 during the critical period of operation was shown to prevent the increase of coagulation factors particularly V and VIII. The antithrombotic effect of Dextran 70 appears to be mediated by its effect on blood flow as well as on platelet function and coagulation factor activity.

It is too early to draw conclusions as to which is the best method of prophylaxis for patients undergoing pelvic surgery and it is doubtful whether any single regimen will have universal acceptance. Further studies are at present in progress and for general use a method which is simple, effective and free of complications is required. Recently, correlation has been found between positive ^{125}I-fibrinogen scans which indicate deep venous thrombosis in the legs and abnormalities of perfusion lung-scans attributable to silent pulmonary emboli in postoperative patients (Lahnborg *et al.*, 1974). These silent pulmonary emboli were significantly reduced by low dose subcutaneous heparin. Further studies are needed to prove that the regimens of low dose heparin and Dextran 70 reduce clinically significant thrombosis and embolism (Chapter 14). Until such definitive studies have been completed prophylactic measures against thrombosis should perhaps be confined to patients who are particularly at risk. In the author's department at present the use of Dextran 70 is preferred except in patients with impaired renal function or poor cardio-pulmonary reserve in which low dose subcutaneous heparin is employed.

References

Allan, T. M. and Stewart, K. S. (1971). ABO blood-groups and superficial puerperal thrombophlebitis. *Lancet*, **1**, 1125

Arthure, H., Tomlinson, J., Organe, G., Adelstein, A. M. and Weatherall, J. A. (1972). In: *Report on Confidential Enquiries into Maternal Deaths in England and Wales, 1967–1969*, 30 (London; HMSO)

Thromboembolism

Ballard, R. M., Bradley-Watson, P. J., Johnstone, F. D., Kenney, A. and Campbell, S. (1973). Low doses of subcutaneous heparin in the prevention of deep vein thrombosis after gynaecological surgery. *J. Obstet. Gynaecol. Brit. Cwlth.*, **80,** 469

Barker, N. W., Nygaard, K. K., Walters, W. and Priestley, J. T. (1941). A statistical study of postoperative venous thrombosis and pulmonary embolism: Predisposing factors. *Proc. Mayo Clin.*, **16,** 1

Bates, M. M. (1971). Venous thromboembolic disease and ABO blood type. *Lancet*, **1,** 239

Bonnar, J., McNicol, G. P. and Douglas, A. S. (1970a). Coagulation and fibrinolytic mechanisms during and after normal childbirth. *Brit. Med. J.*, **2,** 200

Bonnar, J., Prentice, C. R. M., McNicol, G. P. and Douglas, A. S. (1970b). Haemostatic mechanisms in the uterine circulation during placental separation. *Brit. Med. J.*, **2,** 564

Bonnar, J., McNicol, G. P. and Douglas, A. S. (1971). The blood coagulation and fibrinolytic systems in the newborn and the mother at birth. *J. Obstet. Gynaecol. Brit. Cwlth.*, **4,** 355

Bonnar, J. and Walsh, J. (1972). Prevention of thrombosis after pelvic surgery by British Dextran 70, *Lancet,* **i,** 614

Bonnar, J. (1973). Blood coagulation and fibrinolysis in obstetrics. In: *Clinics in Haematology,* 213–233, Vol. 2, No. 1 (A. S. Douglas, editor) (London; Saurders)

Bonnar, J., Walsh, J. J., Haddon, M., Fairweather, J. and Denson, K. W. E. (1973). Coagulation system changes induced by pelvic surgery and the effect of Dextran 70. *Bibliotheca Anatomica,* **No. 12,** *7th European Conference Microcirculation Aberdeen,* 1972, Part II, 351–355

Bonnar, J. (1974). Unpublished data

Browse, N. L. and Negus, D. (1970). Prevention of postoperative leg vein thrombosis by electrical muscle stimulation. An evaluation with [125]I-**Labelled fibrinogen**. *Brit. Med. J.*, **3,** 615

Daniel, D. G., Campbell, H. and Turnbull, A. C. (1967). Puerperal thromboembolism and **suppression of lactation**. *Lancet,* **ii,** 287

Denson, K. W. E. and Bonnar, J. (1973). The measurement of heparin. A method based on the potentiation of antifactor Xa. *Thromb. Diathes. Haemorrh., (Stuttg.)*, **30,** 471

Flanc, C., Kakkar, V. and Clarke, M. B. (1968). The detection of venous thrombosis of the legs using [125] I -labelled fibrinogen. *Brit. J. Surg.*, **55,** 742

Friend, J. R. and Kakkar, V. V. (1972). Deep vein thrombosis in obstetric and gynaecological patients. In: *Thromboembolism: Diagnosis and Treatment,* 131–138 (V. V. Kakkar and A. J. Jouhar, editors) (Edinburgh and London; Churchill Livingstone)

Gibbs, N. M. (1957). Venous thrombosis of the lower limbs with particular reference to bedrest. *Brit. J. Surg.*, **45,** 209

Hall, R. J. C., Young, C., Sutton, G. C. and Campbell, S. (1972). Treatment of acute massive pulmonary embolism by Streptokinase during labour and delivery. *Brit. Med. J.*, **4,** 647

Henderson, S. R., Lund, C. J. and Greasman, W. T. (1972). Antepartum pulmonary embolism. *Amer. J. Obstet. Gynecol.*, **112,** 476

Hills, N. H., Pflug, J. J., Jeyasingh, K., Boardman, L. and Calnan, J. S. (1972). Prevention of deep vein thrombosis by intermitent pneumatic compression of calf. *Brit. Med. J.*, **1,** 131

Hirsh, J., Cade, J. F. and O'Sullivan, E. F. (1970). Clinical experience with anti-coagulant therapy during pregnancy. *Brit. Med. J.*, **1,** 270

Thromboembolism

Jackson, P. (1973). Puerperal thromboembolic disease in 'High risk' cases. *Brit. Med. J.*, 1, 263

Jeffcoate, T. N. A. and Tindall, V. R. (1965). Venous thrombosis and embolism in obstetrics and gynaecology. *Aust. N.Z. J. Obstet. Gynaecol.*, 5, 119

Jick, H., Sloane, D., Westerholm, B., Inman, W. H. W., Vessey, M. P., Shapiro, S., Lewis, G. P. and Worcester, J. (1969). Venous thromboembolic disease and ABO blood type. *Lancet*, i, 539

Kakkar, V. V., Field, E. S., Nicolaides, A. N., Flute, P. T., Wessler, S. and Yin, E. T. (1971). Low doses of heparin in prevention of deep vein thrombosis. *Lancet*, 2, 669

Kemble, J. V. H. (1971). Incidence of deep vein thrombosis. *Brit. J. Hosp. Med.*, 6, 721

Kerber, I. J., Warr, O. S. and Richardson, C. (1968). Pregnancy in a patient with a prosthetic valve, associated with a fetal anomaly attributed to Warfarin sodium. *JAMA*, 203, 223

Lahnborg, G., Bergström, K., Friman, L. and Lagergen, H. (1974). Effect of low-dose heparin on incidence of postoperative pulmonary embolism defected by photoscanning. *Lancet*, i, 329

Lambie, J. M., Barber, D. C., Dhall, D. P. and Matheson, N. A. (1970). Dextran 70 in prophylaxis of postoperative venous thrombosis. A controlled trial. *Brit. Med. J.*, 2, 144

Ludwig, H. (1966). Experimentelle untersuchungen zum diaplazentaren ubertritt von streptokinase. *Geburtsh. Frauenherlk*, 26, 736

Ludwig, H. (1968). *Therapeutische fibrinolyse in der gravidität gynaecol.*, *(Basel)*, 166, 20

Negus, D., Pinto, A. J., Le Quesne, L. P., Broron, N. and Chapman, M. (1968). 125 I-labelled fibrinogen in the diagnosis of deep vein thrombosis and its correlation with phlebography. *Brit. J. Surg.*, 55, 835

Nicolaides, A. N., Dupont, P. A., Desai, S., Lewis, J. D., Douglas, J. N., Dodsworth, H., Fourides, G., Luck, R. J. and Jamieson, C. W. (1972). Small doses of subcutaneous sodium heparin in preventing deep vein thrombosis after major surgery. *Lancet*, ii, 890

Prentice, C. R. M. and McNicol, G. P. (1973). Fibrinolytic therapy. In: *Recent Advances in Thrombosis*, 151–179 (L. Poller, editor) (London; Churchill Livingstone)

Rutherford, R. N., Hougie, C., Banks, A. L. and Coburn, W. A. (1964). Effects of sex steroids and pregnancy on blood coagulation factors. *Obstet. Gynaecol.*, 24, 886

Reports on Confidential Enquiries into Maternal Deaths in England and Wales (1952–1969) (London; HMSO)

Sevitt, S. and Gallagher, N. G. (1959). Prevention of venous thrombosis and pulmonary embolism in injured patients. *Lancet*, ii, 981

Strauss, H. S. and Diamond, L. K. (1963). Elevation of factor 8 during pregnancy in normal persons and in a patient with von Willebrand's disease. *New Engl. J. Med.*, 269, 1251

Tindall, V. R. (1971). The aetiology and pathology of pulmonary embolism. In: *Scientific Basis of Obstetrics and Gynaecology*, 385–414 (London; Churchill)

Todd, M. E., Thompson, J. H., Bowie, E. J. W. and Owen, C. A. (1965). Changes in blood coagulation during pregnancy. *Mayo Clin. Proc.*, 40, 370

Turnbull, A. C. (1960). Prophylaxis by anticoagulants after gynaecological operation. In: *Thrombosis and Anticoagulant Therapy*, 60 (W. Walker, D. C. Dundee and Thomson, editors) (London; Livingstone)

Vessey, M. P., Doll, R., Fairbairn, A. S. and Glober, G. (1970). Postoperative thromboembolism and the use of oral contraceptives. *Brit. Med. J.*, 3, 123

Vessey, M. P. (1973). The epidemiology of venous thromboembolism. In: *Recent Advances in Thrombosis*, 39–58 (L. Poller, editor) (London; Churchill Livingstone)

Thromboembolism

Villasanta, U. (1965). Thromboembolic disease in pregnancy. *Amer. J. Obstet. Gynaecol.*, **93,** 142

Walsh, J. J., Bonnar, J. and Wright, F. W. (1974). A study of pulmonary embolism and deep leg vein thrombosis after major gynaecological surgery using labelled fibrinogen, phlebography and lung scanning. *J. Obstet. Gynaecol. Brit. Cwlth.*, **81,** 311

Westerholm, B., Wiechel, B. and Eklund, G. (1971). Oral contraceptives, venous thromboembolic disease, and ABO blood type. *Lancet,* **94**

Ygge, J. (1969). Changes in blood coagulation and fibrinolysis during the puerperium. *Amer. J. Obstet. Gynaecol.*, **104,** 2

Yin, E. T., Wessler, S., Butler, J. V. and Cole, S. (1973). Plasma heparin—a unique practical submicrogram–sensitive assay. *J. Lab. Clin. Med.*, **81,** 298

340

THROMBOEMBOLISM

INDEX

341

Thromboembolism